Point-of-Care Ultrasound for Emergency Medicine and Resuscitation

OXFORD CLINICAL IMAGING GUIDES

Published and forthcoming

Acute and Critical Care Echocardiography
Edited by Claire Colebourn and Jim Newton

Focused Intensive Care Ultrasound
Edited by Marcus Peck and Peter Macnaughton

Practical Perioperative Transoesophageal Echocardiography, Third edition
Edited by David Sidebotham, Alan Merry, Malcolm Legget, and Gavin Wright

Point-of-Care Ultrasound for Emergency Medicine and Resuscitation
Edited by Paul Atkinson, Justin Bowra, Tim Harris, Bob Jarman, and David Lewis

Point-of-Care Ultrasound for Emergency Medicine and Resuscitation

Edited by

Paul Atkinson

Professor in Emergency Medicine, Dalhousie University,
Saint John Regional Hospital, Saint John, Canada

Justin Bowra

Emergency Ultrasound Program Director, Royal North Shore Hospital;
Adjunct Senior Lecturer, University of Sydney, Sydney, Australia

Tim Harris

Consultant in Emergency Medicine and Pre-hospital Care, Barts Health NHS Trust,
Professor in Emergency Medicine, Queen Mary University of London; London, UK

Bob Jarman

Consultant in Emergency Medicine, Royal Victoria Infirmary, Newcastle upon Tyne;
Visiting Professor, University of Teesside, Middlesbrough, UK

David Lewis

Associate Professor in Emergency Medicine, Dalhousie University,
Saint John Regional Hospital, Saint John, Canada

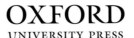
OXFORD
UNIVERSITY PRESS

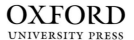

Great Clarendon Street, Oxford, OX2 6DP,
United Kingdom

Oxford University Press is a department of the University of Oxford.
It furthers the University's objective of excellence in research, scholarship,
and education by publishing worldwide. Oxford is a registered trade mark of
Oxford University Press in the UK and in certain other countries

First Edition published in 2019

Impression: 2

Published in the United States of America by Oxford University Press
198 Madison Avenue, New York, NY 10016, United States of America

British Library Cataloguing in Publication Data

Data available

Library of Congress Control Number: 2018962017

ISBN 978–0–19–877754–0

Printed in Great Britain by
Bell & Bain Ltd., Glasgow

To our families, patients, and students.

Foreword

Point-of-care ultrasound (PoCUS) is nothing more than a tool to aid in evaluating hypotheses, narrowing differential diagnoses, and facilitating procedures. My senior physician mentors and instructors have practised the majority of their storied careers without this tool. My students and residents, for the most part, have never practised medicine without it.

Ultrasound is not a new tool. The paradigm shift that occurred during my career was recognizing that a well-trained practitioner could use this tool in a timely fashion at the point of care in a wide variety of locations, ranging from the battlefields of Afghanistan to the shores of Vanuatu. The key was developing excellent image generation skills and their expert integration into clinical problem-solving.

In Vanuatu, it may represent the only imaging modality available to the sole practitioner. This contrasts with the relative availability of formal ultrasound, computed tomography, and magnetic resonance imaging in large first-world teaching centres. Yet even in these well-staffed, affluent environments, this tool has found a niche.

This niche seems to have resulted for a couple of reasons. Firstly, the clinician's willing-ness to use a safe tool at *their* threshold of suspicion to facilitate diagnosis and treatment; PoCUS does not require a telephone call, a consult, or significant delay. Additionally, the low threshold for its use facilitates repeating the evaluation during the course of the illness (abdominal trauma for haemoperitoneum) or adequacy of treatment (a replete inferior vena cava in shock). This tool helps us make good decisions for our patients in a timely fashion. The evidence is growing.

The multinational crew of wonderful editors and authors attests to the wide adoption of PoCUS for the bedside clinician. The tool has evolved from basic applications into areas that could not have been conceived of at the beginning of the journey. This text provides a safe and simple approach to image generation and knowledge integration across the spectrum of clinical environments. The future of this tool is in your hands!

Dr Peter Ross
Immediate Past President, Canadian Emergency Ultrasound Society

Preface

Point-of-Care Ultrasound for Emergency Medicine and Resuscitation (Oxford Clinical Imaging Guides) focuses on the day-to-day utility of clinician-performed point-of-care ultrasound (PoCUS) in emergency medicine and during the resuscitation of critically ill patients. The book aligns with published ultrasound curricula, including those from *The Royal College of Emergency Medicine (UK), The American College of Emergency Physicians, The Canadian Association of Emergency Physicians* and *Canadian Point-of-Care Ultrasound Society, The Australasian College for Emergency Medicine, The College of Emergency Medicine of South Africa, Focused Acute Medicine Ultrasound (FAMUS; UK),* and *The International Federation for Emergency Medicine.*

The traditional separation of 'echocardiography' from 'ultrasound' was due to the historical division of who performed and interpreted the scanning, rather than any particular organic difference in principles. Ultrasound can, of course, be applied to any part of the body, and in modern practice, PoCUS has evolved to become an indispensable clinical tool in the emergency and critical care settings, providing clinically relevant information that impacts patient care.

In this book, we focus on the utility of PoCUS in the diagnosis and management of a wide variety of illnesses and injuries seen in emergency departments, critical care units, hospital wards, and the pre-hospital setting. These include cardiac and extra-cardiac causes of shock and critical illness, as well as other common acute care conditions and procedures. We will address how ultrasound can add value to traditional approaches for key conditions relevant to all clinicians involved in emergency medicine and acute care. The book introduces the concept of PoCUS, provides a practical approach to the practical and technological aspects of scanning, reviews clinical systems, beginning with cardiac ultrasound, before continuing through the chest, abdomen, and pelvis, and finally considers the major vessels, soft tissues, and small parts. The section on procedural ultrasound provides reasoning for, and a practical approach to, the use of PoCUS to make invasive procedures safer for patients and easier for clinicians. We provide an overview of educational principles for PoCUS and how simulation can be integrated into learning and skills maintenance. Finally, we provide further information on the use of PoCUS in paediatric and pre-hospital populations. This book will provide a valuable introduction to PoCUS for the novice, and serve as a useful resource for those who regularly use or teach clinician-performed ultrasound.

Acknowledgements

We would like to thank all the authors and contributors for their hard work, skill, and patience during the writing of this book. We would also like to acknowledge the countless patients, volunteers, physicians, and students who have unwittingly contributed to the body of knowledge in this book, as we first learned and then taught ultrasound throughout our careers.

Table of contents

Abbreviations

AAA	abdominal aortic aneurysm	DPL	diagnostic peritoneal lavage
ACEP	American College of Emergency Physicians	DR	decidual reaction
		DTB	disseminated tuberculosis
ACES	Abdominal and Cardiac Evaluation with Sonography in Shock	DTI	tissue Doppler imaging
		DVT	deep vein thrombosis
ACLS	advanced cardiovascular life support	EAST	Eastern Association for the Surgery of Trauma
ACS	acute coronary syndrome	ECG	electrocardiogram; electrocardiograph
ADHF	acute decompensated heart failure	ED	Emergency Department
AED	automated external defibrillator	EDV	end-diastolic volume
AP	anteroposterior	EF	ejection fraction
APE	acute cardiogenic pulmonary oedema	e-FAST	Extended Focused Assessment with Sonography for Trauma
ARDS	acute respiratory distress syndrome	EGLS	Echo-Guided Life Support
ATFL	anterior talo-fibular ligament	ELS	Echo in Life Support
ATLS	advanced trauma life support	EMS	emergency medical system
BEME	best evidence medical education	EPSS	E-point septal separation
BP	blood pressure	ESV	end-systolic volume
bpm	beats per minute	ETT	endotracheal tube
CAEP	Canadian Association of Emergency Physicians	ETUDE	Evaluation Tool for Ultrasound skills Development and Education
CAUSE	cardiac arrest ultrasound examination	EUP	extra-uterine pregnancy
CBD	common bile duct	EVLW	extravascular lung water
CCA	common carotid artery	4F	fluid–form–function–filling (approach)
CGI	computer-generated image	FASH	Focused Assessment with Sonography for HIV-associated tuberculosis
CHF	congestive heart failure		
CLT	cognitive load theory	FAST	focused assessment with sonography for trauma
cm	centimetre		
CO	cardiac output	FATE	Focus Assessed Transthoracic Echocardiography
CO2	carbon dioxide		
COPD	chronic obstructive pulmonary disease	FB	foreign body
CPD	colour power Doppler	FEEL	Focused Echocardiography in Emergency Life support
CPR	cardiopulmonary resuscitation		
CPUS	clinician-performed ultrasound	FHB	fetal heartbeat
CRL	crown–rump length	FICB	fascia iliaca compartment block
CRT	capillary refill time	FNB	femoral nerve block
CT	computed tomography	FNOF	fractured neck of the femur
CVP	central venous pressure	FoCUS	focused cardiac ultrasound
CW	continuous wave (Doppler)	FP	fetal pole
CXR	chest X-ray	G	gauge
2D	two-dimensional	GCS	Glasgow Coma Scale
DICOM	Digital Imaging and Communications in Medicine	GR	globe rupture
DP	deliberate practice		

GS	gestational sac	OSCE	objective structured clinical examination
HA	hepatic artery		
hCG	human chorionic gonadotrophin	PACS	picture archiving and communication system
(H)EMS	helicopter and ground-based emergency medical services		
		PE	pulmonary embolism/embolus
HPS	hypertrophic pyloric stenosis	PEA	pulseless electrical activity
HR	heart rate	PICC	peripherally inserted central catheter
HTX	haemothorax	PLAX	parasternal long axis
ICP	intracranial pressure	PNS	peripheral nerve stimulation
ICU	intensive care unit	PoCS	point-of-care sonography
IFEM	International Federation of Emergency Medicine	PoCUS	point-of-care ultrasound
		PPV	positive predictive value
IJV	internal jugular vein	PRF	pulse repetition frequency
IUD	intrauterine device	PSAX	parasternal short axis
IUP	intrauterine pregnancy	PTX	pneumothorax
IVC	inferior vena cava	PUL	pregnancy in an unknown location
IVCCI	collapse index of the inferior vena cava	PV	portal vein
		PVD	posterior vitreous detachment
kg	kilogram	PW	pulsed wave (Doppler)
kPa	kilopascal	PZT	lead zirconate titanate
LAD	left anterior descending (artery)	RAP	right atrial pressure
LAST	local anaesthetic severe toxicity	RCA	right coronary artery
LSV	long saphenous vein	RD	retinal detachment
LUQ	left upper quadrant	REBOA	resuscitative balloon occlusion of the aorta
LV	left ventricular		
LVEF	left ventricular ejection fraction	RIF	right iliac fossa
LVOT	left ventricular outflow tract	ROC	receiver operating characteristic
m	metre	ROSC	return of spontaneous circulation
MAC	mitral annulus calcification	RR	respiratory rate
MAPSE	mitral valve annular plane systolic excursion	RUQ	right upper quadrant
		RUSH	Rapid Ultrasound for Shock and Hypotension
MCA	middle cerebral artery		
MHz	megahertz	s	second
MI	mechanical index	SBP	spontaneous bacterial peritonitis
mL	millilitre	SCFE	slipped capital femoral epiphysis
mm	millimetre	SCV	subclavian vein
mmHg	millimetre of mercury	SDOT	standardized direct observation tool
mph	mile per hour	SHoC	Sonography in Hypotension and Cardiac arrest
MRI	magnetic resonance imaging		
m/s	metre per second	SMA	superior mesenteric artery
MSK	musculoskeletal	SMBE	simulation-based medical education
NGT	nasogastric tube	SPC	suprapubic catheter/catheterization
NICE	National Institute for Health and Care Excellence	SSP	supraspinatus
		SV	stroke volume
NPSA	National Patient Safety Agency	SVR	systemic vascular resistance
NPV	negative predictive value	SVV	stroke volume variation
O&G	obstetric and gynaecological	TA	trans-abdominal
ONSD	optic nerve sheath diameter		

TAPSE	tricuspid annular plane systolic excursion	TV	trans-vaginal
TCD	trans-cranial Doppler	UK	United Kingdom
TDI	tissue Doppler imaging	VF	ventricular fibrillation
TGC	time gain compensation	VH	vitreous haemorrhage
THI	tissue harmonic imaging	VT	ventricular tachycardia
TI	thermal index	VTI	velocity time integral
TOE (TEE)	transoesophageal echocardiography	VUJ	vesicoureteric junction
TT	tracheal tube	WHO	World Health Organization
TTE	transthoracic echocardiography	YS	yolk sac
		ZPD	zone of proximal development

Contributors

Dr Miteb Al-Githami, Emergency Medicine Consultant, King Faisal Specialist Hospital, Jeddah, Saudi Arabia

Dr Paul Atkinson, Professor in Emergency Medicine, Dalhousie University, Saint John Regional Hospital, Saint John, Canada

Dr Justin Bowra, Emergency Ultrasound Programme Director, Royal North Shore Hospital; Adjunct Senior Lecturer, University of Sydney, Sydney, Australia

Dr Jim Connolly, Consultant in Emergency Medicine, Great North Trauma and Emergency Centre, Newcastle –upon-Tyne, UK

Dr Chris Cox, Assistant Professor in Emergency Medicine, Dalhousie University, Halifax Infirmary, Halifax, Canada

Dr Stuart Durham, Consultant in Emergency Medicine, Royal Preston Hospital, Preston, UK

Dr Jason Fischer, Associate Professor in Paediatric Emergency Medicine, University of Toronto, Toronto, Canada

Dr James French, Assistant Professor in Emergency Medicine, Dalhousie University, Saint John Regional Hospital, Saint John, Canada

Dr Rip Gangahar, Consultant in Emergency Medicine, Royal Oldham Hospital, Oldham, UK

Dr John Hardin, Emergency Ultrasound Fellow, Beth Israel Deaconess Medical Center; Clinical Fellow in Emergency Medicine, Harvard Medical School, Boston, USA

Dr Tim Harris, Consultant in Emergency Medicine and Pre-hospital Care, Barts Health NHS Trust; Professor in Emergency Medicine, Queen Mary University of London, London, UK

Dr Ryan Henneberry, Assistant Professor in Emergency Medicine, Dalhousie University, Halifax Infirmary, Halifax, Canada

Dr Beatrice Hoffmann, Emergency Ultrasound Program Director, Beth Israel Deaconess Medical Center; Associate Professor in Emergency Medicine, Harvard Medical School, Boston, USA

Dr Bob Jarman, Consultant in Emergency Medicine, Royal Victoria Infirmary, Newcastle-upon-Tyne; Visiting Professor, University of Teesside, Middlesbrough, UK

Sharon Kay, Associate Professor in Echocardiography and Cardiac Imaging, Head of Program CQ University, Northern School, Faculty of Medicine, University of Sydney, Charles Perkins Centre & Kolling Medical Research Institute, Royal North Shore Hospital, Sydney, Australia

Dr Hein Lamprecht, Emergency Physician, Stellenbosch University, Cape Town, South Africa

Dr David Lewis, Associate Professor in Emergency Medicine, Dalhousie University, Saint John Regional Hospital, Saint John, Canada

Dr Osama Loubani, Assistant Professor in Emergency Medicine, Dalhousie University, Halifax Infirmary, Halifax, Canada

Dr Lianne McLean, Assistant Professor in Paediatric Emergency Medicine, The Hospital for Sick Children, University of Toronto, Toronto, Canada

Dr Paul Olszynski, Emergency Physician, Assistant Professor in Emergency Medicine, University of Saskatchewan, Saskatoon, Canada

Dr Nils Petter Oveland, Emergency Physician, Department of Health Studies, Network for Medical Sciences, University of Stavanger, and Department of Anesthesiology and Intensive Care, Stavanger University Hospital, Stavanger, Norway

Dr Brandon Ritcey, Assistant Ultrasound Fellowship Director, University of Ottawa, The Ottawa Hospital, Ottawa, Canada

Dr Michael Rubin, Emergency Physician, The Ottawa Hospital; Emergency Clinical Fellowship Director, University of Ottawa, Ottawa, Canada

Dr Elena Skoromovsky, Emergency Ultrasound Fellow, Beth Israel Deaconess Medical Center; Instructor in Emergency Medicine, Harvard medical School, Boston, USA

Dr Melanie Stander, Emergency Physician, Stellenbosch University, Cape Town, South Africa

Dr Mark Tutschka, Staff General Internist and Intensivist, Saint John Regional Hospital, Saint John, NB, Canada

Dr Matthew L. Wong, Emergency Physician, Beth Israel Deaconess Medical Center; Instructor of Emergency Medicine, Harvard Medical School, Boston, USA

Dr Michael Y Woo, Associate Professor in Emergency Medicine, University of Ottawa, The Ottawa Hospital, Ottawa, Canada

Digital media accompanying the book

Individual purchasers of this book are entitled to **free** personal access to accompanying digital media in the online edition. Please refer to the access token card for instructions on token redemption and access.

The corresponding media can be found on *Oxford Medicine Online* at: www.oxfordmedicine.com/POCUSemergencymed

Videos and figures

There are over 160 videos and 100 annotated figures of point-of-care ultrasound (see example below). These demonstrate and provide instructions on how to perform ultrasound and interpret what you see, for the emergency, acute, and critical care settings.

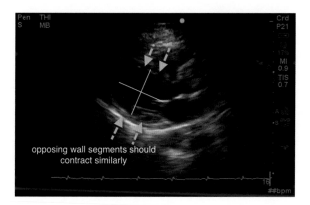

Throughout the book, videos and figures are noted with these symbols, so you can easily find the corresponding material online:

📷 Videos

🖼 Figures

Further reading

Additional further reading lists can be found online—supporting further learning and discovery. This symbol is noted at the end of each chapter to remind you: 📖 Further reading

Share this resource

If you are interested in access to the complete online edition, please consult with your librarian.

Introduction and clinical scenarios

Paul Atkinson and Bob Jarman, with Tim Harris, Rip Gangahar, David Lewis, Justin Bowra, and Hein Lamprecht

Summary

A brief overview summarizes the background and importance of the use of ultrasound in clinical care and the development of ultrasound in emergency medicine and resuscitation.

Understanding the principles and practice of ultrasound:

An introduction to the basic and more advanced facets of ultrasound technology used in emergency and critical care practice is followed by a discussion of the equipment required and the terminology used when scanning.

Clinical scenarios and protocols:

Clinical scenarios help frame the use of point-of-care ultrasound (PoCUS) in the clinical setting, as a tool to help the clinician with initial diagnosis and management of emergencies and in resuscitation. Some of the PoCUS protocols commonly used in emergency medicine and resuscitation are reviewed.

Introduction

There is a long history behind the use of sound waves in medical diagnosis, with the use of percussion in physical examination first described in 1761 by Leopold Auenbrugger, the son of an innkeeper, who had learnt to tap on casks of wine to estimate the volume of their contents. For centuries, percussion, listening for altered reflected sound waves, would assist clinicians to differentiate fluid from air-filled spaces, almost as a crude form of ultrasound. When Rene Laennec first rolled a sheet of paper into a cone to enable him to listen to a patient's chest, the concept of the stethoscope was born. In 1819, Laennac published a manual on his new wooden device and coined terms, such as 'rales', that are still used to this day. John Forbes, writing on the stethoscope in the first English translation of Laennec's manual, stated it to be:

' ... one of the greatest discoveries in medicine ... ' but ' ... that it will ever come into general use, notwithstanding its value, I am extremely doubtful ... '

While the stethoscope continues to play a key role in modern clinical assessment, the widespread integration of ultrasound and echocardiography into education, research, and clinical practice in emergency and critical care medicine, as well as across multiple acute specialties, demonstrates an awareness of the limitations of the traditional physical examination and the success of the clinician-performed 'point-of-care ultrasound' (PoCUS) approach. PoCUS (or alternatively bedside, focused, or clinician-performed ultrasound or echo) is defined as 'ultrasound that is performed by a clinician during a patient encounter to help guide the evaluation and management of the patient'.

While technologies such as computed tomography (CT) and magnetic resonance imaging (MRI) provide impressive imaging of most organ systems, they may not be immediately available to the treating clinician who needs further information at the bedside.

Ultrasound provides the clinician with additional diagnostic and therapeutic information, becoming part of the physical examination, and provides a strengthened link between physician and patient, through the hands-on dynamic nature of this tool.

Ultrasound can, of course, be applied to any part of the body, and in modern practice, PoCUS has evolved to become an indispensable test in the emergency and resuscitation setting. Important advantages are that ultrasound is:

- Readily available at the bedside, eliminating the need for transport to unmonitored areas of the hospital;
- Rapid, giving immediate real-time answers to the clinician performing the examination;
- Reproducible, for monitoring response to treatment;
- Inexpensive (relatively);
- Free of ionizing radiation;
- Versatile, being able to both rule in and exclude multiple different diagnoses.

It is this versatility that, for example, makes ultrasound the ideal imaging modality in the evaluation of the critically ill patient with undifferentiated hypotension. Multiple different aetiologies of hypotension can be considered and investigated, all with the same machine, in a matter of minutes. The limitation, as with many aspects of the physical examination and other bedside tests, is that ultrasound is operator-dependent. Comfort and competence in both image acquisition and image interpretation are essential, as is the knowledge of how to incorporate findings into patient care.

The use of ultrasound in various emergency and resuscitation scenarios has been shown to provide clinically relevant information that impacts patient care, as will be discussed in detail throughout the various chapters of the book.

A review of currently available PoCUS curricula and guidelines highlights that most divide ultrasound applications into core (or basic) and enhanced (or advanced/extended). Core applications cover traditional clinical questions where there is a body of evidence of clinical relevance and that are within the likely skill set of a novice practitioner. In general, *core* clinical PoCUS applications are simple to learn, perform, and interpret; are rapid to perform; answer simple questions, ideally with binary (yes/no) answers; allow learners to consolidate key ultrasound skills, which provide a solid foundation to their practice; and have a significant impact in the area/region being practised due to burden of disease, local resources, or mortality/morbidity considerations.

In emergency medicine, core diagnostic applications have traditionally included the identification of abdominal aortic aneurysm, focused echocardiography during cardiac arrest, and identification of an intrauterine pregnancy (IUP) in the first trimester, as well as assessing for critical pathology in trauma patients. More recently, the scope of answers provided by PoCUS has expanded. *Enhanced* PoCUS applications are those that are more difficult to learn, perform, and interpret; require prior proficiency in a related, more basic core application; answer more complex questions; or may be simple to learn but have less impact in the area/region being practised due to different burdens of disease, local resources, or mortality/morbidity considerations. Enhanced skills for emergency physicians include such problems as identification of pleural fluid and pneumothorax, identification of deep vein thrombosis (DVT), assessment of the inferior vena cava (IVC) for filling status, shock protocols, as well as more traditional ultrasound indications such as cholelithiasis and hydronephrosis. Procedurally, ultrasound guidance has made insertion of central venous catheters safer and has improved success rates for regional nerve blocks.

Critical care physicians practising in intensive care units (ICUs) have traditionally focused on basic and enhanced cardiac ultrasound or echocardiography, assessment of cardiac output, as well as adding complementary modalities such as IVC assessment, guidance for vascular access, and, more recently, thoracic ultrasound.

In everyday practice, clinicians regularly face challenges when trying to identify serious pathology or reduce procedural complications in a timely manner, and as a result, they have continued to develop innovative uses for, and expanded the indications of, PoCUS.

A key feature of PoCUS is that it is not a replacement to traditional ultrasound or echocardiographic practice but is a limited ultrasound examination, usually practised at the bedside of the patient, in suboptimal conditions with time limitations. Hence, the application is focused on answering a clinical question (or set of questions), which can augment clinical care.

In response to the increased number of indications for PoCUS in various clinical settings, several protocols have become established. These combine several ultrasound views and clinical questions, and are aimed at optimizing the approach to the use of PoCUS in certain clinical scenarios and include the *Extended Focused Assessment with Sonography for Trauma (e-FAST)*; *Sonography in Hypotension and Cardiac arrest (SHoC)*; *Rapid Ultrasound for Shock and Hypotension (RUSH)*; *Abdominal and Cardiac Evaluation with Sonography in Shock (ACES)*; *Echo in Life Support (ELS)*; *Echo-Guided Life Support (EGLS)*; *Focused Echocardiography in Emergency Life support (FEEL)*; and *Focused Assessment with Sonography for HIV-associated tuberculosis (FASH)* protocols, among others.

PoCUS now transcends specialty boundaries and has relevance to most clinician groups, and is becoming integrated into undergraduate medical education in some centres. Popularity of use has also been influenced by improved and tailored ultrasound systems: reduction in price and relative size, improved portability and quality, ease of use, and speedy start-up times. We encourage all physicians to review Moore and Copel's list of current PoCUS applications (see 'Further reading', p. 32) in use within various clinical specialties. With a plethora of PoCUS applications available, there are continued challenges to ensure that such PoCUS can be delivered with adherence to good governance principles.

It is essential that opportunities for PoCUS training are available as part of all emergency and critical care training programmes. PoCUS has become a core clinical skill for all clinicians involved in emergency medicine and resuscitation, alongside airway management and electrocardiogram (ECG) and radiographic interpretation.

The book serves as a core text for emergency physicians who wish to apply their PoCUS skills to a wide variety of critical care indications, both cardiac and non-cardiac. It also provides a framework for physicians involved in resuscitation and the management of critical illness to expand their echocardiographic skills beyond the heart, to incorporate the various non-cardiac modalities of PoCUS into their practice.

The book aligns with several international PoCUS curricula, as outlined in the preface.

While the information presented on PoCUS is based on current evidence, with time, new information may change practice. It is essential that PoCUS practice and education develop in line with other general principles of medical practice and education, and considers the following:

- *Training*. While the traditional model of an introductory course or module, followed by a number of supervised determinate scans, may continue in the foreseeable future, a multifaceted approach is needed due to local factors. PoCUS skills are critical to the clinical development of emergency and critical care physicians, and a minimum skill set should be mandatory for all graduating emergency medicine trainees, with additional fellowship training, to provide leaders, researchers, and educators with excellence in PoCUS.

- *Credentialing*. It is essential to ensure that a trainee in PoCUS has demonstrated competency in a particular application, before they can practise independently. Being competent to practise is not just about being able to undertake the application examination, but importantly also understanding the relevance of what the findings mean to clinical practice.

- *Governance*. Once independently practising, the physician sonographer needs to ensure that they keep their skills up-to-date. Peer review and audit have an important role in demonstrating continued competency. Keeping up-to-date with regard to the latest medical research in this area is essential. Regular maintenance of equipment and quality assurance review of ultrasound performance are required.

- *Research*. While there is a growing evidence base supporting the benefits of PoCUS in clinical medicine, much of the literature to date falls short of proving true outcome benefit. It is important that we meet the challenge of conducting well-designed studies to further support our practice.

In this book, we review the approach to the use of PoCUS in the setting of emergency medicine and resuscitation. We hope that the information provided will enhance learning for the reader, but we want to state strongly that, as a clinical skill, ultrasound must be learned 'hands on' and that, as with any skill, experience is key.

Understanding the principles and practice of ultrasound

Purpose

This section will introduce you to the basic and more advanced facets of ultrasound technology used in emergency and critical care practice. It will introduce and explain the equipment required and the terminology used when scanning.

Perspective

The modern clinician has a choice of many types of ultrasound machine, available for use at the point of care. Such equipment is distinguishable from those found in traditional radiological practice, in that they are more simply designed for use at the bedside.

Getting started

The ultrasound machine should ideally be placed in an accessible location for all users where it will not be easily stolen or damaged. There should be power available, so that it can be charged when not in use. Most systems have a battery, so they can be taken to the bedside without needing to always have a power supply available. It may be advantageous to switch the system on, *while taking the machine to the patient*. If your machine takes a long time to boot up after being switched off, you may elect to keep it turned on or in a standby mode. If it is to be kept switched on, keep the freeze button on and turn the screen off to avoid damage to both the probe and screen, respectively.

It is good practice to ensure that, prior to use, you enter the patient details into the machine. These details will be displayed on the screen. If you are performing the scan in an emergency situation, you may decide not to enter all the demographics—often the hospital identification number or surname and initials will suffice. On many systems, you can go back later and complete the details. When you do save any images or clips, these should be identifiable for good governance

and legal reasons—most hospitals will have policies on saving and storing of ultrasound media.

Prior to any scanning, if possible, the patient should be advised on what you are about to do. Patient positioning is important for many applications; however, this is not always feasible in the critical care or emergency environment. For echocardiography, application of electrocardiograph (ECG) leads to the patient (available with most ultrasound machines) allows for the ECG trace to be displayed on the screen at the same time as the ultrasound images. The benefit of this is to correlate the ultrasound image with the timing of the cardiac cycle.

If you are able to control the ambient lighting, this should be reduced to improve the appreciation of details of the image on the screen.

Probe selection and function

The next step is to select the appropriate probe (or transducer) for the type of scan you want to perform. This may involve physically changing the probe's connector (including sometimes needing to turn off the machine) or selecting the appropriate probe via the machine's controls. There are various probes available for PoCUS; these are broadly summarized in Table 1.1. Images of commonly used probes are shown in Figure 1.1.

A probe, or transducer, is an expensive component of the system that essentially converts electrical signals to sound waves, and vice versa. The range of frequencies utilized in medical ultrasound is above the human hearing range, typically 2–15 MHz. This can be split further into two distinct sections—low and high frequency—where the former typically operates in the lower part of the range (2–6 MHz) and the latter in the higher part (6–15 MHz). There is variability between different manufacturers and probe types in what frequencies are adopted—fortunately, these are often written on the transducer (e.g. 5-2 written on a phased array probe means that it operates between 2 and 5 MHz). A probe has a range of frequencies at which it operates, as there is often adoption of harmonic technology, which means that multiple frequencies are used and also the user is able to further manipulate the applied frequencies within the range (discussed in more detail later in this chapter).

Table 1.1 Common characteristics and uses of ultrasound probes

Probe type	Typical operating frequency	Characteristics	Uses in PoCUS
Phased array or sector array	2–5 MHz (low)	This probe has a small, flat footprint and is typically used for cardiac and thoracic indications, due to the ability to scan through the intercostal spaces. It provides a wedge-shaped image in B-mode due to beam steering technology	It is the probe of choice for echocardiography, chest, plus an alternative probe for abdominal, obstetric and gynaecological (O&G) uses
Small curvilinear	2–5 MHz (low)	This probe has a small curved footprint and can be used as an alternative to a phased or sector array probe	As above
Curvilinear	2–5 MHz (low)	This probe has a large curved footprint and provides a wedge-shaped image in B-mode	It is the probe of choice for abdominal and O&G uses. It may be used for thoracic applications. However, the large size of the footprint means that rib shadows often dominate the image
Linear	5–12 MHz (high)	This flat footprint probe comes in a range of sizes, from a small hockey stick shape to a larger traditional shape. They provide a rectangular or trapezoidal-shaped image in B-mode	These probes are excellent for superficial scanning applications such as vascular access, musculoskeletal evaluation, and small parts. Due to the high-frequency operational range, they provide a better resolution

The anatomy of a probe is shown in Figure 1.2. Almost all probes have a cable attaching it to the ultrasound machine, although, in recent times, some manufacturers have adopted the use of wireless technology. There is the main body, designed to be held by the user, which is usually plastic in construction. The part of the probe where the ultrasound beam exits and enters is called the footprint, and this is often made of a rubber-type substance that can be damaged by abrasion or alcohol-based cleaning agents.

Probes are able to produce ultrasonic sound waves due to the presence of a piezoelectric plate. This is often composed of elements of manufactured ceramic material—lead zirconate titanate (PZT). When an electrical voltage is applied to the PZT, it deforms and produces a sound wave. Conversely, when the PZT is deformed by a sound wave, it produces an electrical signal. Many PZT elements are placed side by side in the piezoelectric plate—typically 128, although some linear probes may have twice this amount. There are other components to the probe; however, this is beyond the level of this chapter. Unfortunately, this piezoelectric plate is easily damaged when the probe is dropped; therefore, all users must exercise caution in the often frenetic PoCUS environment.

Ultrasound beam and orientation

The shape of the ultrasound beam produced is technically complex but, for all intents and purposes, should be considered as a flat plane that is very thin (<5 mm) like a blade. The shape of the flat plane depends on the type of probe. Appreciation of this plane is key to understanding the image produced in B-mode and how this relates to the anatomical structures seen. Put simply, whatever the ultrasound 'blade' slices through will be viewed in cross-section on the screen. If the target organ is not 'cut' by the beam, it will not be visualized. Each probe has a notch or groove on one side of the body that corresponds to a marker on the screen. In radiological (i.e. non-echocardiography) uses, the marker is shown

(a)

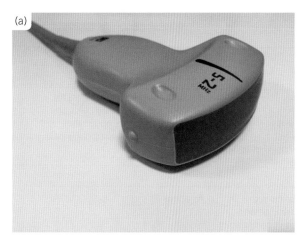

(b)

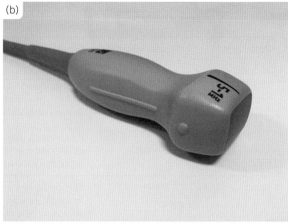

(c)

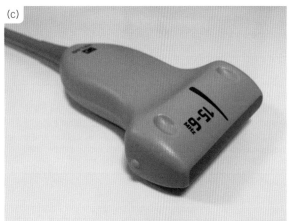

Figure 1.1 (a) A curvilinear transducer (low frequency). (b) A phased array transducer (low frequency). (c) A linear transducer (high frequency).

Reproduced with kind permission from Fujifilm Sonosite.

on the top left of the screen in B-mode. In echocardiography, this marker is denoted on the top right of the screen. In certain echocardiography views, such as parasternal views, the orientation plane used is based on the axis of the heart; the general direction

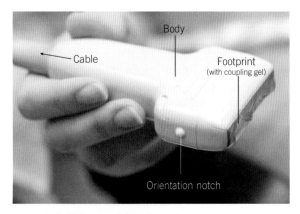

Figure 1.2 Anatomy of a probe.

Image source: iStock.com/zilli.

of the longitudinal plane of the heart is from the right shoulder to the left hip. The essential principle in understanding orientation is that the marker on the screen corresponds to the marker on the probe. The user should orient the probe to ensure they understand which direction on the body is represented on each side of the screen. As a rule, in emergency medicine, we recommend the simplified approach of ensuring that the image on the screen aligns with how the clinician is viewing the patient and how the organs lie anatomically. One exception to this is the parasternal long axis (PLAX) (nicknamed the parasternal 'wrong' axis) where the traditional orientation results in the apex of the heart being represented on the left side of the screen, which, when viewed from the right side of the patient's bed, is inverted anatomically. This is further outlined in Table 1.2 and Figure 1.3 where key orientation principles are highlighted.

Table 1.2 Commonly used plane orientations

Plane orientation	Radiological applications (non-echocardiography)	Echocardiography applications
Longitudinal (sagittal) (Figure 1.3a); (coronal) (Figure 1.3b)	Probe—notch points towards the patient's head end Screen marker position—on the left side of the screen (left side of image corresponds to the patient's head end)	Probe—notch points towards the patient's head end Screen marker position—on the right side of the screen (right side of image corresponds to the patient's head end)
Transverse (horizontal) (Figure 1.3c and d)	Probe—notch points towards the patient's right side Screen marker position—on the left side of the screen (left side of image corresponds to the patient's right side) Procedural: Align probe notch points and screen marker position to ensure near screen is near patient	Probe—notch points towards the patient's left side Screen marker position—on the right side of the screen (right side of image corresponds to the patient's left side)
Subcostal (coronal/4-chamber view) (Figure 1.3e)	Radiological orientation: Probe—notch points towards the patient's right side Screen marker position—on the left side of the screen (left side of image corresponds to the patient's right side)	Cardiac orientation: Probe—notch points towards the patient's left side Screen marker position—on the right side of the screen (left side of image corresponds to the patient's right side)
Parasternal Long Axis (PLAX) (corresponds to the longitudinal axis of the heart) (Figure 1.3f and g)	Alternative radiological orientation: Probe—notch points towards the patient's right shoulder Screen marker position—on the left side of screen (left side of image corresponds to the great vessel part of the longitudinal axis; right side of image corresponds to the apex of the left ventricle)	Preferred cardiac orientation: Probe—notch points towards the patient's right shoulder Screen marker position—on the right side of screen (right side of image corresponds to the great vessel part of the longitudinal axis; left side of image corresponds to the apex of the left ventricle)
Parasternal short axis (PSAX) (perpendicular to the longitudinal axis of the heart) (Figure 1.3h)	Alternative radiological orientation: Probe—notch points towards the patient's right hip (i.e. 90° clockwise to the long axis) Screen marker position—on the left side of screen	Preferred cardiac orientation: Probe—notch points towards the patient's left shoulder (i.e. 90° clockwise to the long axis) Screen marker position—on the right side of screen
Apical (coronal/4-chamber view) (Figure 1.3i)	Alternative radiological orientation: Probe—notch points towards the patient's right side Screen marker position—on the left side of screen	Preferred cardiac orientation: Probe—notch points towards the patient's left axilla Screen marker position—on the right side of screen

Presets

Following selection of a probe to use, you should also select a preset. Most probes will have a selection of these for you to choose, depending on the application you are undertaking. The use of presets allows for you to quickly adapt the various settings on the machine to be optimized for the chosen application; for example, echocardiography presets are optimized to show more of a black/white tissue/fluid differentiation and to refresh the screen rapidly (high frame rate), whereas general abdominal presets are optimized to show different parenchymal architecture, utilizing a wide range of greyscale, and do not refresh the screen rapidly (low frame rate). A wrong choice of preset can seriously affect the quality of your images.

Handling the probe

The way you hold and manipulate the probe is a very important skill that takes some time to learn for most users. You should hold it like a pen, not a paintbrush, to allow fine motor control—essential for small changes in probe position, especially in echocardiography. Also, part of your hand (usually the ulnar border) should be anchored to the patient's body to prevent unnecessary movement or applying too much pressure. There are various movements of the probe that can be undertaken when performing a scan. They are summarized in Table 1.3.

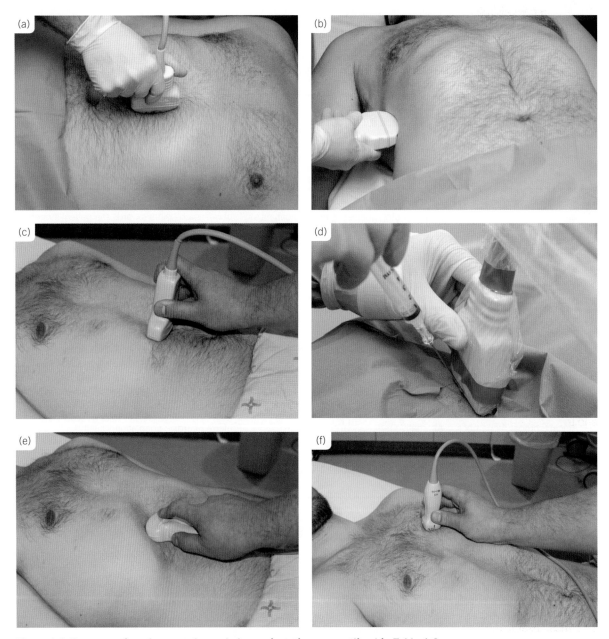

Figure 1.3 Demonstration of commonly used plane orientations, as outlined in Table 1.2.

Parasternal long (wrong) axis

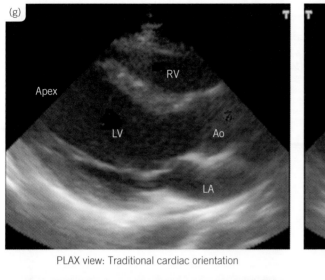

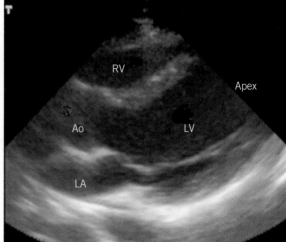

PLAX view: Traditional cardiac orientation

PLAX view: Alternative orientation

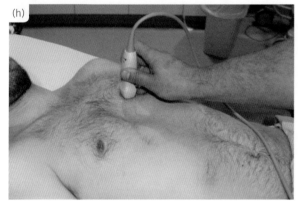

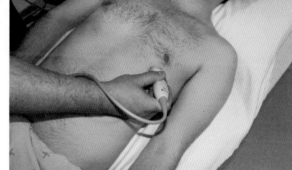

Figure 1.3 (Continued)

Application of ultrasound coupling gel to the footprint of the probe, or the region of the patient being scanned, is essential, as any air between the probe and the patient will result in the ultrasound beam being immediately reflected back to the probe, and not into the patient. If you are struggling to get a good image, always consider whether you have applied enough gel. For applications such as central vascular access, keeping a sterile field is important. The ultrasound probe should be covered with a sterile sheath (although a sterile surgical glove or condom will suffice)—this will be discussed in more detail in Chapter 9.

B-mode

The most useful mode on the ultrasound machine is B-mode; this stands for brightness mode and is sometimes referred to as two-dimensional (2D) scanning (many machines will have either a B-mode or a 2D button). This mode uses the ultrasound information received by the probe to produce a 2D visual representation of the anatomy evaluated—as in Figure 1.4 [a coronal view of the right upper quadrant (RUQ)]. This information is only in greyscale—from black through to white. What is shown as black or white depends on the strength of the ultrasound beam reflected back to the probe—highly reflected areas are represented as white on the screen; areas of no reflection are represented as black on the screen; and areas of partial reflection are shown as grey, with their level of 'brightness' correlating with increasing reflectivity. The position on the screen depends on two things—from which part of the PZT plate the original

Table 1.3 Probe movements

Movement	Description	Image
Rotation	The probe is rotated on its central axis and is beneficial when turning from transverse to longitudinal in vascular access and also between PLAX and PSAX	Rotation
Rocking	The probe is rocked, keeping the angle of the plane constant—this is often towards or away from the marker notch—more intuitive with curvilinear probes, as it uses the natural curve of the footprint	Rocking
Tilting/fanning	Tilting or fanning the probe side to side is beneficial when sweeping the plane through a structure—especially important when performing a PSAX of the heart	Tilting/fanning

Table 1.3 (Continued)

Movement	Description	Image
Pressure	Varying the amount of pressure applied can be beneficial in securing the view—especially relevant to abdominal scanning when this can be used to 'push' bowel gas out of the way	Pressure

ultrasound beam was generated and how long it took for the ultrasound beam to return.

The ultrasound beam generated is not continuous from all parts of the PZT plate. Sets of elements in the plate take it in turn (i.e. in a repeating sequence) to transmit a burst of ultrasound signal. The set of elements then awaits the return of the ultrasound signal. Each set of elements is able to send and receive many times per second. Figure 1.5 shows a simplified model of how the sets of elements send bursts of ultrasound pulses in sequence. In reality, the number of sequences involved is much higher, due to most probes having at least 128 elements. If the sequence is slow to repeat, then the real-time image on the screen may appear to stagger and is not fluid. This is why ultrasound evaluation of moving structures, such as the heart, needs to refresh the B-mode image at least 50 times per second. This is called the frame rate, and some presets, e.g. for echocardiography, are designed for a high frame rate; abdominal presets do not need a high frame rate.

The depth of the reflected ultrasound signal on the screen is related to the time it takes for it to return to the probe; the deeper it is, the longer it takes to return. The ultrasound machine assumes that the speed of sound (ultrasound) in tissues is constant at 1540 m/s. As the signal is required to get to the area of interest and then back, the time taken is halved to give the depth.

Impedance and reflection

Despite the ultrasound machine assuming that the speed of sound is constant in tissues, in reality, it is variable; Table 1.4 highlights the speed of sound in common tissues. Each tissue has an acoustic impedance value

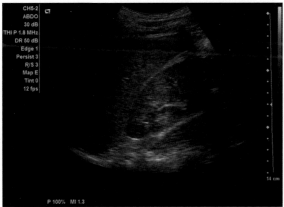

Figure 1.4 B-mode image of a normal coronal view of the diaphragm, liver, and kidney on the right side is shown.

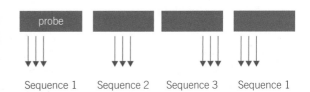

Figure 1.5 Sets of PZT elements send bursts of ultrasound pulses.

Table 1.4 Speed of sound in common tissues

Tissue	Speed of sound in tissue (m/s)
Liver	1578
Kidney	1560
Fat	1430
Water	1480
Air	333
Bone	3190–3406

Data from Duck FA. Physical Properties of Tissue: A Comprehensive Reference Book. London: Academic Press (1990).

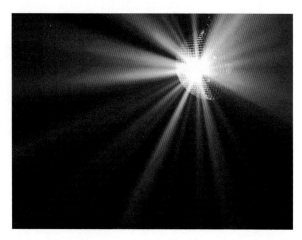

Figure 1.6 Scattering of ultrasound is like light striking a glittering disco ball.

Image source: iStock.com/nikkytok.

(*z*) that is a product of density and acoustic velocity. At the interface between two tissues with differing *z* values, reflection occurs; the larger the difference, the larger the reflection. Hence, soft tissue/air and soft tissue/bone interfaces are large reflectors and will be white (also called echogenic or bright) in B-mode.

There are two main types of reflection:

1. Reflection at broad interfaces between tissues of differing impedance (*z*), e.g. the diaphragm in an RUQ view or fascial planes when scanning for nerve blocks. The direction of reflection is fairly predictable;

2. Scattering by small particles ($\le$ wavelength of the ultrasound signal), e.g. liver appearances on ultrasound. Note the higher the frequency (and therefore the smaller the wavelength), the greater the degree of scattering. The reflections are multidirectional, hence the name scattering; this is similar to when a broad beam of light hits a spherical discotheque ball (see Figure 1.6).

Figure 1.7 shows how the depth and degree of reflectivity result in the B-mode image.

Frequency and attenuation

The depth achievable for a particular probe is dependent on the operating frequency. Frequency is related to the wavelength of the ultrasound generated—the wavelength is the speed of sound in a tissue divided by the frequency. As previously discussed, there are low- and high-frequency probes. High-frequency

sound waves do not penetrate into the tissues very far, and it would be uncommon for a depth of >6 cm to be achievable. Low-frequency sound waves are able to penetrate into tissues further, often up to 30 cm. However, the resolution of the image becomes poorer as the frequency is lowered.

This loss of signal energy with increasing depth is called attenuation. It affects higher-frequency sound waves more than low-frequency, which accounts for the lower penetration. The causes of attenuation include:

- Energy absorption in the form of heat (thermal)
- Scattering of the ultrasound signal by small particles
- Reflection of tissue interfaces.

Different tissues are associated with different attenuation values, with fluid and blood being the lowest and bone being the highest. This is why it is preferable to scan through an area of low attenuation if you want to evaluate a deeper structure, e.g. using a full bladder to see the pelvic parenchyma.

Focus

All ultrasound beams generated have a characteristic whereby they are focused onto a particular point, often by a physical and electronic lens system on the probe. This is called the focal zone. This creates a slight narrowing of the beam that results in a

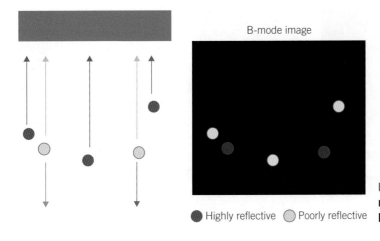

Highly reflective ⬤   Poorly reflective ◯

Figure 1.7 Depth and degree of reflectivity resulting in the generation of the greyscale B-mode image.

tighter concentration of pulses produced by different sets of elements in the PZT plate (see Figure 1.8). Although this is mainly a consideration for the broad plane of the beam, this also applies to the narrow plane. On many machines, the focal zone for the broad plane of the beam is adjustable and should be set for the level of interest. As the focal zone for the narrow plane of the beam is not electronically controllable, it is not adjustable. Some compact PoCUS machines do not have an adjustable focal zone and, as a general rule, the focal zone is set to the centre of the screen.

Resolution

Being able to tell objects apart is key for some PoCUS applications such as nerve blocks or vascular access.

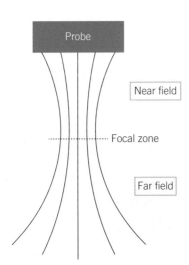

Figure 1.8 Typical beam shape and focal zone.

It is similar to watching television with a high-definition screen—very minute details can be made out. Conversely, watching television with an old standard-definition screen will not provide the same clarity and objects may appear blurred. There are three ways in which B-mode resolution may be improved:

1. By using the highest frequency possible, which is limited by how deeply the structure is located. This improves the ability to differentiate objects in the direction of the ultrasound beam—axial resolution;

2. By focusing the narrowest part of the ultrasound beam—the focal zone—on the area of interest. This improves the ability to differentiate objects side by side—lateral resolution;

3. By ensuring an appropriate frame rate. This will improve the temporal resolution, i.e. the ability of the B-mode to reflect changes in the structures seen with time. In general, the more expected from the machine, the poorer the temporal resolution.

Improving the image

After applying the probe, the image that may appear will often be unsatisfactory. There are many adjustments that the user can do on the console of the machine at the same time as holding and moving the probe. The understanding and manipulation of these controls is called knobology. Controls such as altering the depth range, focal zone setting, frequency adjustment, dynamic range, sector width, overall gain, and time gain compensation (TGC) are important. There

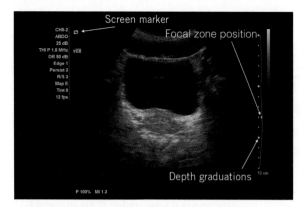

Figure 1.9 B-mode image of the transverse pelvis, showing the screen marker, depth graduations, and the focal zone position.

are also image enhancement tools that can be used, especially in difficult body habitus patients.

As previously discussed, the type of probe and frequency adopted predetermines the maximum depth. However, the machine's console will allow you to change the depth on the screen. It is really important to ensure that the area of interest occupies the main centre of the image in order to get the best resolution. Figure 1.9 shows a B-mode image with the depth graduations on the right-hand side of the image (the large bullet marks are for each 5 cm, and the smaller ones for each cm).

If your machine has an adjustable focal zone, it needs to be set for the area of interest (or just below it) and will improve lateral resolution.

Within the operating frequency range of your selected probe, there will be an opportunity to manipulate the frequency to the top, middle, or bottom of the range. This is often referred to as GEN (for general), RES (for resolution), and PEN (for penetration), respectively. If the area of interest is deep or the patient is obese, then PEN may be the best one to select, and the opposite for more superficial structures in thinner patients. Some machines will allow for the operating frequency to be adjusted throughout the range, as opposed to being limited to the top, middle, or bottom of the range.

Sector width can change the width of the operating beam. Especially in echocardiography applications, if the beam is kept wide, while the machine is also evaluating an area of interest using other modes such as colour flow Doppler, the processor is expected to work hard. This may have an effect on the frame rate—it will be reduced. Therefore, the operator can reduce the width of the sector on some machines, which will reduce some of the processing load off the machine and improve the frame rate, and therefore the temporal resolution (see Figure 1.10).

The dynamic range adjustment is seen in most systems. A full explanation is beyond this chapter. Simply, it is the range between the lowest intensity and the maximum highest intensity returning echoes that a system is capable of displaying. For most applications, the PoCUS user should not have to make many adjustments, as this should be accounted for in the preset settings. On occasion, it may be beneficial to reduce the range to remove background low-level noise echoes. In clinical applications such as echocardiography, using a narrow dynamic range produces a much more black and white image, which is useful to evaluate a moving

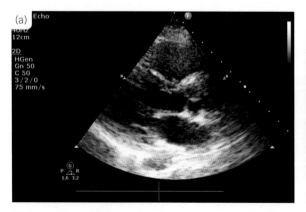
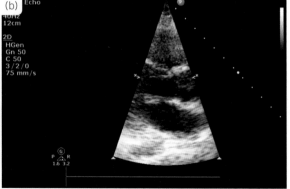

Figure 1.10 (a) Wide sector width. (b) Narrow sector width.

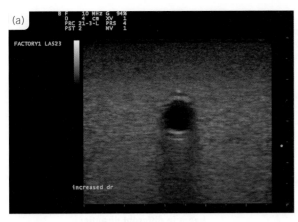

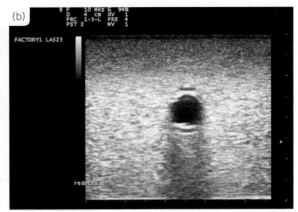

Figure 1.11 (a) Wide dynamic range (more shades of grey displayed). (b) Narrow dynamic range (more black and white displayed).

structure, e.g. the heart. In abdominal sonography of the liver, using a wide dynamic range will show more shade of grey and aid the identification of potential lesions. Figure 1.11 shows different settings of the dynamic range.

Due to attenuation, the signals received by the probe from deeper structures are not as strong as those from superficial structures; the ultrasound machine automatically adjusts for this. However, the level of amplification of the electrical signals received from the probe by the machine can be further adjusted by controls on the console. This does not affect the strength of the signals received by the probe (i.e. sound to electrical) and is a post-receiving feature. This is called gain and can be applied to all signals to increase the level of brightness overall or to a specific range:

- Overall gain causes an increase in the brightness of all signals shown on the B-mode image. It is tempting to increase the gain too high; however, it is important to remember that fluid-filled spaces (e.g. bladder, gall bladder, heart) should be anechoic (black) in B-mode;
- Specific zones of depth are individually adjustable. This may be as simple as two zones (i.e. a near zone close to the probe, and a far zone away from the probe) or multiple zones often as a set of slider controls on the console [called the time gain compensation (TGC)] (see Figure 1.12). The need for control of individual gain of certain depths is to compensate for attenuation of ultrasound

signals with increasing depth. Therefore, it would be expected that the gain for the deeper zones would be higher (although most of the adjustment is undertaken by the ultrasound machine automatically).

Manufacturers have developed tools that can help improve the image and reduce artefacts. A commonly found tool is tissue harmonic imaging (THI); this is where the probe listens for returning echoes of a different frequency to the one transmitted—these are harmonics of the original frequency. The reason for this is to reduce noise in returning echoes of the same frequency as transmitted. THI is especially recommended for patients with large body habitus.

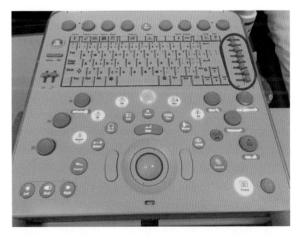

Figure 1.12 Time gain compensation (TGC) sliders on a typical console.

Courtesy of Philips.

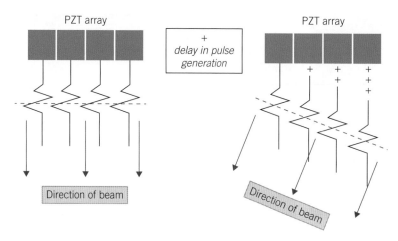

Figure 1.13 Changing the timing of bursts of ultrasound pulses from adjacent PZT elements can direct the beam in different directions.

Another commonly found tool is compound imaging—different manufacturers may call this a variety of trade names. Compound imaging transmits and receives echoes at different angles, as well as perpendicular to the footprint. This can see areas that would be difficult to view, i.e. sidewalls of vessels. Figure 1.13 illustrates how echoes can be directed in different angles from a PZT array.

Other modes

M-mode

M-mode stands for motion or movement mode and is commonly used in applications where evaluation of moving structures is required. It provides excellent temporal resolution of a particular area of the B-mode. Applications include echocardiography valvular and ventricular function and IVC respiratory cycle variation. Select the M-mode setting on the console; this will initially produce a cursor/line on the B-mode image. Most machines will allow the cursor position to be moved to the left or right, over the area of interest. Once positioned correctly, select the M-mode setting again, and all the ultrasound information along the cursor line will be displayed against time. The B-mode image, showing where the cursor position is, will usually be minimized and shown adjacent to the M-mode trace, which looks like a graph (*x*-axis time, *y*-axis ultrasound information along the cursor) (see Figure 1.14). The displayed B-mode is often a still image showing the last view prior to pressing the M-mode setting again; however, in some systems, it will be live (called multi-mode).

Doppler

When transmitted ultrasound signals are reflected off moving targets, the returning signals are affected by the target velocity. This is most commonly used for red blood cell flow evaluation. More specialized applications include movement of tissue in echocardiography (tissue Doppler imaging). This is the same principle as with the audible spectrum of sound; if we hear a police siren coming towards us, it sounds to be at a higher pitch than when it is moving away from us. This is called the Doppler effect, named after the nineteenth-century Austrian physicist. The observed frequency (f_r) is different from the transmitted frequency (f_t), due to movement of the target; f_r is less than f_t when the target is moving away from the probe, and vice versa when the target is moving towards the probe. The degree of change is proportional to the velocity of the target in relation to the

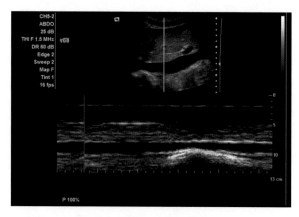

Figure 1.14 M-mode of the proximal IVC.

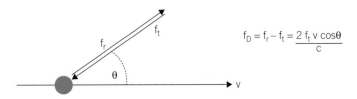

$$f_D = f_r - f_t = \frac{2\, f_t\, v\, \cos\theta}{c}$$

f_D - Doppler shift frequency
f_t - transmitted frequency
f_r - reflected frequency
v - velocity of target
θ - angle between target movement and ultrasound path
c - speed of sound in tissue

Figure 1.15 The Doppler equation.

probe (effectively a stationary source). With red blood cells, the ultrasound signal is scattered, with some of the returning echoes being reflected towards the probe. The observed frequency is not necessarily proportionate to the target velocity, as the target may be moving in a direction perpendicular to the transmitted ultrasound signal. Therefore, to get a true reflection of the movement of targets, the angle of evaluation (θ) is important. When θ is zero, the cosine is 1; when θ is 90°, the cosine is zero. The Doppler equation is shown in Figure 1.15. Clinically, remember to ensure an angle of <60°.

The Doppler principle translates to two usable features on the ultrasound machine: colour flow Doppler and spectral Doppler. The level of detail described is designed to allow for a practical understanding of the key concept, and further reading references for more advanced users are listed at the end of the chapter.

In colour flow Doppler, a colour map is superimposed on the B-mode image. The colour shown reflects the flow velocities for each pixel—typically blue for velocities moving away from the probe and red for velocities moving towards the probe [remember—blue away, red towards (BART)]. The hue level of the colour shown often reflects the velocity; higher velocities are often represented by a paler, greener colour. In turbulent flow, there is often a myriad of colours displayed. However, the settings can easily be adjusted and can mislead users. A typical colour flow image is shown in Figure 1.16.

When the colour flow Doppler modality is activated, a box will appear on the screen. This can be moved, and the size adjusted. The ultrasound machine

will send and receive pulsed waves to ascertain the Doppler information for each part of the boxed area. The larger the boxed area, the more processing the ultrasound machine will need to undertake. Therefore, the smallest box size possible will ensure that temporal resolution is preserved, and thus an adequate frame rate is displayed.

There is another type of colour flow modality that users may encounter—colour power Doppler (CPD). This does not show directional information, like normal colour flow Doppler, but the amplitude of the returning Doppler frequencies is shown as shades of orange/yellow. It is more sensitive than colour flow Doppler for low flow/movement, relatively angle-independent, free of aliasing (more about this later), more accurate in depicting luminal edges, and better at visualizing the continuity of flow. This is used when evaluating vascular anatomy, e.g. evaluation of the carotid artery,

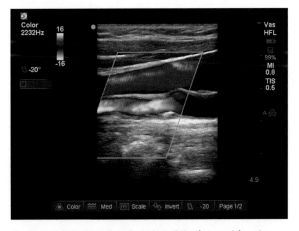

Figure 1.16 Colour flow Doppler of the internal jugular vein and carotid artery (longitudinal section).

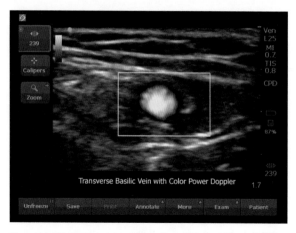

Figure 1.17 **Colour power Doppler of the basilic vein in transverse section.**

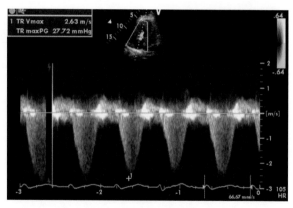

Figure 1.18 **Continuous wave (CW) Doppler image of the tricuspid valve on echocardiography.**

looking at small adjacent branches, and evaluating slow-moving pleural sliding in chest ultrasound. Figure 1.17 shows a typical CPD image.

In spectral Doppler, the aim is to provide quantitative information. This is often represented in graphical format on the screen (with a corresponding adjacent frozen or live B-mode image). Two types of spectral Doppler are commonly used: continuous wave (CW) and pulsed wave (PW). Many ultrasound machines provide calculation packages that can take data from the CW and PW traces and calculate values, e.g. calculating the peak velocity of a regurgitant jet from the tricuspid valve using CW and calculating the velocity time integral (VTI) to estimate the stroke volume (SV) from a PW trace at the aortic valve. Further information on the clinical applications of spectral Doppler will be covered in the relevant echocardiography sections.

In CW Doppler, there is continuous transmission and receiving of ultrasound signals from along a predetermined cursor line—as in M-mode, this is adjustable and appears once you press the CW select button for your machine. Pressing the CW select button again will give you a graph of all the Doppler-detected velocities on the cursor line (see Figure 1.18); there may be a range because not all blood flow in all parts of the cursor line will be travelling in the same direction or at the same velocity. The graph, or trace, given will have time on the x-axis (and will therefore be continually updating) and velocity on the y-axis. Velocities moving towards the probe will be displayed as positive, and vice versa. It also gives audible information too. The

graph will look shaded-in to reflect the variable velocities detected and reflects the pulsed blood flow pattern. In addition, quite high velocities can be detected (which is not the case for PW). However, there is poor spatial resolution, i.e. there is no information provided on what a particular velocity is at a designated location along the cursor.

When selecting PW, a cursor line appears. However, unlike CW, the cursor line has a gate that can be moved up or down the line and can also be widened or narrowed. The orientation of the gate can also be changed to further reduce the angle θ, which will improve the reliability and accuracy of the trace. Pressing the PW select button again will give you a graph of all the Doppler-detected velocities at the cursor line (see Figure 1.19); there will be a narrow range because only the blood flow at the gate region on the cursor line will be sampled. Velocities moving towards the probe will be displayed as positive, and vice versa. The probe does this by transmitting and receiving ultrasound signals to and from this gate; the signals are sent in discrete bursts, with the machine waiting for a period of time (essentially determined by the depth of the gate). The rate at which these bursts are sent is called the pulse repetition frequency (PRF). However, due to the delays in waiting for the signal to return from the gate, the detection of higher velocities is not possible as they exceed the rate at which the PW can process them. Therefore, higher velocities are often shown at an incorrect place on the PW graph/trace—this is called aliasing. Visual comparisons are seen when looking at

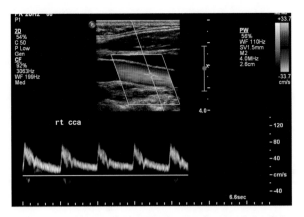

Figure 1.19 Pulsed wave (PW) Doppler image of the right common carotid artery.

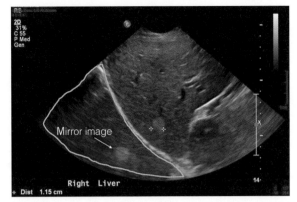

Figure 1.20 Mirror image artefact showing the liver and a haemangioma appearing above, as well as below, the diaphragm.

Courtesy of Hazel Edwards.

a wagon wheel spinning on television; when the velocity of rotation exceeds the camera/television's frame rate, it appears to be going backwards. The maximum Doppler frequency shift that can be detected is half the PRF (called the Nyquist limit). Reducing aliasing can be done by ensuring the PRF is as high as possible; this can be done by ensuring the gate is as close to the probe as possible.

Can you believe what you are seeing?

What you see on the B-mode image is not always a true reflection of the anatomy being evaluated. When this occurs, this is called an *artefact*. This can be significantly misleading to the operator. There are a number of common ultrasound artefacts that you will normally encounter: *mirror image, reverberation, refraction, shadowing, enhancement, edge,* and *comet tail*.

On occasions, the path of the reflecting ultrasound signal is not directed straight back to the ultrasound machine but influenced by adjacent interfaces of high reflectivity. For example, during evaluation of the RUQ, e.g. to assess for free intra-peritoneal fluid in a focused assessment with sonography for trauma (FAST) scan, the diaphragm can act as a reflector of adjacent liver tissue. Due to the longer indirect path, the ultrasound machine assumes it was from an area deeper than it is and the displayed location is different to the actual source. The ultrasound machine assumes ultrasound signals travel in a straight line. This results in the appearance of liver-type tissue above the diaphragm (see Figure 1.20). This is called a mirror image artefact.

Highly reflective surfaces that are parallel to the probe will bounce back the ultrasound signal. However, the surface of the probe has some reflective properties (due to changes in impedance), and this can result in signals bouncing back from the probe surface. This may occur once or more before the signal is received back by the probe. If this occurs, the time taken for signals that have been re-reflected is longer; hence, the ultrasound machine thinks it is located deeper than it is (see Figure 1.21a). Due to attenuation, the more re-reflections that occur are weaker signals than the primary signal received. Figure 1.21b shows this in B-mode. This is called reverberation, or A-lines in thoracic ultrasound.

Refraction errors can occur due to changes in impedance at interfaces between tissues. When the angle of incidence of the ultrasound signal hits the interface at <90°, the angle of refraction will be different. The degree of difference will depend on the difference in z value of the tissues (see Figure 1.22). In reality, this could lead to errors in assuming where structures actually are; in procedural situations, this is very relevant. To avoid refraction errors, the ultrasound signal should be directed to reach tissue interfaces at 90°, i.e. angle of incidence = angle of refraction = 90°.

At tissue interfaces where there is maximal reflectivity, e.g. the interface between soft tissue and bone, there is no discernible signal going beyond the interface. This results in an acoustic shadow. This can sometimes be helpful to identify and distinguish between pathologies, e.g. gallstones cast a shadow, whereas gall bladder

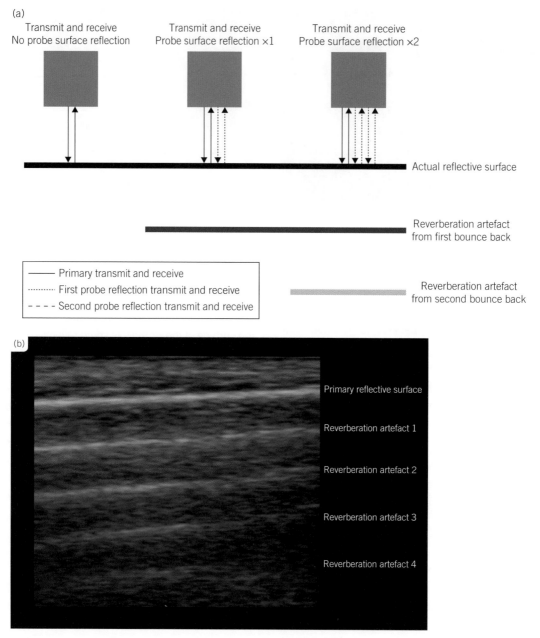

Figure 1.21 (a) Reverberation artefact. (b) Reverberation artefact in B-mode.

polyps do not. The opposite of acoustic shadow is acoustic enhancement. This is seen below areas of low attenuation, e.g. fluid-filled structures. This can aid identification; for instance, a dark (anechoic) lesion will not have acoustic enhancement, but a cystic structure, similar in B-mode appearance, will. Figure 1.23 shows a gall bladder with gallstones, and acoustic shadowing and enhancement can be clearly seen.

When an ultrasound signal hits the side wall of a vessel, it is not always reflected back to the probe and refraction also occurs. This results in a lack of clarity on the B-mode image (see Figure 1.24), with a resultant acoustic shadow distal to the sidewall. The anterior and posterior walls reflect much better and are clearer; therefore, measurements should be taken from those points.

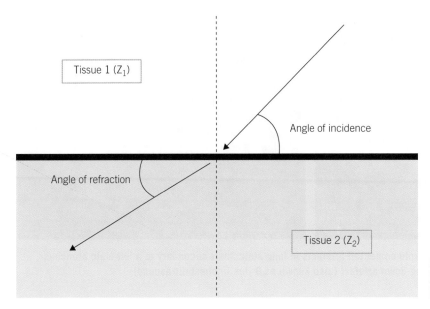

Figure 1.22 Refraction occurring between two tissues with different impedance values.

When small adjacent reflective interfaces encounter ultrasound signals, micro-reverberation may occur. This causes a small attenuating artefact, called a comet tail, to appear (see Figure 1.25a). These should not be confused with a ring-down artefact, which is a non-attenuating, laser-like artefact caused by strong, continuous reflections from exciting trapped fluid surrounded by gas bubbles (see Figure 1.25b).

Is ultrasound safe?

Fortunately, ultrasound involves relatively benign sound waves that are well tolerated without problems. The level of ultrasound energy can be affected by the settings of the machine. There are two main effects associated with ultrasound: thermal and mechanical. The former involves the dissipation of energy into tissues, resulting in warming. In general use, this is not an issue and no tissue damage is caused. There are occasions where small fluid-filled structures may be potentially heated—small changes in temperature may produce permanent damage, e.g. embryos or the eye. All machines display a thermal index (TI), an on-screen indication of the relative potential for tissue temperature rise.

The mechanical index (MI) is an on-screen indication of the relative potential for ultrasound to produce

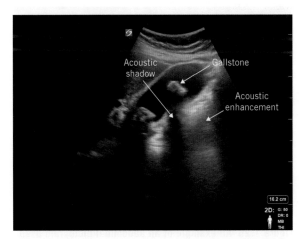

Figure 1.23 B-mode image of a gall bladder with stones.

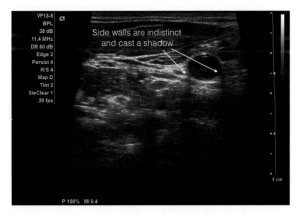

Figure 1.24 B-mode image of an edge artefact of an artery.

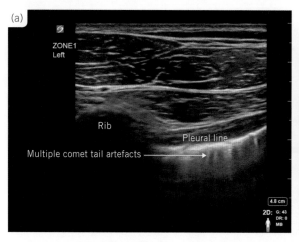

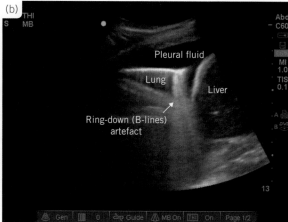

Figure 1.25 (a) B-mode image of multiple comet tail artefacts in lung atelectasis secondary to a left main bronchus mucus plug. (b) B-mode image of a ring-down artefact (also known as B-line in chest ultrasound).

an adverse bio-effect by a non-thermal mechanism such as cavitation.

In general, scanning time should be kept as short as possible, and output levels on the machine should be the least possible to prevent adverse effects. Further guidance is readily available from the British Medical Ultrasound Society website (http://www.bmus.org).

Storing images

You should always try and ensure you save images and clips. This has governance benefits such as being able to review cases, justifying interventions you have undertaken, and also providing valuable teaching material. There are two media forms in which you can save: still image and movie clip. For the former, this is ideal for saving minimally moving structures such as an aortic aneurysm. The freeze button needs to be pressed prior to saving. The image with which you are left, after pressing the freeze button, is not always optimal. Fortunately, ultrasound machines store the immediate B-mode frames prior to the freeze button being pressed. This is called cine-loop. Either via a tracker-ball or pad/ buttons, you can scroll back to the best image available prior to saving. To save the image, the console will have a 'save image' function.

In the case of moving images, such as a view of the heart, it is advantageous to save a video clip, rather than a still image. Most machines will have a 'save clip' feature on the console.

The image or clip should also be annotated prior to saving, as often it can be difficult to know where it was taken. There is usually an 'annotate' or 'text' feature on the console of the machine that will allow you to enter text details, which will be displayed on the screen. On some machines, pictorial representations of body parts (which vary, depending on what probe and preset you have selected) can be used, called pictograms. These come with a movable pictorial representation of the probe placement, so you can change its position in relation to the rest of the pictogram (see Figure 1.26).

Most images are initially stored on the ultrasound machine's hard drive. However, you should endeavour to move these over to a secure area where

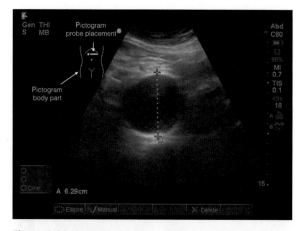

Figure 1.26 An example of an abdominal pictogram used to annotate a B-mode image.

patient-sensitive information can be held. This may be via physically moving the image and video media onto a stick drive and then saving onto a secure server or it can be moved, via wire connections or wirelessly, into radiology picture archiving and communication systems (PACS). The latter usually occurs via Digital Imaging and Communications in Medicine (DICOM) transfer. Most PoCUS machines and hospital radiology PACS systems utilize this as standard. If you want to use anonymized images/clips for teaching purposes, many machines allow for export of media without patient information included.

After the scan

Before you use an ultrasound machine, you would expect it to be clean. You should ensure that you do the same after you have used the machine. Many products are available to clean the probes that do not cause damage; never be tempted to use alcohol-based cleaning products, as they often erode the footprint material. Developing a culture of good practice in your department will ensure that you keep your machine clean and reduce infection transmission risks.

Remember to take the machine back to the designated area, and ensure that it is connected to a power supply to keep the battery charged.

After you examine a patient, you will document your findings in the notes; ultrasound is no different. The report does not need to be lengthy, unless you have lots of relevant findings to document. The structure of a report should be in three parts:

1. Why did you perform the scan?
2. What were your findings?
3. What does this mean to patient care?

This can be written electronically (especially on the machine's reporting module) or written (in the patient notes or on a dedicated proforma). Keeping a log of your scanning activities is important for your own quality assurance and also to demonstrate your regular scope of practice.

Ultrasound machines and probes need servicing (as specified by the manufacturer) and also should have an annual quality assurance review (as dictated by local policy) by a medical physicist.

Clinical scenarios

The following clinical scenarios help to frame the use of PoCUS in the clinical setting as an additional tool to help the clinician with initial diagnosis and management for emergencies and in resuscitation. The cases also provide an overview of some of the PoCUS protocols commonly used in emergency medicine and resuscitation. Further details on the evidence, technique, and further reading for these approaches will be found in greater detail in the rest of the book.

Case 1: Resuscitation—cardiac arrest

A 50-year-old male is brought in cardiac arrest to the Emergency Department (ED). He had been feeling unwell for 24 hours with a fever. His rhythm is that pulseless electrical activity (PEA). Resuscitation is ongoing.

Is there a reversible cause for his cardiac arrest?

PoCUS is less useful in shockable rhythms where the treatment focus is on high-quality, minimally interrupted cardiopulmonary resuscitation (CPR) and defibrillation. However, PoCUS provides immediate diagnostic information on the causes of PEA. If no ventricular activity is seen, then the diagnosis is electromechanical dissociation and the prognosis is less hopeful, similar to asystole. If there is PEA with ventricular movement, then PoCUS may identify the following useful diagnostic information:

- Hyperdynamic activity with systolic ventricular collapse and sometimes an empty [collapsing, anteroposterior (AP) diameter <11 mm] IVC (this is less reliable in a cardiac arrest, as right-sided filling pressures increase consequent to minimal cardiac output), suggesting hypovolaemia or sepsis;

- Pericardial effusion with tamponade and right ventricular (RV) diastolic collapse;

- Dilated right ventricle (greater than left ventricle), hypokinetic right ventricle, often with hyperdynamic left ventricle, and paradoxical septal movement, suggesting pulmonary embolism (PE). An important caveat is if the RV free wall is >4 mm; this suggests hypertrophy and the increased right-sided pressure is not acute;

- Poor left or global cardiac function that may be due to ischaemia, cardiomyopathy, or drugs/medication overdose.

Various echo in life support algorithms, such as the SHoC protocol, describe this approach (discussed in Chapter 2).

Performing the scan

Core cardiac windows performed during the rhythm check pause in chest compressions, minimizing any interruption to CPR, are the sub-xiphoid and/or parasternal cardiac views. Either view should be used to detect pericardial *fluid*, as well as to examine ventricular *form* (e.g. right heart strain) and *function* (e.g. asystole versus organized cardiac activity).

Supplementary views include lung views (for absent lung sliding in pneumothorax and for pleural fluid) and IVC views for *filling*.

Additional ultrasound applications are for endotracheal tube (ETT) confirmation, for proximal leg veins for DVT, or for sources of blood loss (AAA, peritoneal/pelvic fluid).

Should the team continue resuscitation?

There is no published evidence supporting the use of PoCUS to improve mortality in cardiac arrest or shock, but the 2015 Resuscitation guidelines stress the role in diagnosis and prognostication. The absence of ventricular activity is associated with a very poor chance of survival, especially if the end-tidal carbon dioxide (CO_2) is under 1.6 kPa/10 mmHg after two or more cycles of CPR.

Case 2: Trauma

A 34-year-old motorcyclist was in a head-on collision with a wall at 70 mph. Vital signs on arrival: Glasgow Coma Scale (GCS) score 7/15, heart rate (HR) 140 beats per minute (bpm), blood pressure (BP) 90/60 mmHg, respiratory rate (RR) 32/min, capillary refill time (CRT) 6 s.

Is PoCUS able to help in the assessment and management of a patient with blunt polytrauma?

There is now extensive evidence to suggest that PoCUS has a vital role to play in the care of patients with trauma. The FAST scan has been used for the identification of free fluid in the peritoneal cavity and pericardial sac. PoCUS does not seek to identify solid organ injury. The extended FAST or e-FAST exam includes the use of PoCUS additionally in the identification of pneumothorax or haemothorax. The use of PoCUS has now spread to the identification of long bone fractures in the secondary survey phase of assessment (see Chapter 7). Although it is evident that PoCUS is of great utility, it must be realized that this imaging modality only has good sensitivity and specificity with blunt trauma and is to be used cautiously in the assessment of penetrating trauma where the quantity of blood loss is often far less. Even with blunt torso trauma, this modality should be used primarily as a rule-in, rather than a rule-out test, especially when performed by non-expert clinicians. It must be remembered that CT remains the gold standard in the evaluation of patients with polytrauma.

Advanced trauma life support (ATLS) is the most popular system for trauma assessment and management. PoCUS can be integrated as an adjunct to the primary and secondary surveys and can assist with procedures.

Primary survey

Airway

Establishment of a definite airway in the obtunded patient is a priority in management.

PoCUS can assist in the securing of an airway in different ways:

- In endotracheal intubation, for both the insertion of the tube and in early recognition of oesophageal intubation (see Chapter 9);

- In the identification of the cricothyroid membrane, should a surgical airway be required. This is extremely useful when the normal anatomy of the neck is disturbed due to swelling, etc.

Breathing

Assessment of breathing is the next step in the ATLS protocol, and here too PoCUS can contribute greatly.

- *Assessment of lung parenchyma—contusion.* Normal dry, aerated lung demonstrates the A pattern (see Chapter 3). A localized area of contusion will contain blood, which alters the air–fluid balance in that area, and consequently lung tissue may be seen. The appearance is similar to that seen with consolidation of the lung in infection;

- *Assessment of pleural spaces—pneumothorax and haemothorax.* As part of the e-FAST examination, PoCUS can be used to identify the presence of a pneumothorax (loss of lung sliding) or a haemothorax. The sensitivity and specificity of PoCUS for pneumothorax is far greater than those of supine chest radiography and approaches those of CT;

- *Procedural guidance—tube thoracostomy.* PoCUS assists greatly not only with the diagnostics, but also with intervention. It is now accepted that PoCUS should be used routinely to identify and mark the safe area with regard to insertion of a chest drain or for pleural aspiration (see Chapter 9). Several studies have proven that the incidence of organ injury (liver, spleen, heart) with chest drain insertion is significantly reduced with PoCUS.

Circulation

In the case presented at the beginning of this chapter, it is clear that this patient is in shock and that early identification of bleeding is essential if a poor outcome is to be avoided.

PoCUS helps to identify:

- Blood in the peritoneal cavity (see Chapter 4);

- Blood in the pleural cavity (see Chapter 4) and guide drainage (see Chapter 9);

- Blood in the pericardial sac (see Chapter 4) and guide drainage (see Chapter 9);

- Can be used to identify long bone fractures which may contribute to significant bleeding (see Chapter 7).

Fluid resuscitation

PoCUS can facilitate the insertion of wide-bore cannulae, so that fluid replacement can be initiated. This is particularly useful when you have a hypotensive patient with poorly visible/palpable peripheral veins. It can also be used to guide femoral vein cannulation for utilizing rapid infusion devices.

Additionally, evaluation of IVC size and inspiratory collapse (in the spontaneously breathing patient) can be very useful to guide fluid replacement, especially in elderly patients.

Disability

Although PoCUS has not yet gained widespread adoption in the assessment of neurological status, there are a few potential uses:

- To assess for pupil reactivity to light when the pupil is hidden from view by periorbital swelling (see Chapter 8);

- To identify papilloedema (see Chapter 8);

- In the estimation of intracranial pressure (ICP) by measuring the optic nerve sheath diameter (see Chapter 8);

- Trans-cranial Doppler to measure impedance in the middle cerebral artery (MCA).

Secondary survey

The head to toe assessment during the secondary survey can be assisted with PoCUS in the assessment for radiolucent foreign body, e.g. glass fragments (see Chapter 7); shoulder dislocation, rib and sternum fractures, muscle and tendon injuries, haemarthrosis, for fracture/dislocation reduction (see Chapter 7); and for regional/peripheral nerve block guidance (see Chapter 9).

Under normal circumstances, PoCUS should not delay or replace definitive investigations such as CT; however, when a patient is unresponsive to fluid resuscitation, it can greatly assist in determining the location of blood and facilitate early operative management. In addition, for those patients presenting in smaller hospitals without CT or in an austere environment, PoCUS can facilitate early transfer for those patients with positive findings.

Case resolution

The patient described in this scenario had a left-sided white-out on his chest X-ray, and the initial impression was that this was due to a large haemothorax. However, insertion of a chest drain was withheld until an e-FAST exam was performed. The e-FAST scan was negative for free fluid in the RUQ. On the left, the kidney was well visualized with no free fluid, but the spleen could not be identified. The heart was not visualized in either the sub-xiphoid or PLAX views, despite there being no technical factors to account for this. It was recognized that the cause of this non-visualization was likely to be due to the presence of an air-filled organ between the transducer and the heart, and a diagnosis of diaphragmatic rupture was made. A subsequent CT confirmed the presence of the stomach and spleen in the chest. A chest tube was not inserted.

Case 3: Hypotension and shock

A 76-year-old female presents with a 24-hour history of low-grade fever, breathlessness, abdominal pain, and lethargy. Her pulse is 110 bpm and thready, her BP is 90/45 mmHg, her RR is elevated at 28/min, and her SpO$_2$ is 94% on air. She has a history of ischaemic heart disease.

What is the underlying cause of her shock?

Several protocols, such as the SHoC–hypotension protocol, can guide PoCUS assessment of the shocked patient.

- *Core: cardiac views* (sub-xiphoid and parasternal windows for pericardial *fluid*, cardiac *form*, and ventricular *function*); *lung views* for pleural *fluid* and B-lines for *filling* status; and *IVC views* for *filling* status;
- *Supplementary*: other cardiac views; and
- *Additional views* (when indicated), including peritoneal fluid, aorta, pelvic for IUP, and proximal leg veins for DVT.

This PoCUS approach can help differentiate between the various causes of shock during initial resuscitation *(italics for diagnosis made predominantly with echo)*:

- Cardiac—*impaired LV or RV function (ischaemia, cardiomyopathy, depression from sepsis or toxin, cor pulmonale), valvular failure*, arrhythmia;
- Distributive—sepsis, anaphylaxis, neurological, toxicological;
- Hypovolaemic—blood (*trauma, AAA*, gastrointestinal bleed) or fluid loss;
- Obstructive—*PE, pericardial tamponade*, air/gas/fat embolism;
- Cytopathic—sepsis, cyanide or carbon monoxide poisoning.

This will be discussed in detail in Chapter 2 and expands on the findings briefly described earlier for cardiac arrest, but the reduction in time pressure allows a more comprehensive assessment and for additional imaging windows to be obtained.

Cardiogenic shock

- Poor systolic function is suggested by dilated, thin-walled, poorly contractile chambers;
- Poor diastolic function is suggested by small, thick-walled chambers;
- Coronary artery disease and myocardial ischaemia are suggested by regional wall abnormalities, but severe ischaemic cardiomyopathy may appear as global left ventricular (LV) impairment;
- Valvular disease is suggested by obvious regurgitation jets using colour flow, valvular stenosis suggested by thickened, calcified, poorly opening valves with increased velocity with spectral Doppler, diastolic function impaired.

Distributive and hypovolaemic shock

- Suggested by a hyperdymamic left ventricle/right ventricle, in which the ventricular walls contract vigorously and come close to each other in end-systole;
- The IVC may be small (<10–15 mm in AP diameter, measured at end-expiration if spontaneous ventilation, and collapse of >50% with inspiration). IVC size and collapse index should be used cautiously, as dependent on many factors;
- Further PoCUS imaging may reveal the site of blood loss such as AAA or intra-peritoneal blood.

Obstructive

- Massive PE suggested by a dilated right ventricle, poor RV contraction assessed visually or by tricuspid annular plane systolic excursion (TAPSE), and paradoxical septal movement. The LV cavity may be small and hyperdymanic. A free RV free wall of <5 mm suggests the dilatation is acute;
- Pericardial fluid is obvious, but identifying tamponade is harder, systolic collapse of the atria

is suggestive, and diastolic collapse of the right ventricle is diagnostic;

- The IVC is usually large (diameter of >25 mm measured AP) in obstructive shock;

- Lung windows may identify a pneumothorax, which may explain the tension physiology.

Is the patient likely to respond to intravenous fluids?

The goal of resuscitation is to improve the SV and cardiac output (CO) until the point when oxygen delivery is sufficient to reverse tissue hypoxia. The most effective method of improving oxygen delivery to tissues is usually by increasing the CO with intravenous fluids and/or inopressors. However, there is a potential for harm in fluid administration, and it is important, when administering intravenous fluids, that clear end points are targeted. By convention, a patient may be defined as fluid-responsive when a 500-mL bolus of crystalloid delivered over 15 minutes increases the SV by >10–15%.

Using PoCUS, we may assess myocardial performance and obtain information about fluid responsiveness. This is discussed in detail in Chapter 2. Many resuscitative interventions, such as administering catecholamines and positive pressure ventilation, affect preload, afterload, and cardiac contractility, so altering fluid responsiveness.

Inferior vena cava

The simplest PoCUS assessment of fluid tolerance/responsiveness is to use the IVC size and the proportion by which it collapses with respiration. A small (<11–14 mm AP diameter measured within 2–3 cm of the right atrium) and collapsing (>40–50% with respiration, <18–20% with mechanical ventilation, and tidal volume of 8 mL/kg) IVC suggests fluid will not harm, and is likely to benefit, your patient. An IVC diameter of >25 mm suggests pressure–volume overload, and fluid responsiveness is less likely but cannot be ruled out, and more sophisticated tools are required. IVC size and collapsibility are blunt tools in assessing fluid tolerance, rather than fluid responsiveness, but useful guides early in the resuscitation process (see Chapter 6).

Stroke volume

The most direct way to assess fluid responsiveness is to use PoCUS to measure the volume of blood ejected through the left ventricular outflow tract (LVOT), using PW Doppler technology, before and after a bolus of 500 mL of crystalloid delivered over 15 minutes. The VTI records the velocity of red blood cells passing through the LVOT and the time taken for this to occur. The integral of velocity (VTI) with respect to time is distance, in this case the stroke distance. This is discussed in detail in Chapter 2.

Predicting fluid responsiveness

Many ultrasound parameters have been assessed as *predictors* of fluid responsiveness by observing changes in respiration, including CO. Most studies are performed on ventilated patients in intensive care, with little data on spontaneously ventilating patients.

Passive leg raising is a technique that utilizes altered patient position to centralize a small proportion (250–300 mL) of the circulation, so increasing preload. The patient lies either flat or slightly head-up at 30 degrees or so, and the VTI recorded. Then the patient is laid flat and their legs raised 45 degrees in the air, and the VTI is recorded. The larger the increase in SV resulting from this, the more likely the patient is fluid-responsive. An increase of 10% or more suggests fluid responsiveness.

Lung ultrasound to guide fluid therapy

Pulmonary oedema in the lungs is one the earliest and easiest forms of pathology to see with ultrasound. Changes appear earlier than with chest radiographs or clinical signs, so administering fluids until pulmonary oedema, as assessed by PoCUS, has been suggested as a technique to guide fluid resuscitation. An advantage is that it identifies patients who have pulmonary capillary leak early in the process of fluid therapy, who may, in fact, be fluid-responsive but in whom further fluid administration risks impairment of gas exchange and an increase in respiratory work. Multiple B-lines are the sonographic sign of lung interstitial syndrome. The presence of three or more B-lines in two or more sampled lung fields suggests a positive finding. Symmetrical findings suggest pulmonary oedema (see 'Case 4: Breathlessness and acute decompensated heart failure', p. 28 and Chapters 2 and 3 for further explanation).

Case 4: Breathlessness and acute decompensated heart failure

A 68-year-old male with a history of chronic obstructive pulmonary disease (COPD) and congestive heart failure (CHF) presents to the ED with a 2-day history of increasing breathlessness, worse on exertion, but also waking him up at night. He gets incomplete relief from his inhalers. On examination, he is dyspnoeic at rest. His pulse rate is 100 bpm and regular, BP 110/65 mmHg, RR 30/min, and SpO_2 90% on air. He has a widespread expiratory wheeze throughout the lung fields.

What is the cause of his acute decompensation?

Pulmonary oedema, acute exacerbations of chronic lung disease, pulmonary infection, PE, and even pneumothoraces may present with similar clinical syndromes, and there are few disease-specific diagnostic findings. The core SHoC protocol of cardiac, lung, and IVC PoCUS offers the clinician a rapidly performed bedside approach that may assist in differentiating these syndromes.

Cardiac PoCUS is central in the diagnosis and defining the aetiology of heart failure. Valuable information is gained from simple observation of cardiac size (including right atrial size for diastolic heart failure), valves, wall thickness, and wall motion. If these parameters appear normal, then breathlessness is unlikely due to cardiac disease. Impaired systolic function is extremely important, correlating with symptoms and prognosis. Calculating the ejection fraction is time-consuming, but a visual estimation of cardiac function is rapidly performed. Although accurate estimations of ventricular performance require experience, identifying cardiac poor systolic performance, and grading this as normal, impaired, or severely impaired, has been shown to be performed with reasonable accuracy after as little as 1-day training. Assessing diastolic function is more challenging and requires advanced training. Conversely, the finding of a hyperdynamic heart suggests sepsis as a cause for dyspnoea, and a dilated ventricle suggests either chronic lung disease or (massive) PE. Most PEs are too small to embarrass cardiac function, and a normal PoCUS echo certainly does not exclude the diagnosis.

Lung PoCUS can be used to look for lung sliding, A-lines, B-lines, pleural fluid, and lung consolidation. A phased array or curvilinear probe may be used, set to a depth of 12–15 cm. As described previously, occasional B-lines are a normal finding, especially in the lower zones, whereas multiple symmetrical diffuse B-lines are sensitive, but not specific, for pulmonary oedema and appear prior to chest radiograph changes. Three or more B-lines in two or more lung zones bilaterally are commonly used to define an abnormal B pattern, suggesting pulmonary oedema. B-lines may also be seen in acute pulmonary infection, in which they are usually asymmetrical and localized, adult respiratory distress syndrome (rare in the ED), fibrosis, and fluid overload. B-lines are a common finding in lower zones posteriorly. Further work is required to assess the role of PoCUS in the hands of critical care physicians to diagnose acute decompensated heart failure.

Pneumothorax is suggested by the absence of lung sliding and B-lines; pneumonia by focal B-lines, unilateral pleural effusion, and/or lung hepatization; and pulmonary oedema by symmetrical B-lines, especially if identified on anterior windows. B-lines are physiological in the lung bases. Bilateral pleural effusions are also suggestive.

IVC PoCUS can be used to assess filling. A dilated, non-collapsing IVC is a common finding in acute heart failure.

Case 5: Chest pain

A 75-year-old male presents to the ED with intermittent central chest pain. His ECG is normal. Within 30 minutes of presenting, his pain increases and he becomes hypotensive; his ECG is still unremarkable.

Can PoCUS aid in the evaluation of patients with atraumatic chest pain?

Using ultrasound is not a replacement to clinical evaluation, ECGs, and laboratory studies but may reduce the time to diagnosis and narrow the clinician's possible list of differential diagnoses for chest pain. Many chest pain protocols, especially for acute coronary syndrome (ACS) rule-out, require serial ECG and laboratory studies that may result in significant delays. Using ultrasound to aid in the identification of non-ACS causes is helpful.

However, a comprehensive study is seldom achievable in the acute emergency setting, and a focused and pragmatic approach needs to be adopted.

Is it cardiac?

Echocardiography can be used to identify global hypodynamic LV function (and hyperdynamic, e.g. in septic patients), especially when marked. However, the vast majority of chest pain patients will have normal global LV function. Deciding on what is acute and chronic is also difficult.

There is evidence to suggest that, in patients with ACS presenting with chest pain, regional wall motion abnormalities on echocardiography may be seen prior to any ECG changes and raised laboratory studies (e.g. troponin). However, equipment, the environment, time available, and limited echocardiography skills may render this unfeasible for many clinicians. PoCUS echocardiography should be considered as a 'rule-in' tool, not a 'rule-out' tool. Other cardiac pathology, such as pericardial effusion (which may be seen in pericarditis), can be reliably seen, more so when it is large in volume.

In addition, complications associated with acute myocardial infarction and subsequent treatment (e.g. primary coronary artery angioplasty) may be detected by the use of echocardiography in the ED.

Is it non-cardiac?

Not all chest pain is due to cardiac or acute coronary syndromes, and it may be secondary to conditions such as the following:

- Pleural problems (e.g. pneumothorax or pleural effusion) (see Chapter 3);

- Lung visceral problems (e.g. infection/pneumonia or interstitial pulmonary oedema);

- Vascular problems (e.g. thoracic aortic dissection and aneurysm);

- Obstructive problems (e.g. PE).

Performing the scan

Typically, performing the scan can be broken down into two main parts: *focused echocardiography* adopting a mainly qualitative approach, rather than quantitative (i.e. eyeballing), and *extra-cardiac views*. The order that these parts are conducted will be guided by the operator's impression of the likely differential diagnoses.

The cardiac evaluation is described in more detail in Chapter 2. All views may yield important information; however, in reality, they may not be all achievable due to patient positioning, body habitus, and operator familiarity with certain windows. Views to be considered include:

- Parasternal windows (long and short axes);

- Apical windows (2-, 3-, 4-, and 5-chamber);

- Subcostal windows and;

- Specialized windows such as suprasternal (this should only be considered if thoracic aortic pathology is suspected).

The extra-cardiac aspects to the scan include the following:

- Thoracic windows (see Chapter 3) to evaluate pleural and lung viscera pathology;

- IVC ± focused deep vein evaluation (see Chapter 6) to support the diagnosis of thromboembolic disease.

A mixture of high- and low-frequency transducers may need to be adopted, with high frequency for thoracic evaluation of pleural sliding and evaluation of deep veins in the groin/lower limb. A small-footprint, low-frequency transducer, such as a phased array or micro-convex transducer, would be desirable, but not essential for other aspects.

In this case, PoCUS was utilized and a focused assessment of his heart revealed a 5.6-cm thoracic aortic aneurysm on parasternal long and short axes (see Figure 1.27 and Video 1.1 📷). Cardiothoracic referral was expedited.

Case 6: Abdominal pain

A 40-year-old female attends the ED with severe RUQ pain and fever. Her vital signs are normal.

Is PoCUS able to help with the differential diagnosis of atraumatic abdominal pain?

There are many causes of abdominal pain that PoCUS is unable to identify (e.g. peptic ulcer disease), but

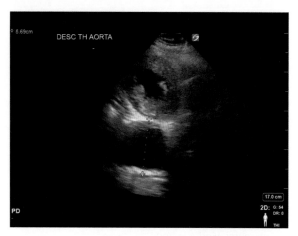

Figure 1.27 B-mode image of the descending thoracic aorta.

PoCUS can assist in the diagnosis of the following conditions:

- Abdominal pain and shock: AAA, free fluid (in ruptured ectopic pregnancy);

- Abdominal pain and peritonitis: appendicitis, cholecystitis, diverticulitis;

- Abdominal pain and RUQ pain: ureteric colic, biliary colic;

- Abdominal pain in children: intussusception, appendicitis;

- Other: bowel obstruction.

In the hands of most operators, PoCUS is able to 'rule in', but not 'rule out', these conditions. Notable exceptions include AAA (most operators can accurately identify a normal-calibre abdominal aorta) and ectopic pregnancy (the sonographic finding of a live IUP can be considered to rule out ectopic pregnancy, unless the patient is on fertility treatment).

Does PoCUS guide disposition in abdominal pain?

Although several studies have demonstrated the accuracy of PoCUS in the above settings, only a limited number have shown that PoCUS alters outcome. PoCUS is most valuable in the shocked patient with abdominal pain (e.g. PoCUS can rule out AAA or identify a live IUP).

Technique

It should be borne in mind that PoCUS is not a 'formal abdominal ultrasound', and simply scanning the entire abdomen is impractical for the busy clinician. Therefore, a clinical assessment and provisional diagnosis is essential *before* scanning. A systematic approach should include the following:

- Begin with a 'scout scan' for free fluid (FAST examination);

- Scan the area of interest (e.g. the abdominal aorta for suspected AAA, pelvis for suspected ectopic pregnancy, gall bladder/common bile duct (CBD)/right kidney for RUQ pain);

- Review areas (if negative scan): formulate a differential diagnosis and scan for these conditions (e.g. AAA mimicking ureteric colic).

Case 7: Back pain

A 72-year-old male patient, with a history of previous renal stones 20 years previously, presents with a 3-hour history of posterior left flank pain. The pain is constant, and he feels dizzy on standing.

Can PoCUS help with the initial differential diagnosis, assessment, and management?

Despite the past history of renal stones, in male patients with abdominal, flank, or back pain over the age of 50 years, the possibility of a symptomatic AAA should always be considered. In addition to this, PoCUS can help to determine if other diagnoses such as biliary or ureteric colic are likely, though this should be a secondary consideration. A useful algorithm is shown in Figure 1.28.

A simple screen of the abdominal aorta for a measurement of the maximum diameter is indicated. An AAA is defined as a dilatation of >1.5 times the normal diameter, or >3 cm in adult patients. As the diameter increases, so does the risk of aneurysmal wall rupture. In symptomatic patients, as in this case, any AAA should be considered as a potential cause for the presentation. An AAA of >5 cm is highly likely to be the cause of the symptoms and should warrant urgent vascular surgical consultation in unstable patients, or immediate further imaging, such as CT, in stable patients (see Chapter 6 for further details).

Gall bladder disease, such as biliary colic (cholelithiasis) or cholecystitis, can be accurately detected or excluded by PoCUS. Details are described in Chapter 4.

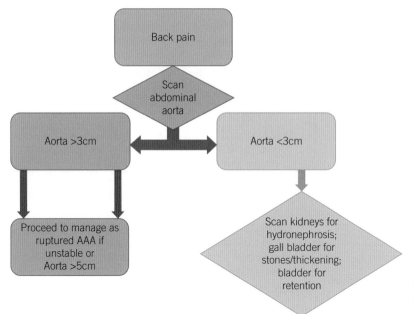

Figure 1.28 An example of a back pain algorithm incorporating ultrasound.

In patients with low back pain and suspected cauda equina syndrome, PoCUS can be used to measure the post-void urinary bladder volume. A small bladder size of <100 mL is helpful in excluding urinary retention. Rarer diagnoses, such as aortic dissection or pancreatitis, may be detected but cannot be excluded by PoCUS.

Case 8: HIV and tuberculosis co-infection—the FASH examination

A 34-year-old female attends the ED [in a high human immunodeficiency virus (HIV)/tuberculosis (TB) prevalence setting] with a fever, while also looking physically wasted.

Is PoCUS able to help to identify tuberculosis co-infection in a patient with underlying HIV infection?

One-third of the world population is infected with TB. Also, TB is the main cause of death in patients infected with HIV, ranging from 5 deaths per 100 000 population in low-prevalence settings to 121 per 100 000 in high-prevalence settings. Disseminated TB (DTB) as first presentation is more common in patients with underlying HIV infection. PoCUS can assist in identifying some of these disseminated locations that are notoriously difficult to diagnose with traditional methods.

In the hands of experienced operators, PoCUS is able to 'rule in', but not 'rule out', DTB if used correctly within the World Health Organization (WHO) guideline, in a high prevalent setting, and in conjunction with other point-of-care diagnostic tests.

Does PoCUS guide disposition?

According to the latest WHO guideline, patients with confirmed HIV infection and associated positive PoCUS findings of DTB might be initiated on their TB antimicrobial regime. However, sputum, body fluid analysis, and chest X-ray imaging must still be performed and reviewed (in many cases as an outpatient). PoCUS impacts positively on ED overcrowding in resource-limited settings, due to expedition of the diagnosis and management.

Technique

PoCUS should only be performed in patients who are confirmed HIV-positive, with confirmed negative GeneXpert TB sputum results to 'rule out' pulmonary TB first.

1. Perihepatic (RUQ) view (similar technique as for FAST scan);
2. Perisplenic [left upper quadrant (LUQ)] view (similar technique as for FAST scan);

3. Pericystic (pelvic) view (similar technique as for FAST scan):
   - The objective is to identify intra-peritoneal fluid and pleural effusions. PoCUS may also guide real-time fluid sampling for laboratory testing.

4. Sub-xiphoid view (similar technique as for FAST scan):
   - *The objective is to identify fluid within the pericardial space.*

5. Spleen sweep (repeat fanning, panning, and rotation of the spleen body with both low- and high-frequency probes):
   - *The objective is to identify multiple micro-abscesses.*

6. Aorta, iliac, and portal vessel sweep (visualize all three vessel groups throughout their abdominal courses in both their respective transverse and longitudinal planes):
   - The objective is to identify multiple, large (>1 cm) lymph nodes.

Positive scans should alert you to the probability of associated DTB. However, some findings (lymph nodes, splenic abscesses, pericardial effusion) are more commonly associated with DTB than others (free fluid). The more positive findings you identify, the higher the probability of a positive diagnosis.

🔖 Further reading

Additional further reading can be found in the Online appendix at www.oxfordmedicine.com/POCUSemergencymed. Please refer to your access card for further details.

American College of Emergency Physicians. *Emergency Ultrasound Guidelines 2008*. Available from: http://www.acep.org.

Atkinson P, Bowra J, Lambert M, Lamprecht H, Noble V, Jarman R. International Federation for Emergency Medicine Point of Care Ultrasound Curriculum. *CJEM* 2015;**17**:161–70.

Atkinson P, Boyle A, Robinson S, Campbell-Hewson G. Should ultrasound guidance be used for central venous catheterization in the emergency department? *Emerg Med J* 2005;**22**:158–64.

Atkinson PR, Bowra J, Milne J, *et al*. International Federation for Emergency Medicine Consensus Statement: Sonography in hypotension and cardiac arrest (SHoC): an international consensus on the use of point of care ultrasound for undifferentiated hypotension and during cardiac arrest. *CJEM* 2017;**19**:459–70.

Blyth L, Atkinson P, Gadd K, Lang E. Bedside focused echocardiography as predictor of survival in cardiac arrest patients: a systematic review. *Acad Emerg Med* 2012;**19**: 1119–26.

Dent B, Kendall RJ, Boyle AA, Atkinson PR. Emergency ultra-sound of the abdominal aorta by UK emergency physicians: a prospective cohort study. *Emerg Med J* 2007;**24**:547–9.

Dipti A, Soucy Z, Surana A, Chandra S. Role of inferior vena cava diameter in assessment of the volume status: a meta-analysis. *Am J Emerg Med* 2012;**30**:1414–19.

Gaspari R, Weekes A, Adhikari S, *et al*. Emergency department point-of-care ultrasound in out-of-hospital and in-ED cardiac arrest. *Resuscitation* 2016;**109**:33–9.

Haydar S, Moore E, Higgins G, Irish C, *et al*. Effect of bedside ultrasoundography on the certainty of physician decision making for septic patients in the Emergency Department. *Ann Emerg Med* 2012;**60**:346–57.

Jones AE, Tayal VS, Sullivan DM, *et al*. Randomized, controlled trial of immediate versus delayed goal directed ultrasound to identify the cause of nontraumatic hypotension in emergency department patients. *Crit Care Med* 2004;**32**:1703–8.

Leung J, Duffy M, Finckh A. Real-time ultrasonographically guided internal jugular vein catheterization in the emergency department increases success rates and reduces complications: a randomized, prospective study. *Ann Emerg Med* 2006;**48**:540–7.

Lichtenstein D, Mezere G, Lagoueyte J, Biderman P, Goldstein I, Gepner A. A lines and B lines: lung ultrasound as a bedside tool for predicting pulmonary artery occlusion pressure in the critically ill. *Chest* 2009;**136**:1014–20.

Moore CL, Copel JA. Point of care ultrasonography. *N Engl J Med* 2011;**364**:749–57.

Preau S, Asulnier F, DEwavrin F, Duricher A, Chagnon J. Passive leg raising is predictive of fluid responsiveness in spontaneously breathing patients with severe sepsis and acute pancreatitis. *Crit Care Med* 2010;**38**:819–25.

Rivers E, Nguyen B, Havstad S, *et al*. Early goal directed therapy in the treatment of severe sepsis and septic shock. *N Engl J Med* 2001;**345**:1368–77.

Schmidt GA, Koenig S, Mayo P. Ultrasound to guide diagnosis and therapy. *Chest* 2012;**142**:1042–8.

Venables H. Practical applications of ultrasound: getting the best out of your ultrasound machine. *Ultrasound* 2011;**19**:50–5.

Via G, Hussain A, Wells M, *et al*. International evidence-based recommendations for focused cardiac ultrasound. *J Am Soc Echocardiography* 2014;**7**:682.e1–33.

Volpicelli G, Elbarbary M, Blaivas M, *et al*. International evidence-based recommendations for point-of-care lung ultrasound. *Intensive Care Med* 2012;**38**:577–91.

2

The heart and resuscitation

Tim Harris, Matthew Wong, James French,
Sharon Kay, and Paul Atkinson

Summary

Cardiac PoCUS is a key investigation for critically ill patients, offering diagnostic information and guiding resuscitation. Use of the '4F' approach provides a structured approach to cardiac PoCUS: *fluid–form–function–filling*.

When to scan (clinical indications):
Core: In cardiac arrest and the patient with undifferentiated shock.
Advanced: Evaluation of chest pain, and shortness of breath for heart failure. Risk stratification of syncope, and guiding treatment in shock and for procedures such as pericardiocentesis and transvenous cardiac pacing.

What to scan (PoCUS protocol):
Core: Sub-xiphoid and parasternal cardiac views in cardiac arrest. In shock, addition of pleural/pulmonary and IVC views. Include abdominal and aortic views when clinically indicated (SHoC protocol).
Advanced: Apical cardiac views, addition of colour Doppler (colour, pulsed and continuous wave), and consider combining with other non-cardiac views, e.g. deep vein views (SHoC protocol).

How to scan (key points on scanning):
Core: Patient and operator positioning. Small movements of the probe.

Advanced: Getting a more 'on axis' scan that allows more accurate assessment of chamber size and function.

What PoCUS adds (what clinical questions does PoCUS answer?)
Core: *Fluid*—is there pericardial tamponade? *Form*—is there an enlarged right ventricle (sign of a massive PE)? Is the left ventricle enlarged (sign of impaired function—may suggest cardiogenic shock)? *Function*—is the heart beating? Should we stop or continue resuscitation? Are there regional wall motion abnormalities? *Filling*—is the IVC small and collapsing, suggesting fluid tolerance, and if so, does the patient need fluid resuscitation?

How to read this chapter

The chapter is the longest in this book. This reflects the challenges of learning cardiac PoCUS echo, the wide range of clinical applications, and the complexity of additional skills, such as colour and spectral Doppler (PW and CW), used in echocardiography. However, by using only B-mode and one or two cardiac windows, clinicians can transform their diagnostic skills in the assessment of cardiac arrest and shock; these constitute core knowledge (also termed Level 1, basic) and is summarized in Part 1. Additional information covered in Parts 2, 3, and 4 will enable the clinician to improve assessment in shock, dyspnoea, chest pain, and syncope, and improve their resuscitation skills.

Readers with previous experience may choose to start at Part 2, while those new to echo may benefit from reading all sections in order to then return to the Part 1 summary section to revise and reinforce their core skill training. To support this approach, some points from Part 1 are repeated in Parts 2 and 3 but are covered in more depth. A selection of summary clinical algorithms are provided in Part 4.

Part 1: Focused cardiac point-of-care ultrasound (echo) core skills summary

PoCUS echocardiography is included as a core competency in most countries and training schemes. Core PoCUS echo focuses on the skills that most clinicians will use in their daily practice and of which they will be able to learn the basics on a 1- to 2-day course. Core echo offers the clinician the skills to determine the aetiology of cardiac arrest and shock, focusing on identifying six echo syndromes or findings:

- Distributive/hypovolaemic shock;
- Obstructive shock due to PE;
- Obstructive shock due to pericardial effusion and tamponade;
- Cardiac shock consequent upon poor myocardial function;
- In cardiac arrest, no ventricular motion may be seen;

- Normal or near-normal RV and LV performance (rare in shock but may help to identify other causes of hypotension or lactaemia or organ failure).

Using ultrasound to assess the aetiology of shock is best viewed as described in Figure 2.1.

There are several algorithms described to provide the novice sonographer with a structured approach to obtaining images; the ACES (see Figure 2.2), Focus Assessed Transthoracic Echocardiography (FATE) (see Figure 2.3), SHoC, and RUSH protocols are all examples, but none have received the near-universal acceptance that the e-FAST approach has for trauma. All use additional windows that may be seen as progressing beyond core training.

Transducer position

The transducer (or probe) most suitable for core echo is the phased array probe, but a curvilinear probe can also be used, particularly for subcostal windows. The phased array probe has a small footprint, allowing it to obtain images through the small intercostal spaces and to be placed high in the epigastrium for subcostal windows. The latter uses the liver as a window. The stomach, also lying in the (left) epigastrium, contains air, which transmits ultrasound poorly, so degrading image quality.

Transducers have a marker on one side to allow the clinician to determine how the transducer is orientated with respect to the viewing screen. Radiologists orientate this marker to the right of the patient, or cranially,

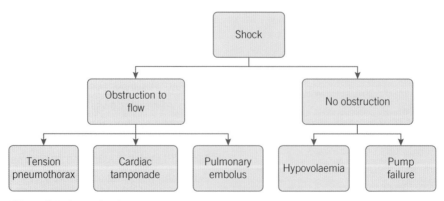

Figure 2.1 The differential diagnosis of shock.

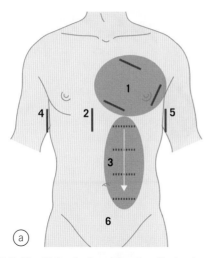

Figure 2.2 The Abdominal and Cardiac Evaluation with Sonography in Shock (ACES) algorithm—an approach by emergency physicians for the use of ultrasound in patients with undifferentiated hypotension. 1. Cardiac views; 2. Inferior vena cava; 3. Aorta; 4 and 5. Right and left flanks for pleural and peritoneal assessment; 6. Pelvic views.

This figure was published in *Emergency Medicine an Illustrated Colour Text*, Paul Atkinson et al., Copyright Elsevier 2010.

with the marker displayed on the left of the screen, as faced by the operator. Cardiologists with their phased array probe orientate the marker to the right of the screen—this is medical convention, just as we examine

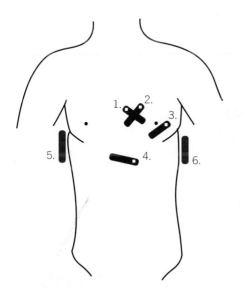

Figure 2.3 The FATE protocol.

Data from Jensen et al., 'Transthoracic echocardiography for cardiopulmonary monitoring in intensive care', *European Journal of Anaesthesiology* 2004;**21**:700–707.

from the left side of our patients. For the subcostal view, a useful approach is to place the transducer in the epigastrium and angle towards the right clavicle; the liver should appear on the left of the screen, as the operator faces it—'if the liver is left screen, you are right'. If the liver appears on the right of the screen, then the transducer is orientated wrongly and should be rotated through 180°.

The positions of the probe on the chest wall for PoCUS echo are described in Figure 2.4. The corresponding cardiac planes are demonstrated in Videos 2.1 to 2.7 ▣. For core PoCUS echo, the subcostal and PLAX views are used, and the remaining views may be considered advanced. These are all discussed in detail in Part 2 of this chapter.

Most of the information you require to function at core training level is obtained from the subcostal view (see Figure 2.4 and Videos 2.6 and 2.7 ▣). The probe is placed just below the xiphoid process, pointing at the left clavicle and using the liver as a window. The probe is placed firmly against the abdominal wall, with pressure applied cranially. The probe is held from above and applied close to the abdominal wall. This is the initial view used most frequently in the early resuscitation phase of critical illness, as diagnostic images are obtained with the patient lying on their back, while parasternal and apical images are best obtained with the patient rotated onto their left side. During a cardiac arrest, the relaxed abdominal musculature maximizes the chance of obtaining good-quality images, while probe placement ensures no interference with colleagues who may be providing airway support or obtaining central access. Views of the IVC are also easily obtained from the subcostal position by rotating and angling the probe vertically.

The second imaging position used in core level training is the PLAX view. The transducer is placed in the third, fourth, or fifth intercostal space, with the probe marker pointing to the right shoulder, so displaying an image of the right ventricle, left ventricle, aortic valve, mitral valve, and left atrium in longitudinal section (see Figure 2.5 and Video 2.1 ▣). The image is not as would be expected from the anatomical cardiac position, and the LV apex is positioned to the left of the screen.

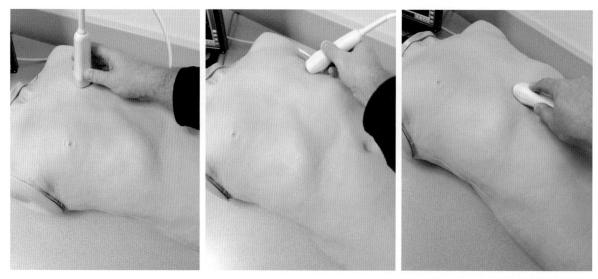

Figure 2.4 **The basic positions for the transducer in cardiac imaging. From top, moving clockwise: 1. Parasternal Long Axis (PLAX); (2. Parasternal Short Axis (PLAX) is shown in Figure 2.8); 3. apical (AP4 and AP5 chamber); and 4. subcostal (SCX) windows. The Focused Assessment by Transthoracic Echocardiography (FATE) protocol incorporates these windows, along with 5. right and 6. left lung bases.** *See Videos 2.1 to 2.7* 🎥.

The fluid–form–function–filling approach

The basic questions to identify the cause of cardiac arrest/shock are:

- *Fluid*: is there pericardial tamponade?

- *Form*: is there an enlarged right ventricle and signs of a massive PE? Is the left ventricle enlarged?

- *Function*: is the left ventricle contracting poorly, suggesting cardiac shock? Is it hyperdynamic, suggesting hypovolaemic or distributive shock? Is the heart beating—should we stop or continue resuscitation?

- *Filling*: is the IVC collapsing, suggesting hypovolaemia, a hyperdynamic heart, and/or fluid responsiveness?

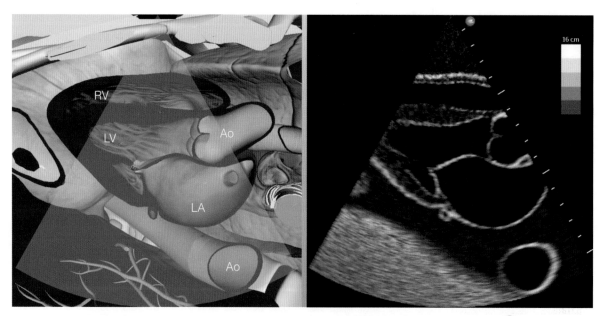

Figure 2.5 **Labelled diagram and computer-generated image (CGI) of ultrasound of PLAX.** *See Video 2.1* 🎥.
Image created on a CAE Vimedix simulator.

Fluid

Question: Is there pericardial tamponade?

Echo findings: pericardial fluid appears as a black rim separating the pericardium from the myocardium. A small volume of pericardial fluid is a normal finding—usually 1–2 mm of fluid seen as a small focal collection. Pericardial fat pads may also appear similar to effusions but are almost always only located anterior to the right ventricle, are not uniformly anechoic, and move with cardiac motion. In a cardiac arrest, it is reasonable to assume any pericardial effusion that surrounds the heart may be causal of the arrest, particularly in penetrating trauma where small (total size of effusion <1–2 cm) effusions developing rapidly can have profound haemodynamic consequences. However, large effusions developing slowly may remain under low pressure and have limited effect on right atrial and ventricular filling, and consequently CO. In shock, the key finding to differentiate a tamponade from a simple pericardial effusion is collapse of the RV free wall in diastole. This is important, as pericardial effusions are common while tamponade is rarer. If BP and lactate levels are normal, then tamponade is unlikely. It is safe to assume that a large effusion is causing tamponade if the patient is haemodynamically unstable (see Figure 2.6 and Videos 2.8 and 2.9 📹).

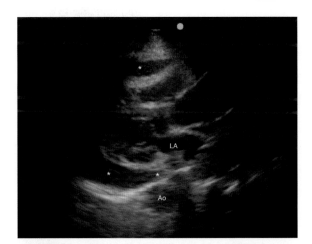

Figure 2.6 Pericardial effusion in PLAX. The fluid (˙) separates the descending aorta (Ao) and the left atrium (LA), following the pericardial sac. *See Videos 2.8 and 2.9* 📹 *and Figure 2.1s* 📷.

Form

Question: Is there an enlarged right ventricle and signs of obstructive shock (from a massive PE)?

Echo findings: there are several findings that suggest the RV afterload is increased by obstruction to flow. Firstly, the right ventricle may be enlarged, most simply assessed by observing if larger than the left ventricle. This is best seen in a 4-chamber apical view, but for Level 1 practitioners, a subcostal or PLAX view is adequate for gross pathology. The latter is simpler to obtain 'on axis', avoiding false-positive or false-negative findings. Further findings include paradoxical septal movement—the septum bows into the left ventricle; suggesting RV pressures exceed those in the left. A very large PE will also embarrass RV function, and the ventricle may be observed to contract poorly. The left ventricle may appear hyperdynamic as a consequence of reduced left-sided preload. The IVC may also be dilated (>20–25 mm measured AP subcostally through the liver) and not alter with respiration, reflecting the high filling pressures to the right side of the heart (see Part 3).

There are many chronic heart and lung diseases, such as chronic obstructive airways disease, pulmonary fibrosis, and valvular heart disease, that cause elevated pulmonary pressures with RV dilatation and impaired performance. However, these are associated with hypertrophy of the RV free wall to >5 mm (measured best in the subcostal or PLAX view).

Question: Is the left ventricle enlarged?

PoCUS does not include any cardiac measurements, but with some experience, clinicians will observe grossly dilated cardiac chambers. The left ventricle may appear enlarged (measured in B-mode in diastole at the level of the mitral valve as larger than 6 cm) with thickened or thinned walls (see Videos 2.14 to 2.17 and 2.21 📹; see discussion in 'Part 3, Acute decompensated heart failure', p. 65).

Function

Question: Is the left ventricle poorly contractile?

Echo findings: there is good evidence that emergency physicians with 1-day training can simply qualitatively assess LV performance as hyperdynamic, normal, mildly impaired, moderately impaired, or severely impaired, based on seeing a number of video images showing different levels of myocardial performance. The most difficult levels to differentiate are normal from mild impairment, but this is not of clinical relevance in the early assessment of shock, as minor LV impairment will not be causal! (See Videos 2.14 to 2.18 and 2.21 📷, with full discussion in 'Part 3, Acute decompensated heart failure', p. 65.)

Question: Is there a hyperdynamic left ventricle, suggesting hypovolaemia or sepsis?

A hyperdynamic ventricular performance is defined as an ejection fraction (EF) of >70%, but at core level, it refers to a heart that is beating rapidly, powerfully, and ejecting most of the blood in systole; indeed, the LV chamber walls may approximate at end-systole. This suggests that the cause of shock is either distributive or hypovolaemic. It can be very difficult to separate these two aetiologies without more detailed cardiac assessment of the volume of ejected blood.

Question: Is the heart beating—should we stop or continue resuscitation?

Echo findings: there may be visible contraction of both ventricles or sometimes just the right ventricle. The absence of any movement of the ventricles is associated with a poor prognosis in cardiac arrest, especially if a treatable cause, such as hyperkalaemia, is excluded. The isolated absence of LV contraction is less well studied but is likely to be similarly prognostic.

Filling

Question: Is the IVC small and/or collapsing with respiration, suggesting the patient benefits from fluid resuscitation? Is the IVC large and fixed with respiration, suggesting right-sided pressure volume overload?

PoCUS findings: the IVC and the proportion it collapses with inspiration (spontaneously ventilating patients, reversed with mechanical ventilation) are a very rough guide to the pressure–volume status of the right side of the heart. If the IVC measures under 11 mm in AP dimension via a subcostal trans-hepatic view in B-mode, then hypovolaemia is likely. The more the IVC collapses with inspiration, the more likely the patient is to increase the SV with a fluid bolus, i.e. to be a fluid responder. There is no single value that identifies fluid responders from non-responders; however, if the IVC

collapses around 40% or more with inspiration, then the patient is likely to respond to fluids by increasing their SV. Most patients with a normal heart will collapse their IVC between 30% and 100% with each breath, as part of their normal physiology.

If the IVC is >20–25 mm in the same AP measurement, then an increase in right heart pressure is suggested, with causes including PE, tamponade physiology, poor ventricular function, or high-volume fluid resuscitation. Thus, a look at the IVC in patients with shock during initial assessment may help divide those with distributive/hypovolaemic shock (high-volume fluid bolus likely to be of benefit for resuscitation) from patients with obstructive or myocardial aetiologies where the main focus of therapy is not on fluids or at least not fluids alone, and other early interventions may be required (see Videos 2.6 and 2.19 📷).

Part 2: Focused cardiac point-of-care ultrasound (echo) and ultrasound-guided resuscitation

Purpose

Why use cardiac point-of-care ultrasound (echo) in emergency care and resuscitation?

Emergency and critical care physicians rapidly integrate information obtained from history, examination, biochemical analysis, and imaging to identify critically ill patients, define the underlying pathophysiology, commence resuscitation, and assess the patients' response to treatment. History and physical examination alone can be misleading. Studies suggest that clinicians are poor at identifying the cause(s) of shock and, in up to a quarter of cases, may not differentiate high from low CO causation. Critically unwell patients may be confused, details of chronic illness may not be available, and they frequently present with a range of non-specific biochemical and ECG abnormalities. The most accurate diagnostic tests (e.g. CT or MRI scans) frequently require transport of the patient to another part of the hospital. Failure to adequately characterize shock states may lead to poor care and excess mortality. Ultrasound is a non-invasive, real-time point-of-care clinical tool, offering anatomical and functional assessment of many organs.

Cardiac PoCUS is the use of bedside ultrasound to display real-time images of the heart, enabling an understanding of both cardiac structure and function and how these are affected by both disease and treatment. This is of particular use in critical illness, as cardiac function is the key determinate of oxygen delivery; matching adequate tissue oxygenation to the patient's needs is the focus of resuscitation. PoCUS may improve accuracy of, and time to, diagnosis and alter management in around two-thirds of patients with shock. However, there are no studies published to date demonstrating an improvement in mortality as a result of PoCUS. In the ED, most patients in shock are thought to benefit from initial fluid resuscitation, although recent data suggest that only 50–70% actually increase the SV by >10–15% with an intravenous fluid bolus. Several studies show only around half of haemodynamically unstable patients admitted to ICUs are fluid responders. PoCUS is associated with more confident haemodynamic management in the ED. As such, several professional bodies recommend that PoCUS be an integral part of critical care assessments.

As emergency and critical care physicians, we perform limited or focused studies integrated into our clinical assessment, so answering specific questions posed by the clinical scenario at hand. There is no internationally agreed term describing this type of sonographic assessment. The terms point-of-care ultrasound (PoCUS), focused cardiac ultrasound (FoCUS), point-of-care sonography (PoCS), or clinician-performed ultrasound (CPUS) have all been proposed. We will use the term 'PoCUS'. This term is used in recognition that we use a range of ultrasound windows and are not bound by traditional specialty training. We choose the windows based on the emerging clinical picture. Thus, a PoCUS assessment of shock may include cardiac, vena cava, and lung windows, along with other specific views such as aortic or abdominal windows.

We suggest that following a systematic 'fluid, form, function, filling' approach will assist as an aide-memoire to learn cardiac PoCUS (see Box 2.1). A structured, systematic approach to image acquisition may reasonably be assumed to reduce error and ensure a sufficient assessment. This qualitative approach can be enhanced with simple measurements, as highlighted in italics.

The primary concern in caring for critically unwell patients is to identify the underlying cause(s) of the presenting illness and provide appropriate resuscitation. This will be discussed in detail below in 'Part 3, Shock', p. 60 and 'Acute decompensated heart

---

Box 2.1 The 'FFFF' approach to cardiac PoCUS

1. Fluid:

  a. Is there evidence of pericardial fluid and tamponade?

2. Form:

  a. Ventricular size and shape. Is there chamber dilatation? Is the left-to-right ventricular size ratio maintained? Are the chamber contours normal? Is the heart size collapsed, suggesting hypovolaemia?

  b. Valves. Are the valves thin and opening normally? Is there calcification or thickening? Is there a regurgitant jet?

3. Function (an approach to physiological and pathophysiological patterns):

  a. Are the ventricular walls thickening evenly and consistently?

  b. Are the ventricular chambers contracting normally, or are the contractions hypo- or hyperdynamic?

  c. Is there global or regional dysfunction, or paradoxical wall motion?

  d. Is there normal valvular movement and opening?

  e. What are the simple measures of function (MAPSE, EPSS)?

4. Filling:

  a. Does the IVC size suggest gross hypovolaemia or evidence of pressure–volume overload?

failure', p. 65. There are many models to assist the clinician in identifying the causes of shock and hypotension. The 'Hs and Ts' are commonly taught in life support courses. Shock may be consequent upon pump failure (myocardial or valvular disease), obstruction to blood flow or cardiac filling (PE, pericardial tamponade, tension pneumothorax), hypovolaemia (blood or fluid losses), or vasodilatation (distributive shock; sepsis or anaphylaxis or neurogenic shock). PoCUS can assist in identifying the disease process or processes contributing to shock (see Figure 2.1). This model may be modified for PoCUS. Here each of the five categories is associated with different PoCUS findings. 'Hypovolaemia' here includes both hypovolaemic and distributive shock, as cardiac findings of hyperdynamic wall motion, high EF, and a small IVC are common to both. In distributive shock, the end-diastolic volumes are often preserved. In many cases of septic shock, there is coexisting hypovolaemia, as patients may have reduced oral intake and increased losses.

In emergency and critical care medicine, most physicians do not perform detailed, comprehensive cardiac studies such as those performed by our cardiology colleagues. Often this level of detail is unnecessary, but also developing and maintaining a sufficient level of competence, e.g. to accurately grade the severity of valvular stenosis, is not feasible for most physicians working in emergency medicine, internal medicine, and critical care.

It is possible to get PoCUS images of sufficient quality to guide care in most ICU patients, with reports that at least one cardiac window can be viewed in 97% of patients in the ICU setting. Experience suggests a slightly lower figure in the ED, as windows are compromised by patient position (e.g. sitting up or agitated with acute dyspnoea) and in spontaneously ventilating patients, but this is less well reported. Pre-hospital, at least one diagnostic-quality window may be obtained in 80–90% of patients, with all cardiac windows being obtained in around one-third. The quality of images may be poorer, and the diagnostic findings consequently less robust.

Although cardiac PoCUS is useful in the management of critically ill patients, there are some potential limitations, particularly in a cardiac arrest. These include technical difficulties acquiring images,

interference from ECG leads, defibrillator pads, chest compression, and other interventions. Transthoracic cardiac PoCUS may also interfere with resuscitative efforts, having been shown to prolong pulse checks, which may lead to decreased coronary perfusion.

Transoesophageal echocardiography (TOE/TEE) may allow clinicians to perform higher-quality PoCUS-informed resuscitation in the scenario of a cardiac arrest where the transthoracic approach is difficult. The American College of Emergency Physicians (ACEP) has produced a guideline for the use of TOE/TEE in the ED for cardiac arrest. It is likely that this technique will become more commonly used over the next few years in this setting. As competency for this technique improves among emergency physicians, other indications, such as diagnosis of aortic dissection, PE, endocarditis, assessment of cardiac function, and more, are likely to develop.

In this chapter, we will discuss how PoCUS guides diagnosis and subsequent therapy. We then will describe the integration of PoCUS into the assessment of acute heart failure, shock, and cardiac arrest.

Perspective

When do I perform focused echo?

The 'ABC approach' to critical illness encourages physicians to focus on rapid identification of threats to life and to correct these, as compared to making a comprehensive assessment. In patients with shock, PoCUS is a key diagnostic test tantamount to the ECG, chest radiograph, and blood gas analysis, and it is easily integrated into the initial assessment. Indeed, in one single-centre randomized trial, integrating PoCUS into the initial assessment improved the probability of a correct diagnosis from 50% to 80% at 15 minutes into resuscitation. PoCUS thus follows the primary survey and focused clinical assessment.

In cardiac arrest scenarios, the team enables parallel assessment. PoCUS may be integrated into the rhythm and pulse check in the first or second cycle for non-shockable rhythms, and arguably after the third cycle in ventricular tachycardia (VT)/ventricular fibrillation (VF). This is because in the former, PoCUS has greater potential clinical benefit, and in the latter, it is less likely to impact management while potentially delaying defibrillation and cardiac compressions.

Differentiating pulseless electrical activity with cardiac contraction from electromechanical dissociation with no cardiac activity offers important prognostic information, with the former suggesting inadequate preload to the left ventricle (PE, hypovolaemia, or pericardial effusion). PoCUS can be performed rapidly and should not interfere with, or delay, external cardiac massage, as even brief interruptions confer worsening prognosis. In well-coordinated resuscitation, the team leader counts down from 5 to 1 to signal a cessation of cardiac massage, allowing team members to simultaneously manage the airway, obtain intravenous (IV) access, check the pulse, and obtain a 10-second recorded echo loop. The subcostal view is first choice, as this allows good-quality images (the upper abdomen is usually very relaxed!) and minimal interruptions to external massage (especially if by mechanical device), requires no patient repositioning, and does not interfere with airway manoeuvres or with attempts at central venous access.

For patients in cardiac arrest from penetrating trauma, PoCUS is the priority investigation, because if there are haemothoraces or pneumothoraces or peritoneal fluid or haemopericardium, the immediate interventions include thoracostomy, thoracotomy, and fluid resuscitation. PoCUS is key to diagnosis. Indeed, in this scenario, echo has been demonstrated to reduce time to diagnosis of pericardial tamponade and to reduce time to thoracotomy, and consequently mortality.

Performing the scan

In what order should cardiac PoCUS windows be performed?

While it is common practice to perform cardiac PoCUS following a prescribed number and order of views, there is no rigid structure that must be followed or number of windows that must be obtained; these will be determined by the clinical picture and findings. A structured, systematic approach may reduce operator stress and error and ensure sufficient images are obtained for diagnosis (see protocols such as ACES, FATE, RUSH, and the 'fluid, form, function, filling' approach advocated in this chapter).

The FATE protocol (see Figure 2.3 in Part 1 of this chapter) consists of:

1. Looking for obvious pathology;
2. Assessing wall thickness and chamber dimensions;
3. Assessing biventricular function;
4. Imaging the pleura on both sides;
5. Relating the information to the clinical context;
6. Applying additional ultrasound, as required.

The FATE protocol (after Jensen, 2004) is based on parasternal long and short axes, apical 4-chamber, subcostal, and left/right mid-axillary line lung base windows. (See 'Obtaining the basic views', p. 34, 35 and Figure 2.3 in Part 1 for explanation.)

However, more advanced practitioners direct their scanning to the clinical presentation. For example, an elderly man collapsing with flank pain and persisting hypotension suggests a leaking aneurysm, so the initial focus would be the abdomen and aorta, while a young postpartum woman with sudden onset of dyspnoea, hypoxia, and hypotension suggesting PE would benefit from an initial cardiac scan focusing on the right ventricle.

Which transducer do I use?

The most appropriate transducer to use depends on the clinical situation and the questions to be answered. The phased array transducer is small, fits between rib spaces, and has software optimized for cardiac studies such as colour (to see turbulent or regurgitant flow) and spectral Doppler (to measure flow velocity and pressure). However, good images are easily obtained with a curved array ('abdominal') transducer from a subcostal view. A curvilinear transducer, particularly with a small micro-convex head, allows better-quality abdominal images, while also offering excellent subcostal images. For example, when treating a patient in traumatic cardiac arrest, the clinician may choose the curvilinear transducer to evaluate for pericardial tamponade (requiring thoracotomy), tension pneumothorax (requiring immediate intercostal catheter placement), or intraperitoneal blood loss (requiring volume resuscitation). Alternatively, when approaching an elderly, shocked (non-trauma) patient, the phased array transducer may be a better choice, as the focus of interest will be on cardiac performance.

Obtaining the basic views

During resuscitation or in a trauma setting, it may be easiest to begin to image the heart using the sub-costal view. Unfortunately, the heart is situated in the thorax, adjacent to several structures that are impermeable to ultrasound beams. The ossified bones of the sternum and ribs reflect ultrasound waves, obscuring structures behind them from view. The lungs diffract sound waves, so generating sufficient artefact to obscure the underlying structures. Patients with chronic obstructive lung disease may have hyperexpanded lungs, making the parasternal and apical views particularly challenging. Rotating the patient into a left lateral decubitus position often improves image quality, but ill patients may not tolerate this.

There are three standard locations on the thorax where the probe is placed (see Figure 2.4, and Videos 2.1 to 2.5 and 2.7 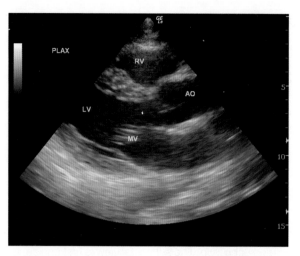 for resulting views):

- The parasternal window;
- The apical window;
- The subcostal window.

From these three locations, there are five common views of the heart that are routinely obtained:

- The PLAX and PSAX views;
- The apical 4-chamber and apical 5-chamber views;
- The subcostal 4-chamber view.

The parasternal long axis (PLAX) window

The probe is placed on top of the sternum, just caudal to the manubrium, perpendicular to the chest, with the probe's indicator angled towards the patient's right shoulder (note this is counter to the general principle of aligning the probe marker with the screen indicator—best remembered as 'parasternal wrong axis'—and derives from the tradition of the sonographer being situated on the patient's left side in cardiology). Slowly glide the probe off the sternum towards the patient's left. Move the probe down each successive intercostal space in a circular motion until the highest-quality images are obtained; there are three parasternal windows known as the high view, on-axis view, and low view. All PoCUS practitioners

Figure 2.7 Labelled ultrasound image in PLAX view. *See Videos 2.1 and 2.23* .

will include the on-axis view; some may also use the additional views to better view the right side of the heart. When these images are aligned with the long axis of the heart, i.e. in a plane running from the cardiac apex to the right shoulder, this is called the parasternal long axis (PLAX) view (see Figures 2.5 and 2.7 and Video 2.1).

The right side of the heart is anterior (near field), and the left side is deep. The mitral valve, aortic valve, and LV cavity are seen in the middle of the field, with the apex to the left of the screen and the ascending thoracic aorta to the right. The probe should be rotated clockwise or counter-clockwise to try to elongate the form of the left ventricle to make it as long as possible. If the transducer is orientated cranially or caudally from the apex, the image is foreshortened and, if not over the central LV cavity, any measurements will underestimate the cardiac dimensions. The angle of the probe and the depth of the field should be adjusted, so that the aortic valve and the mitral valve are in plane and the descending thoracic aorta can be visualized posteriorly beneath the left atrium. This view provides knowledge about the structure and form of the LV cavity, allowing cavity size and wall thickness to be measured and systolic function evaluated. The proximal ascending aorta, aortic valve leaflets, mitral valve leaflets, and posterior pericardium are all clearly seen. Using colour Doppler allows aortic and mitral regurgitation to be assessed (see Video 2.21).

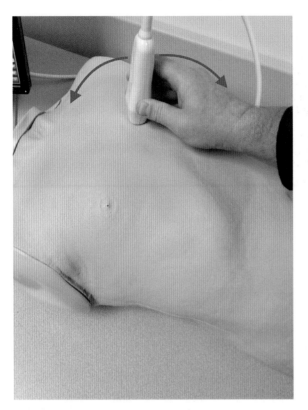

Figure 2.8 Probe positions for the PSAX view.
See Video 2.2 📹.

The parasternal short axis (PSAX) window

Turning the probe clockwise 90°, so the indicator is towards the patient's left shoulder, will image the heart in its short axis, as if the heart apex were in front of the screen and its base behind the screen. Multiple 'slices' across the heart can be made by tilting the probe, aiming to the patient's right to see the base of the heart and to their left to see the apex (see Figure 2.8 and Video 2.2 📹). Moving and angling the probe base towards the patient's right shoulder or towards their left hip will transect the heart at different levels. With the probe base directed under the sternum, the so-called 'Mercedes Benz' view is obtained (see Video 2.2 📹), with images of the aortic valve centrally and the left atrium beneath this, the right atrium to the left, the right ventricle above, and the pulmonary outflow tract to the right. If the probe is directed directly vertically, the left ventricle is imaged at the level of the mitral valve—the 'fish mouth'. This shows the basal LV wall segments (see Video 2.2 📹). Angling the probe a few degrees to the apex then brings the papillary muscles into view, defining the mid cavity of the left ventricle (see Figure 2.9 and Video 2.2 📹). Further angulation to the apex will image the apex and the apical LV segments (see Video 2.2 📹). It may be necessary to slide the probe a short distance along the intercostal space to obtain these images, and to adjust the angulation. The PSAX windows are most useful to assess radial contraction and define myocardial regional wall motion abnormalities. The 'Mercedes Benz' view allows assessment of tricuspid regurgitation and pulmonary pressures, pulmonary artery pressures, and the inter-atrial septum. The probe should

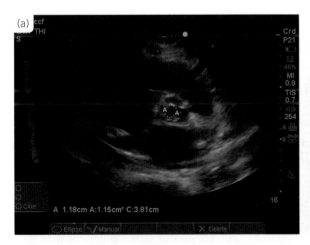
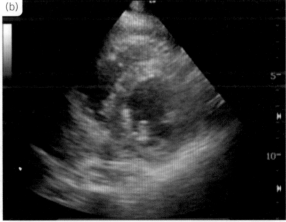

Figure 2.9 (a) PSAX—the 'Mercedes Benz' view, here showing measurement of the aortic valve by planometry.
See Video 2.2 📹. **(b) PSAX—the papillary muscle window, showing papillary muscles and mid-cavity segments of the LV wall.** *See Video 2.2* 📹.

be rotated and fanned to try to create a circular (as opposed to 'D'-shaped or oval) cavity to ensure that the imaging plane is truly perpendicular to the LV cavity.

The apical window

The apical 4-chamber (see Videos 2.3, 2.4, and 2.23) and apical 5-chamber (see Figure 2.10 and Video 2.5) views of the heart are obtained by firstly placing the probe base directly over the LV apex. With the base plate pointing to the right shoulder, the apex can be found by palpating the point of maximal impulse or by self-correction as the probe is moved laterally from the site of the short axis views. To start, place the probe in the fourth or fifth intercostal space, or just under the nipple in a male, in the mid-clavicular line. The indicator is directed towards the patient's axilla, and the probe is slightly rotated counter-clockwise, in a shallow angle almost parallel to the floor. The proper shape of a normal heart in this view has the ventricles in near field and the atria in far field, with the footprint of the probe directly over the apex of the left ventricle. The standard apical 4-chamber view of the heart is so named, because both the atria and the ventricles of both the left and right side are in view. However, fanning the probe base slightly anteriorly (up towards the sternum) will bring the aortic valve into view, which, while not a 'chamber', completes the so-called apical 5-chamber view of the heart. From the apical window, the left side of the heart is visually represented on the right-hand side of the screen. Accidentally flipping the probe is a very common mistake, but there are several ways to detect accidental disorientation. Fanning the probe anteriorly should bring the aortic valve into view, positively identifying the left side. The right ventricle is also distinguished by the moderator band (a band of echogenic material observed to cross the apical right ventricle) and the slightly more apical insertion of the tricuspid valve, compared to the mitral valve on the left. The apical 4-chamber view enables comparison and measurement of the cardiac chambers and assessment of ventricular function, regional wall abnormalities, diastolic function, mitral and tricuspid stenosis/regurgitation, and the atrial septum (see Video 2.24 for an example of tricuspid regurgitation). It is *less* useful to assess wall size, as the ultrasound beam is in parallel with the myocardium. The apical 5-chamber view allows assessment of aortic regurgitation, stenosis, and SV using the VTI (velocity time integral, discussed in the following Part 3 subsections: 'Fluid resuscitation, fluid tolerance, and fluid responsiveness', p. 61; 'Dynamic predictors of fluid responsiveness', p. 62; and 'How does ultrasound assist in guiding fluid resuscitation?', p. 63). Counter-clockwise rotation of the probe from the apical 4-chamber view provides the 2- and 3-chamber images, used to assess wall motion and calculate the EF by the modified Simpson bi-plane methodology. These will not be discussed further here.

The subcostal window

Subcostally, if using cardiac settings, the heart is viewed by placing the probe on the epigastrium, with the probe's indicator towards the patient's left side, and aiming the ultrasound beam towards the patient's left shoulder (see Videos 2.6 and 2.7). (Note that if performing this view using an abdominal setting, as part of a FAST scan, the marker will be orientated to the patient's right and will appear on the left of the screen.) By imaging through the most medial lobes of the liver, the stomach can be avoided. As the heart lies relatively anteriorly in the chest, the technique is to depress the probe on the abdomen, as you aim the probe. Images may be facilitated by asking the patient to breathe deeply, moving the heart inferiorly, and by bending the knees to 90°, reducing the tone in the abdominal wall musculature.

Ensure that a complete sweep, from anterior to posterior, through the heart is made.

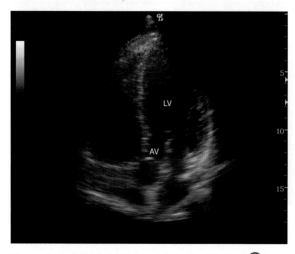

Figure 2.10 Apical 5-chamber view. *See Video 2.5* .

Interpreting the views

'Fluid'

Core:

Identifying and measuring the size of pericardial effusions.

Advanced:

Differentiating pericardial fluid from pleural fluid.

Identifying and measuring the size of pericardial effusions

The outside of the myocardium is surrounded by a two-layered serous pericardium—the visceral and parietal pericardium. Both of these are enclosed inside a more fibrous pericardium, together measuring 1–3 mm thick. Normally, a small amount of fluid provides lubrication between the two layers. The entrance and egresses of the vena cava, as well as the aorta, pulmonary trunk, and pulmonary veins, create two blind-ending sinuses of flexion of the pericardium on the myocardium. Through this, the heart is attached to the sternum anteriorly, the central tendon of the diaphragm inferiorly, and the surrounding mediastinum elsewhere. The thorax pulls tension on the pericardium by its parietal attachments. The intra-pericardial pressures are typically those of the intra-thoracic pressures. The pericardium provides a mechanism for the heart chambers to exert pressure on each other, through a phenomenon known as ventricular interdependence, and protects the heart from nearby structures. When fluid, blood, or other material accumulates in the pericardial space, the intra-pericardial pressures will rise, reducing right atrial, and then ventricular, filling and consequently impeding cardiac function.

Pericardial effusions (see Figure 2.6 and Videos 2.8 and 2.9 📹; see Figure 2.1s 🖼) are common in ill patients and can generally be classified as transudates, exudates, malignant, or haemorrhagic. Because the intra-pericardial pressure is the physiologic basis for pathology, the rate of accumulation of the effusion is the most significant determinant of tamponade physiology, as slow-growing effusions will stretch the pericardium with it. The size of the effusion is usually measured from the edge of the pericardium to the myocardium in the subcostal view, and a comment is usually specifically made if the effusion wraps around circumferentially or whether it is localized to a particular area. Small volumes of pericardial fluid are frequently identified. An effusion of <5 mm is termed trivial, 5–10 mm small, 10–20 mm as moderate, and anything larger than 20 mm as large. The size of the effusion is the sum of the measurements obtained on either side of the epicardium, if circumferential.

Pericardial effusions are predominantly hypoechoic and take the outline of the pericardium that binds it. Epicardial fat pads are a common benign finding that are commonly mistaken for an effusion. Careful assessment demonstrates the diagnostic characteristics of epicardial fat. Simply based on their echo texture, epicardial fat is generally more speckled or granular, while pericardial effusions are homogenous and hypoechoic. However, old blood clots may also assume an echogenic and granular appearance. The epicardial fat pad is attached to the epicardium, moving in a coordinated fashion with the heart, while an effusion will not usually move in conjunction with the heart's systolic and diastolic motions. Additionally, epicardial fat pads are almost always only seen on the anterior surface of the right ventricle, while pericardial effusions may be seen focally or circumferentially.

Differentiating pericardial fluid from pleural fluid

Ultrasonography is very sensitive for detecting pleural effusions, which may not be evident on a chest X-ray. Pleural fluid will layer in the most dependent positions—most patients in the supine or semi-recumbent position will be in the posterior reflections of the hemithorax. To identify pleural effusions, place the probe (phased array or curvilinear) in a coronal plane in the mid-axillary line at the level of the diaphragm. This is similar to the RUQ and LUQ windows of the FAST examination, but scanning slightly more cephalad to include areas just above the diaphragm.

When imaging via PLAX, it can be difficult to determine the precise location of accumulated fluid—pleural or pericardial. If a single contiguous body of hypoechoic fluid can be visualized around both the anterior and posterior parts of the heart, it is self-explanatory that the fluid is a pericardial, rather than a pleural, effusion. However, if there is a significant amount of fluid only posterior to the heart, the question needs to be asked if the fluid is in the pericardium or whether it is actually a left pleural effusion. The landmark that allows differentiation of pericardial and pleural fluid is the descending thoracic aorta, as it is excluded from the pericardium. *Pericardial fluid* collects anterior to the descending aorta, often lying between it and the left atrium. Pleural fluid passes posterior to the descending aorta, non-adjacent to the left atrium. Pericardial and pleural effusions occur concurrently.

Differentiating pericardial tamponade from simple pericardial effusion

In the clinical setting of the shocked patient, the presence of a significant pericardial fluid collection should raise the likely diagnosis of cardiac tamponade. The right atrium has the lowest mean pressure of the entire venous system, allowing blood to flow down the requisite pressure gradient, returning to the heart for circulation. Much like the pressure in the pleural space, the pericardial pressure is normally negative, as fluid and space are held in traction by the fibrous pericardium pulling it outward. In the case of a pericardial effusion with tamponade physiology, fluid accumulates to the point where there is increased pericardial pressure, sufficient to embarrass diastolic filling. Through its series of one-way valves, the chambers of the heart gradually increase the mean intra-cavity pressure, starting from the right atrium, to the right ventricle, to the left atrium, and then finally to the left ventricle. As the pericardial effusion increases in size, it will continue to exert its pressure on all parts of the heart. However, with low intra-cavity pressure, the right atrium is most susceptible to increased pericardial pressures. The most sensitive sign of increased pericardial pressure is collapse of the right atrium during its diastole, which is during ventricular systole. This can be seen as a 'double movement' of the right atrial wall. As pericardial pressure rises, it will reach the point where the pressure on the outside of the right ventricle will be greater than the pressure on the inside of the right ventricle and it will collapse during its diastole. RV diastolic collapse of greater than one-third of diastole can be a characteristic finding for tamponade physiology and has a very recognizable echocardiography pattern. Normally, throughout all phases of the cardiac cycle, the right ventricle has a convex curve to it. However, during tamponade physiology, the right ventricle will indent during its diastolic phase to produce an immediately recognizable pattern.

Ultimately, cardiac tamponade is a clinical diagnosis in the resuscitation setting.

'Form'

Core:

Chamber sizes and ratios.

Advanced:

Ventricular wall thickness;
Mitral valve;
Aortic valve;
Endocarditis.

General assessment of cardiac shape and chamber sizes

There are important differences between the right and left sides of the heart, both anatomically and physiologically. The right side of the heart (the right atrium and ventricle, lying anteriorly to left atria/ventricle) has a much lower pressure than the left side (left atrium and ventricle). The right ventricle has a thinner wall and 'wraps around' the left ventricle, with a crescenteric or 'croissant' shape in cross-section. The left ventricle is thick-walled and circular or 'doughnut'-shaped in cross-section (see Figures 2.7 and 2.8, and Video 2.2). The left ventricle is larger in volume and diameter than the right. As a general rule, the ratio of right-to-left ventricular size is 0.7–1.0 (maximum) and best observed in the apical view. It is important to ensure that the maximum size of each chamber is obtained when visualizing the heart, as some planes may not fully visualize each chamber. Valves should be thin with mobile cusps. During resuscitation, it is sufficient to make a rapid 'eye-ball' assessment of 'form' for large, dilated ventricles versus small, thick ventricles; or a normal versus an increased right-to-left ventricular ratio. In more stable patients, or with advanced scanning, formal measurements may be made. Table 2.1 lists the normal sizes for left heart structures.

Left heart

Assessment of left atrial and left ventricular form

Describing the heart in terms of left versus right can be misleading, as based on embryological changes, the heart is rotated in the chest, with the right side anteriorly

Table 2.1 Normal cardiac chamber dimensions (volumes) (sex differences reported where relevant)

Chamber/measurement (PLAX)	Normal limits in mm (volume in mL)
Left atrium	19–39 (maximum 34 mL/m^2)
Left ventricle (internal diameter, diastole) Right ventricle	Male: 42–58 (62–150 mL) Female: 38–52 (46–106 mL) 33 ± 4 at base, >41 abnormal 27 ± 4 at mid-cavity level papillary muscle, >35 abnormal
Left ventricle (internal diameter, systole)	Male: 25–40 (21–61 mL) Female: 22–35 (14–42 mL)
Inter-ventricular septum, diastole	6–13
LV posterior wall, diastole RV free wall (subcostal view)	6–11 <5 mm

and the left situated posteriorly. The left atrium is a site of frequent pathology and deformation, and is usually enlarged in significant diastolic heart failure and frequently in significant mitral valve disease, LV systolic disease, aortic valve disease, and (indirectly) systemic arterial hypertension (see Figures 2.11 and 2.12) (see Table 2.1 and Figure 2.13 for cardiac measurements). The left atrium is best seen from the PLAX and apical 4-chamber views. A simple guide in the PLAX view is to compare the size of the left atrium to the aorta, so allowing for differing physiological size-related variation. Measurements may be made of the maximum diameter or area using B-mode (now recommended, as opposed to M-mode) from inner wall to inner wall (see Table 2.1 and Figure 2.13). Volumes are measured using the Simpson's modified bi-plane method, as discussed in Stroke volume and cardiac output. All cardiac dimensions and, in particular, the left ventricle can vary with changes in race, body surface area, and gender, and so the table only offers a rough guide.

The mitral valve

Critically unwell patients often have heart murmurs. PoCUS can assist in identifying significant underlying disease that is severe enough to require treatment or to factor in during resuscitation. The mitral valve consists of one (larger) anterior and one (smaller) posterior valve leaflet, both of which are easily seen from the parasternal, apical, and sub-xiphoid windows (see Figure 2.7, and Videos 2.1, 2.3, 2.4, and 2.6). The primary function of the valve is to prevent back flow of blood during ventricular systole. Mitral valve regurgitation (see Figure 2.14, and Videos 2.11 and 2.12),

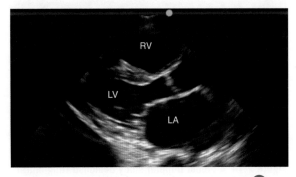

Figure 2.11 Left atrium, left ventricle, and pleural fluid in PLAX view.

Figure 2.12 Left atrial enlargement. *See Video 2.10* .

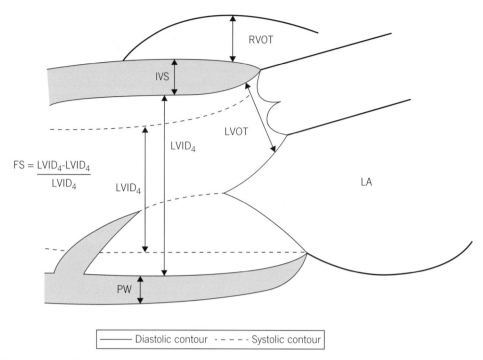

RVOT

IVS

LVOT

LVID$_4$

$$FS = \frac{LVID_4 - LVID_4}{LVID_4}$$

LVID$_4$

LVID$_4$

LA

PW

——— Diastolic contour - - - - - Systolic contour

Figure 2.13 Normal left-sided cardiac measurements.

prolapse, stenosis, and therefore mitral valve replacement, are all common. The leaflets are semicircular in shape, with a saddle-shaped annulus, and are tethered by tendinous cords to the papillary muscles in the LV cavity, and when the mitral valve leaflets come together to coapt during ventricular systole, they form a gentle curve that resembles a canted smile. When they coapt, the leaflets should come together completely and competently. However, sometimes the

valve leaflet tips, after coming together, will translate into the left atria past the annular apparatus in PLAX, which can indicate mitral valve prolapse. This may be an incidental finding on echo, but it is rarely relevant to resuscitation.

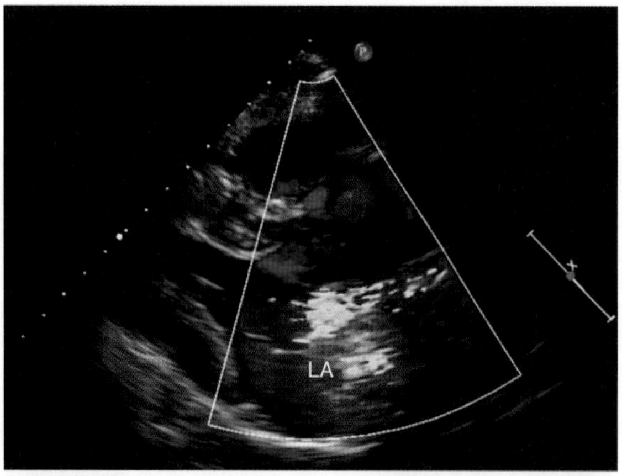

In the early filling phase of diastole, the mitral valve opens and the anterior mitral valve leaflet should touch, or come within 5–7 mm of, the inter-ventricular septum. The opening of the mitral valve is impaired by valvular disease and poor LV function. If there is no obvious valvular calcification, the opening is macroscopically normal, the anterior and posterior leaflets coapt together in end-diastole, and colour Doppler shows no regurgitation, then valvular disease that is significant to affect resuscitation is extremely unlikely.

Mitral annulus calcification (MAC) is a common degenerative finding that can involve the annulus and sometimes the leaflet itself. When sufficiently dense, it casts an acoustic shadow downfield, similar to renal or biliary calculi. MAC is commonly associated with old age, hypertension, diabetes, ischaemic heart disease, and renal disease, and is generally benign. MAC less commonly involves the distal-most tips of the leaflets and generally does not cause significant mitral stenosis.

Figure 2.14 A colour Doppler study demonstrating mitral regurgitation filling the enlarged left atrium (LA).
See Videos 2.10 to 2.12 .

Although now rare in wealthy nations, rheumatic valve disease commonly involves mitral valve stenosis. Rheumatic mitral stenosis has some similarity to MAC, in that it causes leaflet calcification, but the pathology really comes from fusion of the valve commissures, significantly decreasing the effective orifice area of the mitral valve. Because of the restricted flow, the pressure inside the left atria will mount during its systole and the anterior mitral valve leaflet will develop a characteristic hockey stick shape, as it balloons apically with the distending pressure (see Video 2.10 ⬤). Quantifying the severity of mitral stenosis is beyond PoCUS assessment.

Mitral regurgitation is a common finding in PoCUS (see Figure 2.14 and Video 2.10 ⬤). Mitral regurgitation with pulmonary oedema requires rapid identification and assessment for repair. Causes include degeneration, secondary to LV dilatation, papillary muscle rupture, rheumatic fever, and infection. The acutely incompetent mitral valve allows a retrograde jet of blood to flow into the left atrium and pulmonary veins to the lungs during systole (see Videos 2.10 to 2.12 ⬤).

Doppler colour studies focus on the different frequencies of ultrasound waves being reflected by moving red blood cells. Different colours are applied to different velocities. Blood moving towards the transducer is viewed as red, and that away blue (blue away, red towards—'BART'). Higher velocities appear yellow or green. The motion of blood through the cardiac chambers in systole and diastole can thus be followed, and regurgitant jets identified. In the apical 4-chamber or PLAX view, a colour Doppler window can be placed over the entire left atrium to look for regurgitant jets (see Figure 2.14 and Videos 2.10 and 2.11 ⬤). If there is blood flow coming back through the mitral valve during systole when it should be closed, that is evidence of mitral valve insufficiency. The width, length, and velocity of that jet can be measured to quantify the severity of the insufficiency, but the specific characteristics are beyond the PoCUS exam. Larger, longer, and faster regurgitant jets are more severe than thinner, shorter, and slower jets. Even valves that appear to come together completely can have degrees of incompetence, so it is worthwhile to make colour flow Doppler part of your standard scanning protocol.

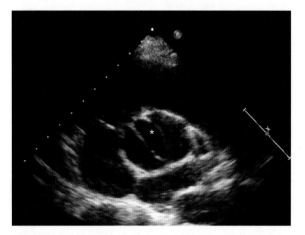

Figure 2.15 Aortic stenosis as a result of: (a) bicuspid aortic valve (*) and (b) thickened aortic valve leaflets. AV, aortic valve.

Aortic valve

Aortic valve disease is also common (see Figures 2.15 and 2.16 and Video 2.14 ⬤). The three semilunar leaflets are made of the endocardium and connective tissue, and are supported by a more rigid annulus. The three cusps are almost equal in size and come together to coapt during diastole. In the reflections of the base of the leaflets and the ascending aorta, the left and right coronary arteries take off, which name the leaflets: the right coronary cusp, the left coronary cusp, and the non-coronary cusp. From the PSAX view, the aortic valve is said to have the shape of an inverted 'Mercedes Benz' sign and the number of valve

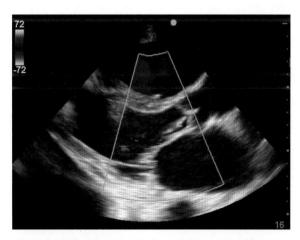

Figure 2.16 Aortic regurgitation, with regurgitant jet seen with colour Doppler. *See Videos 2.13, 2.22, and 2.23* ⬤.

leaflets can be identified (see Figure 2.15, and Videos 2.13, 2.22, and 2.23 ⬤▶).

Bicuspid aortic valves occur in 1–2% of the population, more common in females (see Figure 2.15). The M-mode PLAX view through the aortic valve leaflets loses the characteric 'box' shape in a bicuspid valve. The three leaflets may be visualized in the PSAX 'Mercedes Benz' window or using M-mode in PLAX. Sclerosis of the aortic leaflet valves is very common in older age, but it may be seen in accelerated forms in younger patients with bicuspid aortic valves or underlying connective tissue disease. As the valves thicken, they may have difficulty opening and closing properly, which decreases the effective valve area and impedes the flow of blood as it tries to leave the left ventricle. Over time, this can cause increased intra-cavity pressures, with resultant hypertrophy, dilatation, and systolic dysfunction. Because the flow of blood is related to the radius of the aortic valve orifice to the fourth degree, small changes in aortic valve opening greatly increase the resistance encountered by blood flow and result in increasing the velocity of blood through the valve.

In PLAX, the aortic valve leaflets should be seen coming together in the same plane as the mitral valve. The leaflets should be thin, freely mobile, of equal length, and coapting neatly together during diastole. Particularly echogenic aortic valve leaflets should raise concern for possible aortic stenosis.

As in mitral incompetence, colour flow Doppler studies may suggest aortic regurgitation, with back flow through the valve in diastole. These are best performed in PLAX and apical 5-chamber windows (see Figure 2.16). The best measurement of the severity of an aortic regurgitation jet is obtained from the apical windows, as the ultrasound waves are most parallel with the outflow and the (now) regurgitant inflow. Again, wider, longer, and faster jets suggest more severe disease.

Aortic stenosis may be assessed from the apical 5-chamber view. The velocity of blood flow is measured in the LVOT (using PW) and also in the aorta distal to the aortic valve (maximal velocity, using CW). Higher pressure gradients across the valve result in higher velocities.

In the context of resuscitation, if the aortic blood flow velocity using CW Doppler in the apical 5-chamber view is under 1.5 m/s, the valve is macroscopically normal, and there is no visible regurgitation, then significant aortic valve disease is highly unlikely. More detailed valvular studies are beyond the context of PoCUS.

Endocarditis

Among the many causes of mitral and aortic valve regurgitation, the diagnosis of endocarditis should be carefully considered. Infected masses of platelets, fibrin, inflammatory cells, and infective organisms have a few characteristics that are amenable to diagnosis by echocardiography. While vegetations are usually similar in sonographic texture to the regular myocardium, they tend to be mobile and move independently of the nearby structures, may be irregularly shaped, and usually accumulate on the upstream side of the valve or structure to which they are attached. The differential diagnosis should also include a non-infected mass such as a myxoma, papillary fibroelastoma, or lipoma, but the clinical context and historical clues may influence the pre-test probability. Transoesophageal studies are more sensitive at identifying vegetation than transthoracic studies.

Right heart

Assessment of right ventricular size

The dimensions of the right atria are not routinely measured during PoCUS, but from the apical 4-chamber view, anything larger than 55 × 44 mm in the major and minor dimensions during diastole is considered abnormal. The right atrial pressures may be estimated from the size and collapse index of the IVC (IVCCI). Starting from a subcostal window, the IVC is viewed in long axis as it enters into the right atrium. The middle hepatic vein will typically also feed into the IVC, just caudal to the right atrium, and just caudal to that, the IVC is measured from edge to edge during normal respiration and with forced inhalation—'sniff'.

The American Society of Echocardiography and the European Society of Cardiovascular Imaging have standardized the reporting of right atrial pressure measurements (see Table 2.2). Validation for these figures is limited, and they are best regarded as rough estimates, with study data suggesting, in fact, correlation with the central venous pressure (CVP) is not precise.

Table 2.2 IVC collapse index as a guide to central venous pressure

CVP (mmHg)	IVC diameter (cm)	Collapse with Sniff (%)
Low: 3	<2.1	>50
Normal: 8	<2.1	<50
	>2.1	>50
High: 15	>2.1	<50

Adapted from *Journal of the American Society of Echocardiography*, 23, 7, LG Rudski *et al.*, 'Guidelines for the Echocardiographic Assessment of the Right Heart in Adults: A Report from the American Society of Echocardiography Endorsed by the European Association of Echocardiography, a registered branch of the European Society of Cardiology, and the Canadian Society of Echocardiography', pp. 685–713, Copyright 2010, with permission from American Society of Echocardiography; and Data from ASE / EACI 2015 Guidelines, *JASE* 2015;**28**:1–39.

The structure and physiology of the right ventricle are more complex than the left ventricle. If the left ventricle is roughly the shape of a standing flower vase, the right ventricle is closer in resemblance to a hand that goes to grasp it. The right ventricle wraps around the outside of the left ventricle along the right side and anterior aspects, with blood entering it from the right atrium near the vena cava, with an outflow tract parallel to, and twisting around, the aorta. Unlike the smooth cavity of the left ventricle, the right ventricle is trabeculated and interrupted in the middle by the moderator band that runs obliquely through it.

Because the pulmonary arterial circulation has a much lower resistance than the systemic arterial circulation, with correspondingly lower systolic and diastolic pressures, the right ventricle pumps blood with a much thinner amount of myocardium, compared to the right. In states of chronically increased pulmonary hypertension, the right ventricle will hypertrophy and thicken, but generally the free wall of the right ventricle, when measured at end-diastole from a subxiphoid window, will be 5 mm or less. Hypertrophy to 6–7 mm can occur in a few days, but further increases take weeks to months.

The lower intra-cavity pressures of the right ventricle see the shared inter-ventricular septum normally bowed concave into the right ventricle chamber, reflecting the outward distending pressure of the left ventricle. However, in states of RV pressure or volume overload, the right heart will dilate and exert an abnormal amount of pressure on the shared inter-ventricular septum. In cases when the intra-cavity pressure on the right exceeds that of the left, the inter-ventricular septum will flatten or even bow backwards into the left ventricle and the right ventricle will dilate. The right ventricle is normally <41 mm at its base, when measured from the apical 4-chamber view, which is roughly two-thirds the size of the left ventricle at the same level (see Table 2.1). A simple approach is to compare the RV and LV cavity size in the apical 4-chamber view; the right ventricle should be smaller than the left ventricle, and the ratio should be under 0.7.

'Function'

Core:

Qualitative assessment of ventricular systolic function.

Advanced:

Quantitative assessment of ventricular systolic function;

Regional wall motion abnormalities;

Diastolic function.

Left ventricular systolic function

Estimating LV systolic function is key to the evaluation of the circulatory system in patients in shock and dyspnoea and the most common reason for a comprehensive echocardiogram to be requested. It correlates with symptoms, prognosis, and complications in a wide range of cardiovascular disease, including ischaemic heart disease and cardiomyopathy. Proper evaluation requires not only skill in image acquisition, but also sufficient experience in normal and abnormal exams to get a sense of pathology.

Measuring the overall systolic performance of the left ventricle is actually related to multiple different interconnected physiologic principles. In resuscitation, the focus is on the CO—the product of SV and heart rate.

Qualitative assessment/estimated ejection fraction

An experienced clinician's gestalt ('eye-ball') of the overall EF is considered the 'gold standard' of techniques. This is an assessment of how much smaller the left ventricle becomes in systole. While expert echocardiographers may be able to accurately report an exact EF, PoCUS users commonly report semi-quantitative assessments, described as 'severely' (EF <30% male/female), 'moderately' (EF 30–40% male/female), or 'mildly' (EF male 41–51%, female 41–53%) impaired, and normal (male >52%, female >54%). The term hyperdynamic is often used in critical care and implies an EF of >70%. Using this semi-quantitative assessment, PoCUS sonographers have demonstrated high levels of agreement with cardiologists, with the poorest agreement in differentiating mild impairment from normal contraction—where, in fact, there is likely little impact on management decisions.

Quantitative assessment of ejection fraction

In comprehensive echo reports, systolic function is most often recorded as the EF. LVEF is the percentage of the LV diastolic volume ejected during systole. The most accurate, simplest way to assess systolic performance is using the methods described by Simpson. The end-diastolic and end-systolic ventricular sizes are traced and the EF calculated by [end-diastolic volume (EDV) – end-systolic volume (ESV)/EDV × 100], using built-in software. The measurements can be made using just the apical 4-chamber (monoplane) or (better) also the 2-chamber view (bi-plane). End-systole and end-diastole are best identified by ECG, with diastole identified by the R wave and systole by the end of the T wave, but may be approximated by scrolling through a recorded loop, identifying the maximum and minimum dimensions or positions of the aortic (close end-systole, start diastole) and mitral valves (close end-diastole, start systole). The method relies on a clear view of the endocardial border and no foreshortening of the chambers, and also assumes the LV cavity to be cylindrical.

EF requires careful interpretation. It loses accuracy in atrial fibrillation and with wall motion defects not apparent in the views used to make the measurements. EF is also not synonymous with SV. Dilated left ventricles, compared to smaller ventricles, can eject the same volume of blood with a smaller percentage change in size. Similarly, a small-volume ventricle, e.g.

in hypovolaemia, ejects a larger proportion of blood to maintain the same SV. Given its limitations, EF is less useful to guide resuscitation in the emergency or critical care setting.

Simplified quantitative assessment of left ventricular function

Fractional shortening

There have been many attempts to try to make the estimation of EF more quantitative, reproducible, and easy. One common technique is to measure the change in diameter of the LV cavity as it contracts radially, usually in PLAX using an M-mode beam at the mid-papillary level. The percentage change in the 2D chamber diameter is called 'fractional shortening'. It is susceptible to off-angle imaging, is inaccurate in the setting of a regional wall motion abnormality, and does not consider the rotational or longitudinal contraction of the left ventricle. For these reasons, it is rarely used and is not recommended.

E-point septal separation

E-point septal separation (EPSS) allows rapid, approximate assessment of LV systolic function. When viewed from a PLAX view, the closeness of the anterior leaflet of the mitral valve to the septum correlates with overall systolic performance. As cardiac performance falls, so does the velocity and volume of blood passing through the mitral valve, leading to decreased mitral valve opening. In hyperdynamic and normal hearts, the tip of the anterior leaflet almost touches the septum at end-diastole. If the distance from the tip of the anterior leaflet is within 5 mm of the inter-ventricular septum, LV function is considered normal. A distance of >7 mm has been suggested as 87% sensitive and 75% specific for identifying an EF of <50%, and a distance of >18 mm suggestive of EF of >30%, assuming normal mitral valve function. One MRI study suggested the following formula to calculate EF:

$$EF = 75.5 - (2.5 \times EPSS \text{ in mm})$$

Measurements are made in M-mode or, less accurately, in B-mode (see Figure 2.17 and Video 2.25 📹). Off-axis measurements, regional wall motion abnormalities, mitral valve disease, and aortic regurgitation

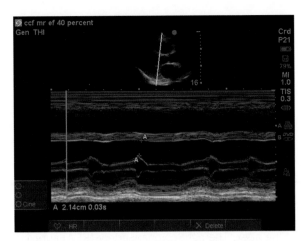

Figure 2.17 Mode of measurement of E-point septal separation.

may all adversely affect the interpretation. Like fractional shortening, EPSS essentially assesses radial contraction of the left ventricle, adding to potential inaccuracies. The ease and reproducibility of the technique should not preclude a more global assessment of LV systolic performance.

Mitral valve annular plane systolic excursion

Longitudinal contraction of the left ventricle from its base to apex is an important contribution to the overall performance of the left ventricle. The mitral valve annular plane systolic excursion (MAPSE) technique involves M-mode measurement of the movement of the mitral annulus longitudinally, and its values correlate with overall systolic function (see Figures 2.18 and 2.19). Values of >1.3 cm in males and 1.1 cm in females suggest normal LV function, 0.6–0.9 cm moderate impairment, and <0.6 cm severe impairment. With the apex of the heart just under the footprint of the probe, an M-mode beam is placed over the lateral annulus of the mitral valve and then tracked over time.

Stroke volume and cardiac output

A related concept, SV is the volume of blood ejected by the left ventricle into the aorta with each systole and, as such, is measured in millilitres. This is less commonly assessed in formal echocardiography but is a fundamental part of shock assessment and PoCUS. As such, it is discussed below in 'Inferior vena cava ultrasound as a guide to fluid therapy', p. 63.

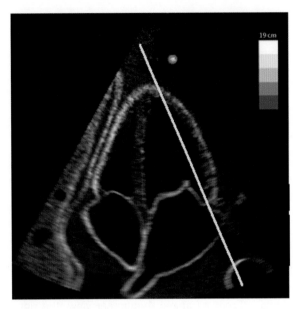

Figure 2.18 MAPSE: B-mode, showing the position of the cursor.

Image created on a CAE Vimedix simulator.

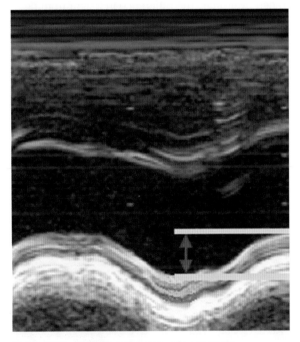

Figure 2.19 MAPSE: estimation using M-mode.

Assessing right ventricular systolic function

As reflected by its peculiar geometry, the mechanics of systolic function are different on the right than on the left side. The left heart typically squeezes blood in three ways: longitudinal contraction, radial contraction, and torque. Conversely, the right ventricle contracts mostly longitudinally, meaning most of the systolic function of the right heart comes from the base and apex of the heart coming closer together. This is a result of the directionality of the myocardial fibres of the right ventricle.

While RV systolic function is typically estimated by gestalt, similarly to LV function, there have been many attempts to objectively quantify its performance. One of the most common methods is to measure the distance that the base of the right heart descends during systole, exploiting the fact that systolic function is predominantly longitudinal. While this method is not without limitation, it is an easy measurement to perform and is highly reproducible. From an apical 4-chamber view, the right ventricle is focused on by angling the probe medially. Then an M-mode beam is placed over the lateral annulus of the tricuspid valve, and its excursion is traced over time. The difference in height from peak to trough is the tricuspid annular plane of systolic excursion (TAPSE) (see Figure 2.20). Measurements of <17 mm are considered abnormal, but a normal TAPSE measurement does not exclude right heart systolic dysfunction.

Regional wall motion abnormalities

Regional wall motion abnormalities are difficult to assess and require considerable experience; as such, this may be considered beyond the scope of PoCUS

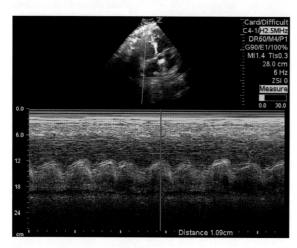

Figure 2.20 M-mode TAPSE.

for most users. Detailed regional wall motion assessment requires apical 2- and 3-chamber views, in addition to PLAX/PSAX and apical 4-chamber images. These were mentioned, but not fully described in the introduction, as these are rarely part of a PoCUS assessment.

Regional differences in LV performance follow from the coronary distributions and are of greatest value in the assessment of coronary artery disease. In general, the left anterior descending (LAD) artery supplies the basal and mid-anterior wall segments, the anterior half of the inter-ventricular septum, and most of the apex. The right coronary artery (RCA) supplies the right ventricle and most of the inferior wall, and the basal inferior wall, but often shares distribution with the LAD artery for the mid-inferoseptal wall and the apical inferior apex. The circumflex artery or the LAD artery supplies the anterolateral segments of the ventricle, while the circumflex of the RCA may cover the basal and *inferolateral* segments. These echocardiographic segments correlate with the more familiar regions of distribution on ECGs. For instance, a patient with a proximal LAD artery occlusion, causing an anterior ST-segment myocardial infarction, will have wall motion abnormalities in the anterior segments basally, at the mid level, and apically, and likely involving the anterior inter-venticular septum as well (see Figures 2.21 and 2.22).

However, there are also several important causes of wall motion abnormalities that are not caused by coronary artery disease such as Takotsubo cardiomyopathy, intracranial haemorrhage, or even regional myocarditis.

Echocardiographically, there are 17 segments of the left ventricle: six basal segments, six middle segments, four apical segments, and then one apical 'cap' at the very tip (see Figure 2.22). In the long axis, the left ventricle is divided into three parts. The basal level is the region from the mitral valve annulus to the start of the papillary muscles. The mid level is the region that covers the papillary muscles and ends at their base. The apical segment starts from there and continues to the apex. The apex is then capped with its own final segment. These views are amenable to the PSAX window and can be optimized by either angling or/and translocating the probe basally or apically.

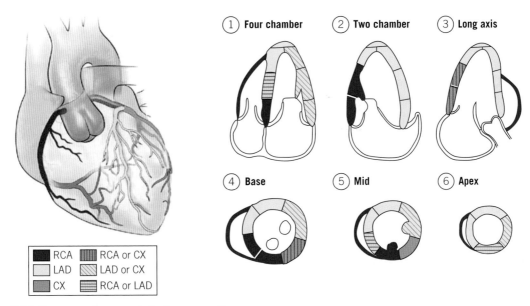

Figure 2.21 Coronary artery supply to the myocardium.

Reprinted from *Journal of the American Society of Echocardiography*, 28, 1, Lang, Roberto M., *et al.*, 'Recommendations for cardiac chamber quantification by echocardiography in adults: an update from the American Society of Echocardiography and the European Association of Cardiovascular Imaging', pp. 1–39, Copyright © 2015, with permission from the American Society of Echocardiography and Elsevier.

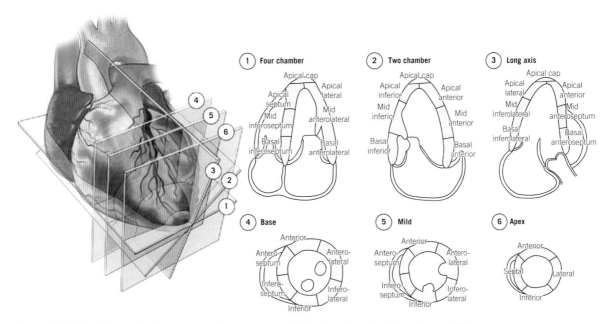

Figure 2.22 The left ventricular segments for assessment of regional wall motion abnormalities.

What would be called anatomically the 'posterior' wall of the left ventricle is actually named the 'inferior' wall. For rotational consistency to delineate anterior from inferior, each of the levels is further divided into segments relative to an imaginary line perpendicular to the inter-ventricular septum (see Figure 2.22).

Healthy myocardium thickens by around 40–50% during contraction. When viewed in short axis, the endocardial border will process inwards radially towards the centre, which serves to reduce the LV cavity size to generate the SV. As the myocardium will also contract longitudinally, deficits in contractility can also be appreciated in the long axis. Ischaemic or infarcted myocardium does not thicken as much (hypokinetic segments; see Video 2.26 ▸), and in more pathologic states, it will not move at all (akinetic segments; see Video 2.27 ▸) or it will move to the opposite of the intended direction (dyskinetic segments). Akinetic segments may appear thin, often representing infarcted muscle. Dyskinetic segments are also usually thinner than normal and show further thinning or stretching during systole. Dyskinetic segments were formally described as aneurysmal if constantly deformed during all phases of the cardiac cycle, but the term is no longer used for echo findings.

There are many potential sources of error in assessing wall cardiac motion. Dysfunctional myocardium adjacent to normal myocardium may be tethered and pulled along during systole, so mimicking normal function when, in fact, it does not exist. Patients with aberrant conduction, as in bundle branch blocks or those with pacemakers, will exhibit variable timing of contraction that may mimic a wall motion abnormality. Significant coronary artery disease may exist with no regional wall abnormalities.

Assessing diastolic function

Diastolic function is a key determinate of overall cardiac performance, has prognostic importance in a wide range of diseases, and is central to the discussion of fluid resuscitation. In diastolic heart failure, impaired ventricular relaxation sees higher filling pressures; elevated LV end-diastolic pressures are thus required to achieve a given CO. While systolic function is apparently obvious to see, diastolic function cannot be so readily appreciated. The sonographic skills required to assess diastolic dysfunction require dedicated experience and training but are required for a PoCUS assessment of acute dyspnoea, as around half of all cardiac failure patients have preserved EF.

The easiest sonographic assessment for diastolic failure is to observe for increased left atrial size; this is most simply estimated by comparing this to the descending aorta in the PLAX view. Diastolic heart failure rarely causes acute dyspnoea as a sole cause with a normal left atrial size. The inter-atrial septum may also be observed to bulge towards the right atria in the apical view, as left side pressures increase.

However, these findings assume there are no other causes of increased left atrial size and that the diastolic heart failure is not acute. Diastolic dysfunction is complex to assess with depressed systolic function, in atrial fibrillation, with moderate or severe MAC, in mitral stenosis, in moderate or severe mitral regurgitation, with a prosthetic mitral valve, in the presence of left bundle branch block, and in a paced rhythm.

There are two steps to defining diastolic function. A normal (preserved) EF is identified. Firstly, assess the E/A ratio and then the following four variables:

- Annular e' velocity (septal e' <7 cm/s; lateral e' <10 cm/s); tissue Doppler;
- E/e' ratio (septal >15; lateral >13; average >15);
- Left atrial volume index (>34 mL/m^2);
- Peak tricuspid regurgitation velocity (>2.8 m/s).

If the E/A ratio is ≤0.8 and E is <50 cm/s, grade I diastolic dysfunction is identified. If the E/A ratio is ≥2, then grade III diastolic dysfunction is diagnosed. If the E/A is ≤0.8 and E is >50 cm/s or E/A is <0.8 to <2, then LV diastolic function is abnormal and the four variables above are used. If abnormal values identified for 4/4, 3/4, 3/3, or 2/3 are found, then grade II diastolic dysfunction exists. If only two criteria are available, then left atrial pressure and diastolic dysfunction cannot be determined.

The principal function of diastole is to fill the left ventricle with preload, so impaired diastolic filling can be most easily inferred by monitoring the flow of blood from the left atrium into the left ventricle. From an apical 4-chamber view, a PW Doppler gate (3 mm) can be placed between the mitral valve leaflet tips, which will provide a tracing of blood velocities as it traverses the mitral valve (see Figure 2.23). Diastolic ventricular filling consists of two components; initially, blood enters passively during early ventricular relaxation—the E wave; and secondly, blood is ejected during atrial systole—the A wave. The E wave is normally 1–2 times larger than the A wave, reflecting the fact that most LV filling is a result of ventricular relaxation, not atrial contraction, in the normal young population. Patients in atrial fibrillation will not have an A wave at all. The E/A ratio will reverse in the natural progression of ageing.

As diastolic function worsens and the LV end-diastolic pressure rises, the atrial–ventricular pressure

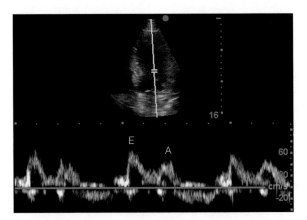

Figure 2.23 The Doppler gate placed between mitral valve leaflets and the resulting E and A waves.

gradient will decrease, limiting blood flow during early relaxation. This form of impaired relaxation manifests as a decreased E wave.

As diastolic function degrades further, the left atrial pressure increases and the left atrium pressure will rise, so the E wave velocities will become higher. The increased left atrial pressure restores the atrial–ventricular pressure gradient, so resulting in a 'pseudo-normal' E to A wave pattern (see Figure 2.24). To distinguish pseudo-normal E/A wave patterns from normal E/A wave patterns, additional information is gleaned from the LV tissue itself, using tissue Doppler. Further information can be inferred by measuring the amount of time it would take the E wave to intersect the abscissa of zero velocity, but this technique is beyond the scope of PoCUS.

In all of the applications of Doppler discussed so far, the focus has been on blood as it travels through valves and chambers. However, the same Doppler principles can be applied to measuring myocardial movement. The velocity of LV tissues as they relax during diastole correlates with diastolic performance. Measuring the speed of moving myocardium requires special software toggling on the ultrasound machine, as the myocardium moves more slowly than blood; this is called tissue Doppler imaging (TDI, or DTI).

With TDI software turned on, velocities are recorded by placing the PW Doppler sampling gate on the medial or lateral portion of the mitral valve annulus in an apical 4-chamber view, with the Doppler gate as parallel to the longitudinal axis as possible. Measurements are made in mid expiration and measured over 3–5 cardiac cycles.

In systole, the annulus moves towards the apex— the S' wave; in diastole, it moves away from the apex in two phases—the 'e' (early diastolic filling) and 'a' (atrial contraction) waves (see Figure 2.25). The e' septal annular velocity should be >7 cm/s, and the e' lateral annular velocity >10 cm/s. Velocities above this rule out diastolic dysfunction. Analysis of the e' velocities is central to diastolic analysis. As diastolic functions get worse, e' velocities steadily decrease, and unlike E waves, there is no pseudo-normalization pattern. TDI readings are affected by basal wall motion abnormalities, mitral valve disease, and valve replacement.

The ratio of the E wave velocity to the e' velocity is also a useful measure of diastolic function. As LV

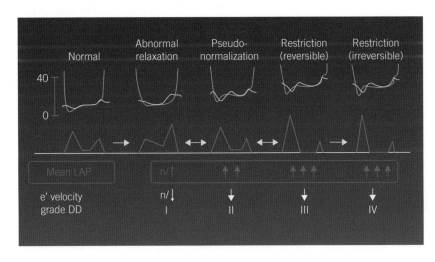

Figure 2.24 The patterns of E and A waves found in progressive diastolic dysfunction.

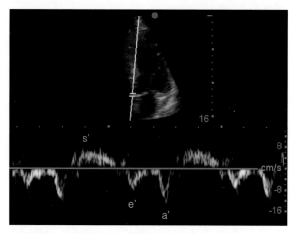

Figure 2.25 Septal tissue Doppler mitral annulus readings.

filling pressures begin to rise, the E wave will increase slightly, while the tissue Doppler velocities of the mitral valve will steadily decrease. An E/e′ of <8 suggests normal LV filling pressures, but elevated values should be used in conjunction with criteria outlined earlier to define diastolic dysfunction. The E/e′ ratio approximates the pulmonary capillary wedge pressure.

Chronic elevations in filling pressures will also result in atrial enlargement. And the magnitude of atrial enlargement correlates with symptoms. The simplest measurement is to use the PLAX to measure the left atrium. The measurement should be taken during end-ventricular systole, just before the mitral valve leaflets open, to measure the atrium at its largest. Standard measurements for males are between 3.0 cm and 4.0 cm, with females being slightly smaller at 2.7–3.8 cm. More accurate assessment includes tracing the atrial area in the apical 4-chamber view or calculating the volume using two different apical views, adding the apical 2-chamber view, similarly to calculating the ventricular ESV and EDV to assess EF using Simpson's methodology (abnormal >34 mL/m²).

Thus, a normal left atrial size (left atrial volume <34 mL/m²) and septal/lateral wall TDI values above 7 (septal)/10 (lateral wall) cm/s effectively rule out diastolic heart failure.

'Filling'

Filling refers to the assessment of a patient's preload and is assessed by integrating information obtained from the previously described cardiac windows, in conjunction with views of the IVC size (see Box 2.2) and variability, and lung views for interstitial and air-space fluid. This is discussed in 'Shock', p. 60 and 'Acute decompensated heart failure', p. 65.

Part 3: Resuscitation—cardiac arrest, shock, and acute heart failure

Resuscitation: cardiac arrest

Purpose

PoCUS can be used during cardiac arrest resuscitation to look for cardiac activity, assess for reversible causes, and assist with guiding resuscitative efforts.

Perspective

Is PoCUS able to help with the differential diagnosis of pulseless electrical activity?

PoCUS has clinical utility in the diagnosis of PEA resulting from mechanical, reversible conditions, including severe hypovolaemia, cardiac tamponade, PE, and tension pneumothorax. All of these conditions require clinical correlation. However, the use of PoCUS rapidly narrows the differential.

Note that, in addition to cardiac PoCUS, additional views, such as lung or pleural windows for pneumothorax or pleural fluid (see Figure 2.11), visualizing the IVC for extreme low or high right-sided filling pressures, the proximal lower limb veins for thrombosis, a sweep of the aorta for an aortic aneurysm, and assessing the peritoneal space for fluid, may be

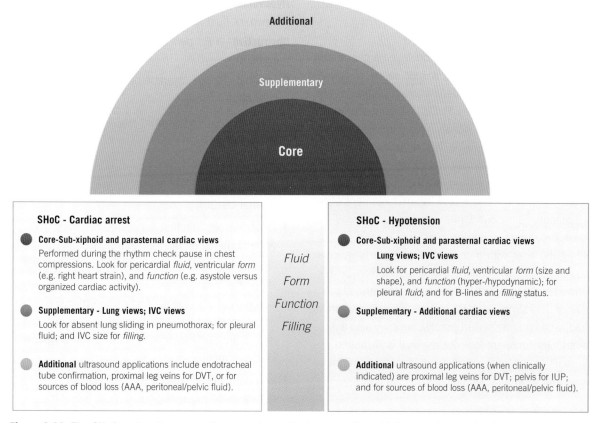

SHoC - Cardiac arrest

- **Core-Sub-xiphoid and parasternal cardiac views**
  Performed during the rhythm check pause in chest compressions. Look for pericardial *fluid*, ventricular *form* (e.g. right heart strain), and *function* (e.g. asystole versus organized cardiac activity).

- **Supplementary - Lung views; IVC views**
  Look for absent lung sliding in pneumothorax; for pleural fluid; and IVC size for *filling*.

- **Additional** ultrasound applications include endotracheal tube confirmation, proximal leg veins for DVT, or for sources of blood loss (AAA, peritoneal/pelvic fluid).

Fluid
Form
Function
Filling

SHoC - Hypotension

- **Core-Sub-xiphoid and parasternal cardiac views**
  Lung views; IVC views
  Look for pericardial *fluid*, ventricular *form* (size and shape), and *function* (hyper-/hypodynamic); for pleural *fluid*; and for B-lines and *filling* status.

- **Supplementary - Additional cardiac views**

- **Additional** ultrasound applications (when clinically indicated) are proximal leg veins for DVT; pelvis for IUP; and for sources of blood loss (AAA, peritoneal/pelvic fluid).

Figure 2.26 The SHoC protocol summary for assessing patients presenting with hypotension or shock.

indicated. Various echo in life support algorithms, such as the SHoC protocol, describe this approach (see Figure 2.26).

Does PoCUS predict or effect outcome in cardiac arrest?

There is no published evidence showing the use of PoCUS to improve mortality in cardiac arrest or shock. Clinicians are clearly using PoCUS in cardiac arrest and resuscitation, and are changing their management and diagnosis with the information obtained. Observational data suggest that PoCUS is a useful tool to assist in clinical decision-making for the termination of resuscitative efforts, although it is not independently reliable to predict outcome. A single-centre randomized trial of non-trauma patients with shock demonstrated that early ultrasound improves the accuracy of correct diagnosis for the aetiology of shock. A small study exploring the role of IVCCI and myocardial contractility, as assessed by echo, in patients

with sepsis found diagnostic changes were made in around 1 in 5 patients and management changes (mainly around fluid dose or use of inotropes) in around half.

Performing the scan

Can PoCUS assist with procedural guidance during resuscitation?

PoCUS can assist with the guidance of some procedures during resuscitation. These include:

Airway—confirmation of ETT placement, right main stem tracheal tube placement, and identification of the site for emergency cricothyroidotomy;

Breathing—guidance of chest drain insertion;

Circulation—guidance of central venous access and arterial catheter placement; guidance of pericardiocentesis; confirmation of external pacing capture or the position of a temporary pacing wire (see Video 2.30 ▶).

Shock

Purpose

Shock is a common presentation to emergency and critical care physicians, with a wide range of causes and high mortality. Early identification, diagnosis, and therapy improve outcomes. PoCUS is the most powerful tool available to the resuscitation team to assist in diagnosis, to guide fluid resuscitation, and to influence vasodilator, inotrope, and/or vasopressor choices.

In this section, we will explore the role of ultrasound in the diagnosis of shock and the management of resuscitation. Ultrasound may be used to assess the heart, IVC, lungs, abdomen, and large vessels, so providing the user with a comprehensive cardiovascular assessment of the patient. These scans may be performed at differing skill levels—an inexperienced practitioner may simply look for pericardial/intra-peritoneal fluid, while a more skilled practitioner may also assess ventricular function, look for regional wall motion abnormalities, identify diastolic dysfunction, and use echo measurements of SV to guide fluid therapy.

Perspective

Pathophysiology and integrated PoCUS in shock

Shock may be defined as a life-threatening generalized maldistribution of blood flow, resulting in failure to deliver and/or utilize adequate amounts of oxygen, leading to tissue hypoxia. The diagnosis of shock is made from clinical, physiological, and metabolic assessment, with evidence of impaired tissue perfusion, new organ failure, lactaemia, inadequate CO, and hypotension.

The most commonly used approach to classifying shock fits neatly with PoCUS assessment: cardiogenic (pump fails), distributive (pipes leak), hypovolaemic (pipes empty), obstructive (pipes or pump blocked), or cytotoxic (pump and pipes OK).

The most widely seen diagnostic patterns are as follows (*italics for diagnoses made predominantly with echo*) and will be discussed in detail later in the chapter:

Cardiac—*impaired LV or RV function* (*ischaemia, cardiomyopathy, depression from sepsis or toxin, cor pulmonale*), *valvular failure*, arrhythmia;

Distributive—sepsis, anaphylaxis, neurological, toxicological;

Hypovolaemic—blood (*trauma, AAA*, gastrointestinal bleed) or fluid loss;

Obstructive—*PE, pericardial tamponade*, air/gas/fat embolism;

Cytopathic—sepsis, cyanide or carbon monoxide poisoning.

The initial cardiac and IVC findings are as follows:
Cardiogenic shock:

- Poor systolic function is suggested by dilated, thin-walled, poorly contractile chambers, low VTI (< 15, normal 15–25);
- Poor diastolic function suggested by small, thick-walled chambers; dilated left atrium > 34 ml; impaired e' < 7/10 cm/s (septal/free wall annular velocity);
- Coronary artery disease and myocardial ischaemia are suggested by regional wall abnormalities, but ischaemic cardiomyopathy may appear as global LV impairment;
- Valvular disease suggested by obvious regurgitation jets using colour flow, valvular stenosis suggested by thickened, calcified, and poorly opening valves with increased velocity with spectral Doppler.

Distributive:
- Suggested by a hyperdymamic left ventricle/right ventricle, in which the ventricular walls contract vigorously and come close to each other at end-systole;
- IVC may be small (<10–15 mm AP diameter), measured at end-expiration if spontaneous ventilation, and collapse of >50% with inspiration). IVC size and collapse index should be used cautiously, as dependent on many factors.

Hypovolaemic:
- This is usually hard to differentiate from the distributive pattern of echo findings.

Obstructive:
- Massive PE suggested by a dilated right ventricle, poor RV contraction assessed visually or by TAPSE, paradoxical septal movement. The LV cavity may be small and hyperdynamic due to inadequate preload;

- Pericardial fluid is obvious, but identifying tamponade is harder, systolic collapse of the atria is suggestive, and diastolic collapse of the right ventricle diagnostic;

- The IVC is usually large (>25 mm measured AP) in obstructive shock (as well as in valvular and chronic lung disease).

The diagnosis of shock is often complex, involving several factors that contribute to inadequate tissue perfusion. PoCUS allows the practitioner to identify and respond to these differing factors and identify the dominant and secondary factors causing the shock state.

Fluid resuscitation

The primary goal of resuscitation is to correct the deficit in tissue oxygen delivery of the patient. The primary treatment modalities are to increase oxygen delivery with supplementary oxygen, increase the haemoglobin level, and increase CO. The latter may be achieved with fluid loading or inotropes.

IV fluids may be prescribed to prevent the discomfort of thirst in a patient held nil by mouth or simply to replace fluid lost, e.g. in gastroenteritis, or we may prescribe fluids to resuscitate. The explicit goal of fluids in shock resuscitation is to improve SV and CO until the point until oxygen delivery is sufficient to reverse tissue hypoxia. However, there is potential for harm in fluid administration and it is important, when administering IV fluids, that clear end points are targeted.

Fluid resuscitation, fluid tolerance, and fluid responsiveness

Fluid and oxygen administration are the most common interventions in critical care and emergency medicine. The most effective method of improving oxygen delivery to the tissues is usually by increasing CO with IV fluids, and this is the first step in most resuscitations. The benefit of fluid administration also has decreasing marginal gains, even within its therapeutic window. To help interpret the risks and benefits of fluid administration, the physiology of venous return and preload–SV (Frank–Starling) curves should be revisited (see Figure 2.27).

The Frank–Starling relationship—if on the steep part of Frank–Starling curve, then fluid bolus increases SV/CO, but on the flat part, there is no or little increase in SV and a large increase in extravascular lung water (EVLW).

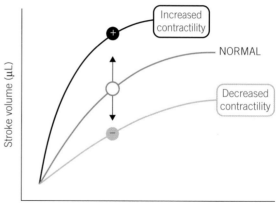

Figure 2.27 The Frank–Starling curve, showing the relationship between preload and stroke volume/cardiac output.

Under low preload conditions, there is a lot of marginal gain for administering IV fluids. Fluid responsiveness exists when fluid administration increases the SV by > 10–15%, moving up the Frank–Starling curve (see Figure 2.27). While there is no part of the Frank–Starling curve with a negative slope (for a normal heart), it is important to remember that, at the top of this curve, additional fluid administration barely increases the SV and risks tissue oedema and compartment syndromes, which may reduce tissue oxygenation—the dilemma being that both under- and over-resuscitation with IV fluids risks suboptimal oxygen delivery. By convention, a patient may be defined as fluid-responsive when a 500-mL bolus of crystalloid delivered over 15 minutes increases the SV by >10–15%.

Under normal resting conditions, healthy people operate on the lower end of the Frank–Starling curve, but in response to exercise or illness, the CO can be increased by increasing sympathetic tone, circulating volume/preload, myocardial contraction, and heart rate. Humans are fluid-responsive in health. Fluid tolerance describes the state when IV fluids may safely be given without the risk of tissue oedema, as predicted by the Marik–Phillips curve.

Determining whether a patient is fluid-responsive is key to initial resuscitation. This may be achieved

61

by delivering a fluid bolus and assessing the beneficial effects of improving BP, CO/SV, and oxygen delivery, as well as the adverse effects such as increasing EVLW with falling saturations and increasing oedema. Using PoCUS, we may measure the SV before and after a fluid bolus. However, many resuscitative interventions, such as administering catecholamines and positive pressure ventilation, affect preload, afterload, and cardiac contractility, so altering our assessment of whether more IV fluid is needed. If clinicians rely on delivering a fluid bolus each time they seek to assess fluid responsiveness, there is a risk of fluid overload. By predicting which patients are fluid-responsive, we avoid recurrent fluid challenges.

IVC diameter is associated with hypovolaemia, and patients with a small IVC diameter and hypotension are likely (but not certainly) fluid-responsive. The caveat is that if the heart is extremely efficient, e.g. an athlete with meningococcaemia, then this could represent the plateau of the Frank–Starling curve.

IVC diameter is best measured a few centimetres below the junction of the hepatic veins and ICV, in B-mode, and at end expiration, i.e. maximum size.

Dynamic predictors of fluid responsiveness

Cardiac performance is the relationship between CO and preload; changes with respiration inform clinicians on cardiac performance. Dynamic assessment of the cardiovascular system for fluid responsiveness involves two variables: measurement of volume, flow, or pressure, and how this changes with respiration or other form of augmentation. Larger variations with respiration imply a cardiovascular system more likely fluid-responsive. Cyclical variations of intra-thoracic pressure throughout respiration alter cardiac preload. As intra-thoracic pressure increases (inspiration if mechanically ventilated and expiration if spontaneously ventilating), so the juxtacardiac pressures increase, with consequent rise in right atrial pressure (RAP), impeding RV filling; this reduces RV SV, causing a decrease in LV preload and resulting in a decrease in LV SV and systolic BP.

Inspiration also increases pulmonary afterload, as intra-pleural pressure compresses the pulmonary capillaries. These effects are usually insignificant but may have an impact if RV failure is present. In this case, there may be significant changes in the measured parameter with respiration, so suggesting fluid responsiveness when, in fact, the patient is already on the flat part of the Frank–Starling curve.

Similarly, (spontaneous) inspiration squeezes blood from the pulmonary vessels to the left side of the heart, so transiently increasing LV filling and SV. Inspiration also increases intra-thoracic pressure and reduces LV afterload. A biphasic response may thus be seen with inspiration, increasing then reducing LV SV.

The changes in cardiac performance with respiration are proportionally greater in hyperdynamic hearts and lower in those with myocardial depression. This is because the 'flatter' fluid dose–response curve associated with poor LV function is associated with elevated RV, right atrial, and IVC pressures.

Unfortunately, the natural variation in our respiratory cycle and the large range of factors affecting the tidal volume (individual variation, chronic lung disease, acute lung disease, acidosis, pain, anxiety) mean that, to date, only patients undergoing controlled and passive mechanical ventilation with tidal volumes of 8 mL/kg or greater can be reliably assessed by most dynamic measurements. Common measurements include pulse pressure variation, SV variation (SVV), and IVCCI. If ventilator volumes are <8 mL/kg, the resultant effects on the SV are too small to be reliably assessed and may need to be transiently increased to allow preload responsiveness to be determined. Similarly, any spontaneous breathing activity will interfere with measurements.

Many ultrasound parameters have been assessed as *predictors* of fluid responsiveness by observing changes in respiration, including LVOT VTI, aortic Doppler flow, aortic peak flow velocity, carotid/brachial/femoral VTI, and brachial artery peak velocity variation. The evidence from small studies in mechanically ventilated patients is encouraging, but in spontaneously ventilating patients, there are limited data to support their use.

A more recent dynamic measure of fluid responsiveness is to use passive leg raising (discussed in 'Inferior vena cava ultrasound as a guide to fluid therapy', p. 63). This is the only dynamic preload marker with evidence to support its use in spontaneously ventilating patients. However, the studies were small, used selected patient cohorts, and were single-centre, so their results may not be generalizable.

How does ultrasound assist in guiding fluid resuscitation?

The key to successful fluid resuscitation is to understand where the patient sits on the Frank–Starling curve. The clinician delivers IV fluid until the SV is maximized, after which further fluids do not increase the SV and may risk harm. What PoCUS does not provide us with is an answer to whether the patient requires further fluid administration; this is provided by reassessing the effects of improved tissue oxygenation over time, using a range of clinical tools, including:

- Lactate clearance (although the optimal rate is not yet known) and normalization;

- Evidence of improving end-organ function such as urine output, improved mental status, improved peripheral perfusion, and improved biochemical measures of function;

- Measures of the adequacy of oxygen delivery and utilization.

Resuscitation using goals of oxygen delivery or utilization is termed goal-directed therapy. The benefit of early goal-directed therapy in shock has also been suggested in one randomized trial and several large observational studies. Three recent large multicentre trials suggested that, for most patients with severe sepsis, a simpler clinical approach with early antibiotics and high volume of fluid may be sufficient, without set cardiac goals. These trials used CVP as a fluid goal in the intervention arms, and this is known to be a very poor guide for fluid assessment and as a guide to further fluid administration. More work is required to assess whether more measured titration improves outcomes.

However, there are data to suggest fluid overload is associated with increasing mortality and morbidity, and that early resuscitation is associated with improved outcomes. Since cardiac PoCUS is non-invasive and fluid overload confers risk, it makes good clinical sense to support titrated fluid therapy, especially in patients with cardiac disease who may reach the top of the Frank–Starling curve with smaller volumes of fluid or when higher volumes are infused with evidence of continued tissue hypoxia/organ failure.

Clinicians often withhold fluid resuscitation from patients with severe sepsis and a history of cardiac failure, out of fear of overzealous administration of fluid, precipitating acute cardiac failure. Thus, identifying a hyperdynamic heart due to reduced vascular resistance that is fluid-responsive may provide confidence for the clinician to continue fluid administration, even after the BP has normalized, should there be ongoing evidence of tissue hypoxia. Conversely, the clinician may identify patients with sepsis-induced myocardial depression, in whom a more restrictive fluid regime and early catecholamines may be of benefit. These issues have not yet been teased out in current sepsis trials.

Performing the scan

There are three components to assist the clinician in assessing fluid responsiveness:

- IVC ultrasound;

- Lung ultrasound;

- Focused echo.

Inferior vena cava ultrasound as a guide to fluid therapy

Ultrasound of the IVC is attractive, as it is simple to teach and rapidly performed (see Video 2.6 📷). A detailed description on how to scan the IVC can be found in Chapter 6. IVC size is affected by cardiac performance, intra-pleural pressure, and intra-abdominal pressure, as well as intra-vascular volume. Interobserver reliability of this technique is moderate at best. There are some data to suggest that, at the extremes of intra-vascular volume, the IVC size may be a useful aid in fluid assessment. An IVC of <10–12 mm suggests the patient is intra-vascular-deplete and likely fluid-responsive. An IVC diameter of >25 mm suggests pressure–volume overload and fluid responsiveness is less likely but cannot be ruled out, and more sophisticated tools are required.

The IVCCI describes the proportion of the IVC that collapses with respiration (inspiration if breathing spontaneously and expiration if mechanically ventilated). It is commonly expressed as a percentage, with the difference between the maximum and the minimum IVC size divided by the maximum.

Small studies suggest that IVCCI can identify fluid-responsive patients undergoing mechanical ventilation. One study defined changes in IVC size as [(maximum diameter – minimum diameter)/minimum diameter] ('IVC distensibility') and identified 18% as separating fluid responders and fluid non-responders with 90% sensitivity and specificity. A second study used a different calculation [(IVC maximum – IVC minimum)/mean IVC diameter]. In this study, an IVCCI of 12% separated non-responders with a positive predictive value (PPV) of 93% and a negative predictive value (NPV) of 92%. However, data for spontaneously ventilating patients are mixed, presumably as the variation in intra-thoracic pressure varies with tidal volume, and this changes during resuscitation (as acidosis, pulmonary oedema, and pain are corrected) and between individuals.

IVCCI is commonly described as a predictor of CVP. However, since CVP is known to have little or no value in assessing fluid responsiveness or intra-vascular volume, this will not be discussed further. Echo may be used to estimate pulmonary artery occlusion pressure. The technique is described earlier in the chapter (see 'Assessing diastolic function', p. 56) (the ratio of E to e' waves).

Using lung PoCUS to guide fluid therapy in shock

Pulmonary oedema in the lungs is one the earliest and easiest forms of pathology to see with ultrasound. Lung ultrasound identifies patients with evidence of pulmonary oedema/acute respiratory distress syndrome (ARDS) in whom fluid administration may be harmful. This is discussed in Chapter 3.

A-lines in the anterior upper lung fields predict a pulmonary wedge pressure of <18 mmHg and so, if present, suggest the absence of pulmonary oedema. Conversely, the appearance of B-lines in the upper lobes suggests the onset of hydrostatic oedema (see Chapter 3).

Using advanced cardiac PoCUS to guide fluid therapy

Fluid responsiveness may be assessed using changes in SV, CO, aortic peak velocity, LVOT VTI, and LV end-diastolic area, all of which may be simply calculated (see Figure 2.28 and Video 2.28 📹).

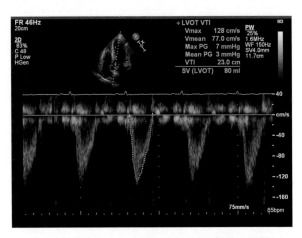

Figure 2.28 Measurement of the left ventricular outflow tract velocity time integral with pulsed wave Doppler.

The evidence that echo can be used to guide fluid responsiveness is contentious. One systematic review, which included studies using several CO monitors, concluded echo-based parameters were an excellent tool to guide fluid resuscitation.

SV is calculated by measuring the volume of blood ejected through a defined area—the LVOT. This may be assumed to be a cylinder with the size fixed in systole and diastole. The AP diameter is measured in PLAX 1–2 frames post-systole (mid systole) at the point where the aortic cusps insert into the aortic annulus.

The area of the LVOT is calculated using:

$$\text{LVOT area} = \text{Pi} \times \left(\text{LVOT diameter} / 2\right)^2$$

The volume of blood passing through the LVOT is measured using PW Doppler technology. This records the velocity of red blood cells passing through the LVOT and the time taken for this to occur. The integral of velocity (VTI) with respect to time is distance, in this case the stroke distance. The PW Doppler gate is set to 3 mm and placed around 5 mm proximal to the LVOT in the apical 5-chamber view (see Figure 2.14). The envelope of the VTI is traced using the cursor (see Figure 2.28), and the stroke distance obtained. Most PoCUS equipment will do this if including a phased array transducer and cardiac software package. Then:

$$\text{SV} = \text{LVOT area} \times \text{VTI}$$

As with all PoCUS, this is highly operator-dependent. Error is introduced if the LVOT is measured poorly and if the ultrasound beam does not align with the LVOT.

As SV and measurements may vary, the average of 3–5 readings is used. If the patient is in atrial fibrillation, then 5–10 measurements are taken and averaged.

However, since the LVOT is part of the cardiac skeleton, the area will change little, if at all, with each intervention. Most clinicians simply measure the VTI and use this as a surrogate of the SV. The normal VTI range is around 15–25 cm. In cardiac shock, the VTI may fall to <12 cm, and in hyperdynamic high-output, low-systemic vascular resistance (SVR), or fluid-overloaded cardiovascular systems, it may be 25–40 cm. Ideally, the numbers should be corrected for body surface area, but as the figures are used as a comparator to assess fluid responsiveness, as opposed to definimg circulation, this is rarely done in practice.

The interobserver reliability is reported as being <15%. In patients undergoing mechanical ventilation, VTI changes with respiration predict fluid responsiveness similarly to pulse pressure and SVV. VTI changes to a passive leg raise may also predict fluid-responsive patients.

To avoid the need for a fluid challenge, cardiovascular changes with respiration may be used to predict who will increase their SV with fluid administration. Changes in aortic peak velocity and VTI, as measured by echo, have been explored in this role. In the former, a delta peak velocity of 12% identified fluid responders with a sensitivity of 100% and a specificity of 89%. A 2012 systematic review identified only one study that looked at echo-assessed SVV with respiration as a predictor of fluid responsiveness. A receiver operating characteristic (ROC) curve suggested 9% SVV as best cut-off, and at this level, sensitivity to identify fluid responders was 100% and specificity 88%. The need for sinus rhythm, mechanical ventilation, and large tidal volumes limits these techniques.

Passive leg raising is a technique that utilizes altered patient position to centralize a small proportion (250–300 mL) of the circulation, so increasing preload. The patient is sat up at around 30 degrees, and a measurement of the CO performed. The patient is then laid flat, and their legs raised 30–45° in the air. The larger the increase in SV resulting from this, the more likely the patient is fluid-responsive. An increase of 10% or more identifies fluid responders with a sensitivity of 86% and a specificity of 85% in mechanically ventilated patients. A second small study identified that an increase in VTI of >12.5% with passive leg raising predicted fluid responders in spontaneously ventilating patients.

Passive leg raising has numerous limitations, including patient discomfort and increased respiratory distress, and is explored in only small single-centre studies. The changes in VTI consequent upon passive leg raising are short-lived, often under 3 minutes, and so measurements must be made rapidly.

Pulmonary embolism

PoCUS is insensitive to diagnosing PE, but it is very useful for prognosis and to guide therapy. PoCUS can assist in the diagnosis of PE only when of sufficient size to impair RV performance or cause acute dilatation, and it is a clinical diagnosis inferred from clinical assessment, combined with PoCUS findings. The PoCUS findings are:

- Acute RV dilatation (RV:LV ratio >0.8), with the RV free wall <4–5 mm suggesting acute dilatation and >5 mm suggesting chronic dilatation from longer-standing pulmonary hypertension;

- Poor contraction, as assessed by visual inspection or TAPSE (<17 mm at RV free wall in apical 4-chamber view);

- McConnell's sign (the apical contraction in the 4-chamber view appears preserved, with the mid and basal segments poorly contractile) has been cited as specific for PE, but recent work disputes this;

- Acute RV hypertension. PoCUS can be used to estimate RV systolic pressure by measuring the peak velocity of tricuspid regurgitation, combined with an estimate of the CVP (see Table 2.2). A pulmonary systolic pressure of >55 mmHg is very unlikely to be acute.

See Videos 2.19 and 2.20 📹, demonstrating an enlarged right ventricle.

Acute decompensated heart failure

Purpose

Acute decompensated heart failure (ADHF) remains common and has an appreciable mortality, with 9.4% of patients likely to die in hospital and 30% within 1 year. Determining the aetiology of an acutely dyspnoeic patient is a frequent diagnostic dilemma, with clinical assessment rarely sufficient to diagnose and characterize the cause. Pulmonary oedema, acute exacerbations of chronic lung disease, pulmonary infection, and PE may present with similar clinical syndromes, and there are few disease-specific diagnostic findings.

Heart failure exists when an abnormality of cardiac function or structure leads to inadequate oxygen delivery for the needs of the metabolizing tissues, despite normal filling pressures or at the expense of elevated filing pressures. Cardiac failure may be consequent upon (most commonly) poor systolic function, diastolic dysfunction, or abnormalities of valvular function, the pericardium, the endocardium, heart rhythm, or conduction.

Lung PoCUS alone is likely insufficient to confirm a diagnosis of ADHF, and cardiac PoCUS is also required. Lung PoCUS is more sensitive than chest radiographs to diagnose ADHF (see Chapter 3).

Perspective

Echo is the diagnostic modality of choice to identify the pathophysiology causing cardiac failure. Valvular lesions and left and/or right heart muscle disease are readily identified. Echo provides detailed knowledge of cardiac anatomy and function, and is central to determining the aetiology of heart failure. Valuable information is gained from simple observation of cardiac size, valves, wall thickness, and wall motion. If these parameters appear normal and if mitral annular tissue Doppler velocities are also normal, then breathlessness is unlikely due to cardiac disease.

Systolic heart failure is characterized by a reduced EF (<45%) consequent upon impaired myocardial contraction (normal EF >55%). As myocardial contractility decreases and EF falls, the cardiovascular system compensates for reduced myocardial contraction by ventricular dilatation—a higher volume is ejected for the same wall movement, heart rate, and preload, with salt and water retention. Common causes include coronary artery disease, cardiomyopathy, muscular dystrophy, toxins, valvular disease, hypertension, arrhythmias, and thyrotoxicosis.

Cardiac failure consequent upon diastolic dysfunction is better termed heart failure with preserved EF. The key abnormality in heart failure with preserved EF is impaired ventricular filling (see 'Assessing diastolic function', p. 56). This may be due to increases in wall thickness or rigidity, leading to elevated filling pressures. CO falls with reduced EDV, but the proportion of ejected blood—the EF—remains preserved and may be elevated. Diagnosis requires the presence of signs and symptoms of congestive heart failure, normal or mildly abnormal LV function (often defined as an EF of >45%), and evidence of abnormal LV relaxation, filling, diastolic distensibility, or diastolic stiffness. Common causes of diastolic failure include hypertension/aortic stenosis with LV hypertrophy, diabetes, constrictive pericarditis, restrictive cardiomyopathy, and age.

Common echo findings in patients with acute heart failure include a dilated left ventricle in end-diastole (>60 mm) and systole (>45 mm), regional wall abnormalities, impaired ventricular contraction on visualization, reduced EF (EPSS, MAPSE), valvular stenosis or regurgitation, pericardial effusion, impaired relaxation on tissue Doppler, and a dilated IVC (>25 mm measured at the junction of hepatic veins and the IVC) (see Video 2.29 ⏺).

Many current studies of PoCUS to diagnose ADHF rely on a combination of cardiac, IVC, and lung windows. One study suggests that the inclusion of PoCUS increases the proportion of patients with a diagnosis of ADHF in the initial ED assessment. ADHF is suggested by an IVCCI of <20%, multiple B-lines in lung windows, and impaired systolic or diastolic function. Studies on ADHF are hampered by no clear gold standard and the final diagnosis often being made outside the ED. Not all studies have included a cardiology-performed echo, and often this is performed following acute treatment. Signs of fluid overload, such as IVCCI, are also not specific to cardiac causes and may result from fluid overload as a result of other pathologies such as acute renal impairment.

Part 4: Summary algorithms

The SHoC protocol provides a guide to PoCUS in critically ill patients. It provides an approach based upon the likelihood of an underlying pathology and the key questions to be asked, according to the clinical presentation. Here we outline how the SHoC protocol can be used in cardiac arrest, hypotension/shock, and dyspnoea. Figure 2.26 outlines this approach.

Integrated PoCUS in the management of cardiac arrest (SHoC-cardiac arrest)

PoCUS can be integrated into an ABC approach for the management of cardiac arrest. Although cardiac PoCUS is the primary focus, a combination of cardiac and extra-cardiac views may be required. **Core** cardiac windows performed during the rhythm check pause in chest compressions, to avoid interruption to CPR, are the *sub-xiphoid* and *parasternal cardiac views*. Either view should be used to detect pericardial *fluid*, as well as examining ventricular *form* (e.g. right heart strain) and *function* (e.g. asystole versus organized cardiac activity). **Supplementary** views include lung views (for absent lung sliding in pneumothorax and for pleural fluid) and IVC views for *filling*. **Additional** ultrasound applications are for ETT confirmation, for proximal leg veins for DVT, or for sources of blood loss (AAA, peritoneal/pelvic fluid).

PoCUS assists in identifying reversible causes and offers some guidance on prognosis. Its use should not impede cardiac massage and defibrillation. Images are integrated into the 10-second pulse/rhythm check and recorded for review. PoCUS may also assist with confirmation of ETT placement and guidance for venous catheterization.

Key questions and approach:

The heart:

- **C**irculation—is there electrical activity and ventricular mechanical activity?

  - Is there a pericardial effusion and tamponade?

  - Is there a dilated right ventricle suggesting massive PE? (remembering that the right ventricle will dilate progressively in prolonged arrest and that a RV free wall of >5 mm suggests long-standing pulmonary hypertension)

  - Is there a hyperdynamic left ventricle and an IVC of <10–12 mm?

  - Is there poor ventricular contraction suggesting cardiac disease with some CO?

  - Is there LV standstill suggesting a poor prognosis?

- PoCUS may assist in identifying CPR quality and guiding procedures such as transvenous pacing (see Video 2.30 🎥).

Beyond the heart:

- **A**irway—look anteriorly in the neck for evidence of oesophageal intubation.

- **B**reathing—if concerned about tension pneumothorax, obtain anterior chest wall images for lung sliding.

- **C**irculation—look for AAA. Look for free fluid—trauma, ruptured ectopic pregnancy, intra-abdominal catastrophe?

PoCUS integrated into the assessment of shock and resuscitation (SHoC-hypotension)

The order of the views may be directed by clinical suspicion or following a prescribed algorithm. As resuscitation progresses, a more detailed scan may be required, focusing on fluid loading and fluid responsiveness. The SHoC-hypotension protocol comprises: (a) **core views:** (1) cardiac views (sub-xiphoid and parasternal windows for pericardial **f**luid, cardiac **f**orm, and ventricular **f**unction), (2) lung views for pleural **f**luid and B-lines for **f**illing status, and (3) IVC views for *filling* status; (b) **supplementary views:** additional cardiac views; and (c) **additional views** (when indicated), including peritoneal fluid, aorta, pelvic for IUP, and proximal leg veins for DVT.

1. **Core views:**
   a. *Cardiac and IVC*—use as many or few windows as required for diagnosis.

   - Is there a pericardial effusion and tamponade?

   - Is there a dilated right ventricle, suggesting massive PE (remembering that the right ventricle will dilate progressively in prolonged arrest and an RV free wall of >5 mm suggests long-standing pulmonary hypertension)?

   - Is there a hyperdymamic left ventricle, suggesting hypovolaemia or sepsis? Is this supported by an IVC of <10–12mm or collapsing >50% with respiration?

- Is there impaired LV or global ventricular function, suggesting cardiogenic shock, underlying cardiomyopathy, or myocardial depression, with supporting evidence provided by an IVC of >25 mm or collapsing >20% with respiration?

  b. *Lung windows:*

  - Is there evidence of (tension) pneumothorax (see PoCUS—an integrated approach to dyspnoea, p. 68)?

  - Are there bilateral symmetrical B-lines (>3 per field), providing evidence for pulmonary oedema and suggesting cardiogenic shock, fluid overload, or ARDS? Are there unilateral B-lines, suggesting infection or pulmonary infarction?

2. Supplementary and (c) additional views:

  a. *Abdominal:*

  - Is there evidence of AAA?

  - Is there abdominal free fluid—ascites or blood from a ruptured ectopic or intra-peritoneal blood vessel?

  b. *Peripheral venous system:*

  - Is there evidence of DVT to support a provisional diagnosis of PE?

PoCUS—an integrated approach to acute dyspnoea

Common causes of dyspnoea include pneumothorax, pleural effusion, sepsis, heart failure, PE, and acidosis. Again the SHoC algorithm provides a likelihood-based approach to PoCUS for dyspnoea (see Figure 2.26).

Core SHoC views (cardiac, lung, and IVC)

Lung views:

Anterior chest wall:

- Normal lung fields (lung sliding, scattered B-lines with two or less per window, A-lines, lung sliding): *PE, sepsis, acidosis*;

- Pneumothorax (absent lung sliding, absent B-lines, absent lung sliding, lung point);

- Pulmonary oedema (interstitial fluid with >3 symmetrical pathological full-field B-lines, pleural effusion), absent anterior A-lines;

- Infection (one-sided or asymmetrical B-lines, consolidation with heparinized lung, air bronchograms).

Posterior chest wall at costal margin:

- Pleural effusion, suggesting cardiac failure, infection, malignancy.

Cardiac views:

- Pericardial effusion—if identified, evidence of tamponade with collapse, RV free wall diastolic collapse;

- Hyperdynamic left ventricle, suggesting sepsis;

- Enlarged, hypodynamic right ventricle, reduced TAPSE ± hyperdynamic left ventricle, suggesting massive PE;

- Reduced global/LV function ± dilated chambers, suggesting reduced systolic function;

- If abnormal LV size ± poor function, apply colour box over aortic/mitral valve to demonstrate if valvular incompetence;

- Tissue Doppler septal/lateral mitral annulus >8–10/10–12 cm/s—normal diastolic function; less than this, diastolic dysfunction present and further evaluation with E and A waves; E/e' ratio 8–12 moderate, >12–15 severe; atrial size >34 mL/m² suggests significant diastolic dysfunction.

IVC views:

- IVC is problematic in acute dyspnoea, as intra-thoracic pressures complicate size and collapse index. If AP diameter >25 mm or collapse index <20%, elevated right heart pressures are likely.

Additional views:

Peripheral venous system:

- Is there evidence of DVT to support a provisional diagnosis of PE?

🗐 Further reading

Additional further reading can be found in the Online appendix at www.oxfordmedicine.com/POCUSemergencymed. Please refer to your access card for further details.

Part 2: Why use cardiac point-of-care ultrasound (echo) in emergency care and resuscitation?

Perera P, Mailhot T, Riley D, Mandavia D. The RUSH exam: Raid Ultrasound in SHock and in the evaluation of the critically ill. *Emerg Med Clin North Am* 2010;**28**:29–56.

Via G, Hussain A, Wells M, *et al*. International evidence-based recommendations for focused cardiac ultrasound. *J Am Soc Echocardiogr* 2014;7:**682**.e1–33.

Part 2: When do I perform focused echo?

Jones A, Tayal V, Sullivan M, Kline J. Randomised, controlled trial of immediate versus delayed goal-directed ultrasound to identify the cause of nontraumatic hypotension in emergency department patients. *Crit Care Med* 2004;**32**:1703.

Part 2: In what order should cardiac PoCUS windows be performed?

Lichtenstein D, Meziere G. Relevance of lung ultrasound in the diagnosis of acute respiratory failure. The BLUE Protocol. *Chest* 2008;**134**:117–25.

Part 2: 'Fluid', 'form', 'function', and 'filling'

Atkinson PR, Bowra J, Milne J, *et al*. International Federation for Emergency Medicine Consensus Statement: Sonography in hypotension and cardiac arrest (SHoC): An international consensus on the use of point of care ultrasound for undifferentiated hypotension and during cardiac arrest. *CJEM* 2017;**19**:459–70.

Holst JM, Kilker BA, Wright S, Hoffmann B. Heart failure with preserved ejection fraction: echocardiographic VALVE protocol for emergency physicians. *Eur J Emerg Med* 2014;**231**:394–402.

Lang R, Bandano L, Mor-Avi V, *et al*. Recommendations for the cardiac chamber quantification by echocardiography in adults: an update from the American Association of Echocardiography and the European Association of Cardiovascular Imaging. *J Am Soc Echocardiogr* 2015;**28**:1–39.

Part 3: Can cardiac PoCUS be done without interfering with current guidelines for cardiac resuscitation?

Blyth L, Atkinson P, Gadd K, Lang E. Bedside focused echocardiography as predictor of survival in cardiac arrest patients: a systematic review. *Acad Emerg Med* 2012;**19**:1119–26.

Gaspari R, Weekes A, Adhikari S, *et al*. Emergency department point-of-care ultrasound in out-of-hospital and in-ED cardiac arrest. *Resuscitation* 2016;**109**:33–9.

Part 3: Pathophysiology and integrated PoCUS in shock

Atkinson PR, Milne J, Diegelmann L, *et al*. Does point-of-care ultrasonography improve clinical outcomes in emergency department patients with undifferentiated hypotension? An international randomized controlled trial from the SHoC-ED Investigators. *Ann Emerg Med* 2018;**72**:478–89.

Via G, Hussain A, Wells M, *et al*. International evidence-based recommendations for focused cardiac ultrasound. *J Am Soc Echocardiogr* 2014;**7**:682.e1–33.

Part 3: Fluid resuscitation

Lamina B, Ochagavia A, Monnet X, Chemla D, Teboul J. Echo prediction of volume responsiveness in critically ill patients with spontaneous breathing activity. *Intensive Care Med* 2007;**33**:1125–32.

Part 3: Dynamic predictors of fluid responsiveness

Scmidt GA, Koenig S, Mayo P. Ultrasound to guide diagnosis and therapy. *Chest* 2012;**142**:1042–8.

Part 3: Inferior vena cava ultrasound as a guide to fluid therapy

Zhang Z, Xu X, Ye S, Xu L. Ultrasonographic measurement of the respiratory variation in the inferior vena cava diameter is predictive of fluid responsiveness in critically ill patients: systematic review and meta-analysis. *Ultrasound Med Biol* 2014;**40**:845–53.

Part 3: Using advanced cardiac PoCUS to guide fluid therapy

Mandeville JC, Colebourn CL. Can transthoracic echocardiography be used to predict fluid responsiveness in the critically ill patient? A systematic review. *Crit Care Res Pract* 2012;**2012**:513480.

Part 3: Pulmonary embolism

Casazza F, Bongarzoni A, Capozi A, Agostoni O. Regional right ventricular dysfunction in acute pulmonary embolism and right ventricular infarction. *Eur J Echocardiogr* 2005;**6**:11–14.

Part 3: Acute decompensated heart failure

Volpicelli G, Elbarbary M, Blaivas M, *et al.*; International Liaison Committee on Lung Ultrasound (ILC-LUS) for International Consensus Conference on Lung Ultrasound (ICC-LUS). International evidence-based recommendations for point-of-care lung ultrasound. *Intensive Care Med* 2012;**38**:577–91.

3

The chest

Justin Bowra, Osama Loubani, and Paul Atkinson

Summary

When to scan (clinical indications):

Core: In trauma or acute dyspnoea for 'pleural space' pathology—pneumothorax (PTX) or haemothorax (HTX)/pleural fluid (e.g. as part of the Extended Focused Assessment in Trauma (e-FAST) examination.

Advanced: In dyspnoea for lung pathology—pulmonary oedema/interstitial syndrome; consolidation. Also for pleural thickening.

What to scan (PoCUS protocol):

Core: The most elevated area of the lung (for PTX), base of the lung (for HTX/pleural fluid).

Advanced: Ideally as much of the lung as possible, but at least three areas on either side (representing upper lobes/middle lobe and lingula/lower lobes).

How to scan (key points on scanning):

Core: Curved probe on FAST/lung present. Depth 15 cm initially, then reduce depth to assess lung sliding. 'Filters' (tissue harmonics and compounding) ideally turned off. M-mode may assist for PTX; turning on filters may assist for HTX/pleural fluid.

Advanced: Following core scans, turn filters off and adjust focal depth for B-lines. Then change to linear probe on superficial/musculoskeletal preset for fine detail (pleural space and subpleural consolidation); consider colour flow Doppler to differentiate pleural fluid from thickening and to differentiate the causes of consolidation.

What PoCUS adds (clinical reasoning—how results change practice):

Core: Is there air (PTX) or fluid (e.g. HTX) in the pleural space?

Advanced: Is there pleural fluid or thickening? Is there pulmonary fibrosis or oedema? Is there acute lung injury, pneumonia, infarcted lung, or malignancy? What is the overall pattern of the findings?

Introduction

The presence of air scatters sound waves, thereby destroying any ultrasound image beyond that point. So it may seem counterintuitive to examine the lung using PoCUS. However, certain pulmonary and pleural disease processes can be identified readily using PoCUS, as summarized in Table 3.1. Lung, or more correctly thoracic, PoCUS, has now become a core application in emergency and critical care medicine, offering diagnostic advantages over both the clinical examination and traditional bedside investigations. While ultrasound may not have replaced the stethoscope as the initial tool to help with assessment for thoracic disease, it has been shown to be more reliable for the early diagnosis of common critical conditions. The thorax should be scanned on both sides of the chest and should include anterior, lateral, and posterior views. The diaphragm is a key landmark to outline the inferior

Table 3.1 Point-of-care ultrasound (PoCUS) of the chest and related diagnoses

Ultrasound visualizes	Possible diagnoses
Presence versus absence of 'lung sliding' (sliding of visceral pleura on parietal pleura with respiration)	Pneumothorax (absent sliding) Lack of ventilation, e.g. main stem or oesophageal intubation (absent sliding) Pneumonia (sometimes reduced sliding) Adhesions
Defined anechoic area (fluid) in pleural space	Pleural effusion/haemothorax
Various lung artefacts such as B-lines	Pulmonary oedema (found in cardiogenic oedema, ARDS, and pneumonia) or fibrosis
Abnormal lung parenchyma (hepatization)	Pulmonary consolidation (e.g. pneumonia)
Abnormal (e.g. thickened) pleura	Pleural disease such as mesothelioma

border of the thorax, while the ribs and costal cartilages should be used to identify the level of the pleura.

The typical sonographic appearance of the lung is artefactual. In other words, normal lung tissue is not visible on ultrasound because the lung–pleura interface is so echogenic and the ultrasound 'lung image' deep to the pleural line is actually made up of a combination of pleural reflections, reverberation artefacts, and various degrees of sound wave propagation, depending on the airspace filling. Normal lung findings on ultrasound (see Figure 3.1) include the presence of pleural sliding, the scatter of sound waves deep to this, A-lines (horizontal reverberation artefacts between the probe and pleural line), and occasional B-lines (reverberation artefacts generated within the lung) (see Figure 3.2). Other normal findings include Z-lines (see Figure 3.3) and the lung curtain (obliteration of the view of deep field structures by the respiratory movement of the lung into the near field). Detailed descriptions of various lung lines follow in each subsection and are summarized in Table 3.2.

Air versus fluid

As the lung parenchyma or pleural space increases in fluid content, more ultrasound waves will be transmitted, and the pattern seen on the screen will change from the normal 'A-pattern' appearance, through the 'B-pattern' with increasing numbers of B-lines (see Figure 3.2), to consolidation (see Figure 3.4), and finally the anechoeic appearance of fluid collections

(see Figure 3.5). This is outlined in Table 3.3. It is important to note that lung pathology that does not reach the pleura will not be identified by ultrasound.

Pneumothorax

Purpose

PoCUS can detect PTX with a high degree of certainty. There are several ultrasound findings characteristic of moving lung abutting the chest wall, as will be discussed in Image interpretation, 'Normal appearance', p. 77. When moving pleura and lung parenchyma are seen abutting the chest wall, PTX can be excluded *at that site*. When air is present between the lung and chest wall, these characteristic features are abolished, and in the appropriate clinical setting, PTX can be diagnosed.

Perspective

PTX may occur in a number of clinical settings. While PoCUS can be used for the diagnosis of PTX in any clinical situation, including small asymptomatic PTX, we will focus in particular on the trauma patient and the critically ill patient.

PTX is common in thoracic trauma. In large population studies, nearly 20% of patients suffering from blunt thoracic trauma develop PTX. A significant number of potentially preventable deaths occur in this population, due to a missed or delayed diagnosis of

(a)

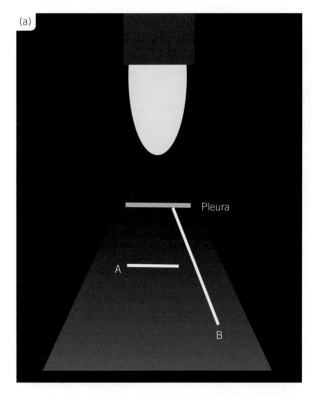

Pleura

A

B

(b)

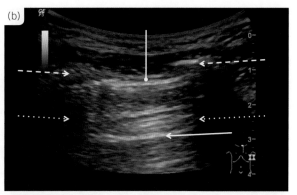

Figure 3.1 Normal lung. (a) Schematic drawing of a B-mode ultrasound image of the chest, showing the pleural line, A-line, and B-line. The intercostal space is delimited by two shadows that represent rib shadows. (b) A B-mode ultrasound image of the chest (depth 4 cm). Note the image is framed by a costal cartilage on the left and a rib on the right of the image (dashed arrows) and rib shadows (dotted arrows). The pleural line (oval arrow) is visible deep to the costal cartilages. Deep to the pleura is an A-line (solid arrow).

(a)

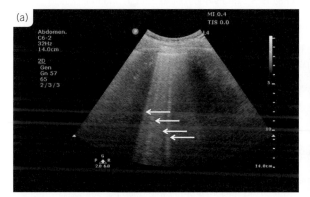

(b)

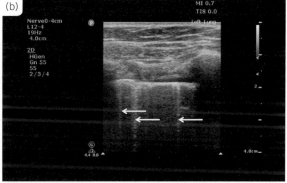

Figure 3.2 B-pattern—the term used when multiple B-lines (arrows) are seen. Note that the B-lines (arrowed) arise from the pleural line and extend to the end of the screen. (a) Four B-lines (arrowed) demonstrated using the curved probe. (b) Three B-lines (arrowed) demonstrated using the linear probe.

PTX. In the critically ill patient, PTX is also relatively common. As many as 6% of ICU patients develop PTX during their ICU stay. This increases to as much as 15% in ICU patients receiving mechanical ventilation.

A missed or delayed diagnosis of PTX can lead to tension PTX. Even in the absence of tension PTX, a missed diagnosis of PTX worsens clinical outcomes, as evidenced by nearly doubled hospital stays in the critical care population.

Why not use traditional diagnostic modalities?

Although CT is the gold standard for diagnosing PTX, physical exam and CXR tend to be employed initially due to their portability, ease, and speed. The sensitivity and specificity of physical examination findings are poor. Auscultation, chest tenderness, and tachypnoea carry sensitivities of between 40% and 80% and specificities of between 78% and 97% in the thoracic trauma population.

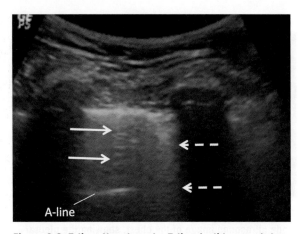

Figure 3.3 Z-line. Note how the Z-line (solid arrows) does not erase the A-line below nor does it extend to the end of the screen. By contrast, the confluent B-lines (dashed arrows) obliterate the A-line.

CXR has been the favoured imaging modality for pneumothorax for much of the past century. CXRs are most often obtained in the supine position in trauma and critically ill patients because of the impracticality and potential danger of sitting up the patient or making them stand. Unfortunately, supine CXRs are poor at detecting PTX. In ICU patients, one-third of PTX are missed on initial supine CXR. In thoracic trauma, supine CXR has sensitivity of between 21% and 75% for detecting PTX.

How good is ultrasound at diagnosing pneumothorax, and how does it impact clinical care?

PoCUS is superior to both physical exam and CXR and rivals CT in the detection of PTX. Three separate

---

Table 3.2 The chest and its 'lines' (see also Figure 3.1)

A-lines	*A-lines* are horizontal, regularly spaced reverberation artefacts that are not related to any pathology. They represent the ultrasound waves reflecting off the pleural lining, rather than returning directly back to the probe. This finding can be seen in normal lungs (see Figure 3.1 and Videos 3.1 to 3.3 🎥) and in PTX (see Videos 3.4 to 3.7 🎥). Equally, they may also be absent in either condition. Therefore, their presence or absence does not differentiate between normal lung and PTX.
B-lines	*B-lines* are bright vertical lines that are caused by fibrosed lung interstitium or by air and fluid intermingling in the lung interstitium. Note that *three or more B-lines per intercostal space are termed 'B-pattern'* (see Figure 3.2 and Videos 3.8 to 3.12 🎥). The B-pattern is considered to be pathological, unless found only at the lung bases, and is due to the 'interstitial syndrome' (see below). The B-pattern has previously been termed *lung rockets* or *lung comets*, but an international consensus conference in 2009 dropped these terms to standardize the terminology.
	B-lines have several key characteristics:
	1. B-lines arise at the pleural line, distinct from subcutaneous emphysema, which generates similar artefacts above the pleural line (referred to as E-lines).
	2. B-lines are vertical and spread to the edge of the screen, in contrast to other vertical 'comet' artefacts that extinguish after a short distance such as Z-lines. For this reason, a probe with deep penetration is necessary to properly identify B-lines.
	3. B-lines are extremely bright, even by comparison with the bright scatter of air in lung.
	4. B-lines abolish the horizontal 'A-lines' found in 'dry' lungs.
	5. B-lines are synchronous with lung sliding.
	6. Finally, B-lines can be quite difficult to appreciate, unless 'filters', such as compounding and tissue harmonics, are switched off (see Videos 3.8 and 3.9 🎥).
Z-lines	These are comet tail artefacts that arise from the pleural line like B-lines, but they do not reach the end of the screen. They are found in apparently normal lungs and have no known significance (see Figure 3.3).
E-lines	These are comet tail artefacts that are *superficial* to the pleural lining. Seen in subcutaneous emphysema or in the presence of echogenic foreign bodies.
V-line	The vertebral (V) line is seen in supine patients in the presence of pleural fluid (or basal consolidation) (see Figure 3.5). The posterior thoracic cage (vertebral bodies and posterior ribs) is seen as an echogenic line extending cephalad to the diaphragm, due to transmission of ultrasound waves through fluid to the posterior thoracic cavity. Also known as the spine sign.

meta-analyses on the detection of PTX by PoCUS in a mixed population (trauma, critical care, and post-procedure) have demonstrated pooled sensitivities of 90.9%, 89%, and 78.6%, respectively, and pooled specificities of 98.2%, 99%, and 98.4%, respectively. The range of accuracy among these three meta-analyses is likely due to the heterogeneity in the population and differences in the gold standard determination of PTX.

The use of PoCUS for detection of PTX has received the greatest amount of investigation in the trauma population, with at least 13 prospective studies examining the sensitivity and specificity of PoCUS in this setting. These studies have consistently shown PoCUS

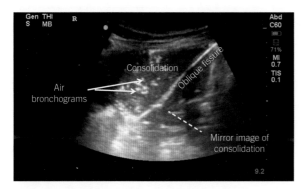

Figure 3.4 Right middle lobe pneumonia with hepatization. On ultrasound, the consolidated lung resembles a solid organ (compare with the image of the spleen in Figure 3.5). Air bronchograms appear as bright areas (arrowed) within the consolidated lung. A mirror image of the consolidated lung (dashed line) appears below the oblique fissure.

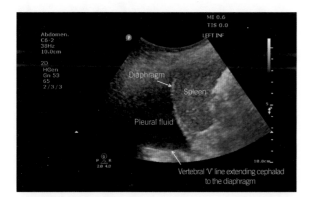

Figure 3.5 Pleural effusion, seen here as anechoic fluid, cephalad to the diaphragm. The *vertebral (V) line* or *spine sign* confirms the presence of pleural fluid on this image.

Image courtesy of Dr Richard Lennon.

to have a sensitivity of between 82% and 100% and a specificity of between 94% and 100%—far exceeding those of CXR. It is worth noting here that two separate prospective studies of PoCUS in trauma demonstrated rather dismal sensitivities of 47% and 53% for the detection of PTX—values discordant with other published trials. Closer inspection of these papers demonstrates that all of the missed PTX in both trials were considered small, and in only one case did a missed PTX require drainage.

The literature also demonstrates that PoCUS provides the diagnosis of PTX in trauma in a fraction of the time a CXR does—2.3 minutes versus 19 minutes, respectively.

The literature regarding PoCUS in the critically ill, while less extensive than for trauma patients, has also consistently shown PoCUS to be superior to CXR. PoCUS in the critically ill patient has a sensitivity of 95–100% and a specificity of 84–96.5%.

Performing the scan

Image generation

Visualization of the pleural line, and specifically determining if there is pleural sliding, is the ultimate goal of image generation, as the pleural line serves as a reference point for the various signs used to detect PTX. As will be discussed at greater length in Image interpretation, 'Normal appearance', p. 73, the normal pleural line is an echogenic dynamic line at the interface of the chest wall and the aerated lung.

Probe selection and machine settings

Very small PTX are best seen using a high-frequency linear probe (5–12 MHz). However, a low-frequency probe (curvilinear or sector) demonstrates all but the smallest PTX and is better able to demonstrate certain artefacts (such as B-lines, discussed in greater detail in 'Image interpretation, B-lines', p. 77), and also to distinguish the lung from nearby structures such as the liver and spleen. Therefore, begin scanning with a curved probe, and switch to a linear only if one suspects a very small PTX. (See Videos 3.5 to 3.7 🎥 for the same very small PTX visualized using a linear, curved, and sector probe, respectively.)

Set the depth at 10–15 cm initially (this allows visualization of B-lines to the edge of the screen, as

Table 3.3 Degree of lung/pleural aeration and typical ultrasound findings, after Lichtenstein (please note that the percentages quoted are rough estimates only)

Degree of aeration	Pathology	Ultrasound appearance
100%	Pneumothorax	Bright scatter due to air. A-lines often seen (see Video 3.4 📹). Lung point may be seen in small PTX (see Videos 3.5 to 3.7 📹). However, no B-lines, no lung sliding, and no lung pulse
98%	Normal	Bright scatter due to air. A-lines often seen. Also lung sliding and lung pulse (see Figure 3.1 and Videos 3.1 to 3.3 📹). Occasional B-lines may be seen
95%	Interstitial syndrome (thickened interlobular septae)	Multiple B-lines (see Figure 3.2 and Videos 3.8 to 3.12 📹)
80%	Ground-glass (alveolar oedema)	B-lines become more confluent (see Video 3.13 📹)
10%	Alveolar consolidation	Irregular anechoic areas that abut the pleural surface (see Video 3.14 📹)
5%	Atelectasis	Hepatization and air bronchograms may be seen (see Figure 3.4 and Video 3.14 📹)
0%	Effusion	Anechoic collection (see Figure 3.5)

Data from Lichtenstein D. *Whole Body Ultrasonography in the Critically Ill*, 4th edition. Springer; 2010.

will be discussed in Image interpretation, 'Normal appearance', p. 77). If your machine has a focal zone control, ensure that the focal zone is set at the level of the pleural line. If lung sliding (visible movement of the lung surface/visceral pleura on the parietal pleura) is not readily apparent, reduce the depth until the echogenic pleural line is in the middle of the screen (in practice, usually 4–5 cm; see Videos 3.1 to 3.7 📹).

Many point-of-care machines have a lung preset. If this is not available, use an abdominal (or FAST) preset with compounding ('multibeam') and tissue harmonics *turned off*, as these settings can filter out artefacts useful in lung ultrasound such as B-lines (see Videos 3.8 and 3.9 📹).

Patient position, surface anatomy, and key landmarks

The examination is best performed in the supine or semi-recumbent position. Although counterintuitive to practitioners accustomed to sitting a patient up for CXR, it ensures that pleural air moves to the most accessible part of the anterior chest, rather than being obscured by the clavicle.

If only PTX is sought, then it should suffice simply to place the probe at the highest point of the chest, which, in the supine position, is just above the diaphragm on either side. On the right, this will be in the mid-clavicular line (see Figure 3.6). On the left,

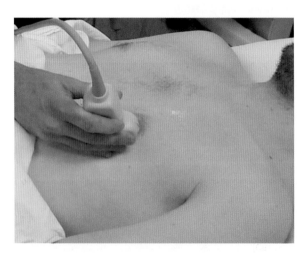

Figure 3.6 Placement of ultrasound probe for pneumothorax. If only a pneumothorax is sought, the probe is placed at the highest point of the chest—*just cephalad to* the diaphragm on either side.

this will be more lateral to avoid the heart. However, if other pathology is sought (such as lung contusions and HTX in chest trauma), it is wise to scan several zones, to image each lobe of the lungs. To do so, place the probe sequentially on the upper chest in the mid-clavicular line, on the lower chest in the mid-clavicular line (more lateral on the left to avoid the heart), and as posterior and inferior as possible, just above the diaphragm. These sites roughly correspond to those originally described by Lichtenstein as the upper BLUE point (upper lobe), lower BLUE point (middle lobe/lingula), and PLAPS point.

Alternatively, one may use Volpicelli's 8-zone approach (four zones on each side). (see Figure 3.7)

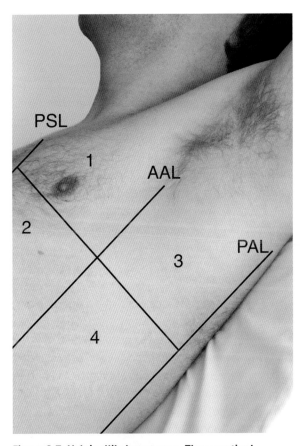

Figure 3.7 Volpicelli's lung zones. Three vertical lines (parasternal line/PSL; anterior axillary line/AAL; posterior axillary line/PAL) and one unnamed horizontal line (approximately halfway between the clavicle and costal margin) divide each anterior and lateral chest wall into four zones—zone 1: upper anterior; zone 2: lower anterior; zone 3; upper lateral; zone 4: basal lateral.

At each site, place the probe in the sagittal axis (probe marker superior). Again, this may seem counterintuitive when one considers that rib shadows will obscure the lung, but, in fact, the ribs are essential landmarks for identifying the pleural line below and between them. Firstly, identify the ribs/costal cartilages on the screen by their echogenic (bright) leading edge and prominent acoustic shadows. Slide the probe cephalad (towards the patient's head) or caudad (towards the feet) until the rib shadows are positioned at either end of the image (see Figure 3.1). The echogenic pleural line will be found approximately 0.5 cm below the rib line at the interface between the water-rich chest wall and the air-rich lung parenchyma. This is the reference point for all subsequent imaging.

Image interpretation

Normal appearance

Once the pleural line is identified, the normal ultrasound findings of the lung parenchyma abutting the chest wall are sought, namely: (a) very bright scatter below the pleural line due to air in the lung; (b) 'lung sliding' (visceral sliding on the parietal pleura); (c) *sometimes* B-lines or other vertical artefacts collectively termed 'comets'; and (d) lung pulse (transmitted arterial pulsation visible through lung tissue).

Lung (pleural) sliding

Lung sliding represents the normal respiratory movement of lung parenchyma against the chest wall—specifically, it is the movement of the visceral pleura on the parietal pleura. In B-mode, lung sliding is seen as a glistening movement at the pleural line, in stark contrast to the still chest wall above (see Videos 3.1 to 3.3 ▶). M-mode (literally *motion mode*) can also be used to detect lung sliding and has the advantage of being able to document lung sliding in a single image. In M-mode, the movement of lung parenchyma, located below the pleural line, appears as a grainy image, while the still chest wall above the pleural line appears as static straight lines. This gives the appearance of grains of sand on a beach and has been termed the *seashore sign* (see Figure 3.8). When lung sliding is abolished, as in PTX, the lack of movement above and below the pleural line gives static straight lines throughout the image, giving the appearance that has been termed the *stratosphere* or *barcode sign* (see Figure 3.9). In

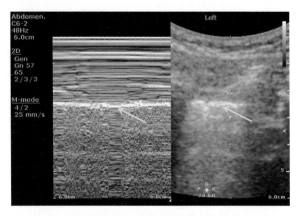

Figure 3.8 M-mode image of normal lung, demonstrating lung slide, often described as the *seashore sign*. Movement of lung parenchyma, located below the pleural line (arrowed), appears as a grainy image, while the still chest wall above the pleural line appears as static straight lines.

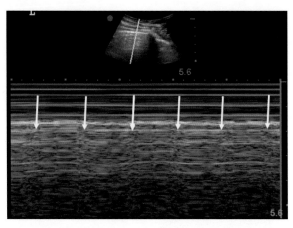

Figure 3.10 M-mode image of normal lung, demonstrating the *lung pulse sign* (regularly spaced vertical lines, arrowed).

normal lungs, lung sliding is least at the apex of the lung and increases towards the base of the lung.

B-lines

B-lines are also important in the differentiation of normal lung from PTX. B-lines are a form of reverberation artefact formed at the interface of objects with very different acoustic impedance. In the chest, B-lines arise from the lung, rather than the pleural line, and are thought to be due to reverberation of sound waves at the intermingling of air and fluid (or air and fibrous tissue) in the lung interstitium (see Figure 3.2 and Videos 3.8 to 3.12 📹) (see Table 3.2 for further details).

Lung pulse sign

Like B-lines and lung sliding, the *lung pulse sign* is also present in normal lung, but absent in PTX. This represents pulsation from the heart and arteries, transmitted through the lung tissue to the surface of the lung. In B-mode imaging, this may appear as a regular 'twinkle' of movement at the pleural line that is independent of lung sliding and synchronized with the patient's heartbeat (see Video 3.17 📹, in which lung pulse is seen, even during a breath-hold). In M-mode imaging, lung pulse appears as a regularly spaced vertical line (see Figure 3.10).

Abnormal appearance

In PTX, air intervenes between the parietal pleura (chest wall) and visceral pleura (lung parenchyma). Because ultrasound waves are scattered by air, the lung parenchyma can no longer be visualized, abolishing the normal findings of lung sliding and B-lines (see Figure 3.11 and Videos 3.4 to 3.7 📹).

The disappearance of lung sliding in PTX was first described in horses. Initial reports in the medical literature showed the absence of lung sliding to have a sensitivity and specificity of 100% for the detection of PTX. A similarly high sensitivity and specificity of 98.1% and 99.2% has been demonstrated in the thoracic trauma population.

However, in the critically ill population or patients with chronic lung disease, absence of lung sliding has

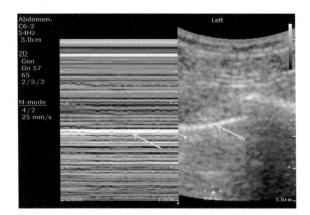

Figure 3.9 M-mode image of pneumothorax, which appears as static straight lines above and below the pleural line (arrowed)—the *stratosphere* or *barcode sign*.

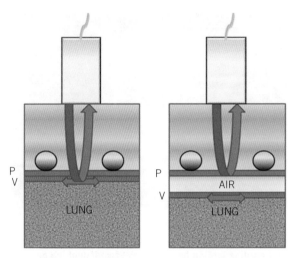

Figure 3.11 Schematic drawing of pneumothorax. Air in the pleural space separates the visceral (V) and parietal (P) pleura, preventing visualization of pleural sliding on PoCUS.

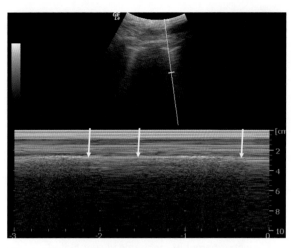

Figure 3.12 M-mode image of the *lung point*, which represents the appearance of the normal lung edge adjacent to the pneumothorax. Note the alternation (arrowed) between the normal seashore sign and the abnormal stratosphere sign.

poor *specificity* for the detection of PTX—between 78% and 91.2%, though an excellent *sensitivity* is maintained. This poor specificity is explained by the fact that lung sliding is abolished by any factor that prevents lung expansion—unilateral bronchial intubation, ARDS, pneumonia (see Video 3.12 📹), pleurodesis, fibrosis, cardiopulmonary arrest, or high-frequency ventilation—all of which are common in critically ill patients. As such, the presence of lung sliding can be used to rule out PTX, but the absence of lung sliding does not definitively diagnose PTX.

Similarly, the absence of B-lines cannot be used to diagnose PTX in the critically ill population, as the specificity of this sign in the critically ill is only 60%; therefore, 40% of critically ill patients with the absence of B-lines will still have PTX.

Because of the inability of lung sliding and B-lines to definitively diagnose PTX in the critically ill, another sign—the *lung point*—is used. The lung point is an extremely specific sign for the presence of PTX. First described by Lichtenstein, the lung point represents the appearance of the normal lung edge adjacent to PTX (see Figure 3.12 and Videos 3.5 to 3.7 📹). On B-mode imaging, findings of PTX (no sliding or B-lines) are seen on one side of the screen, with a sudden change to the normal pattern of lung sliding (and occasional B- or Z-lines) indicating normal lung ventilation. The lung point moves with respiration, as the

ventilated lung pushes the 'bubble' of air represented by the PTX (see Videos 3.5 to 3.7 📹).

While the lung point is not always seen in PTX, its presence nearly always indicates PTX—in other words, the lung point has a poor sensitivity (66%), but a high specificity (100%). The poor sensitivity of this sign may be explained by the simple observation that there will be no lung point in a large PTX because the lung is completely collapsed and therefore does not abut the chest wall.

Pitfalls—factors that hinder interpretation

False positives for pneumothorax

- Underventilated lung: as noted in previous section, 'Abnormal appearance', any lung that has decreased or no ventilation may resemble PTX, as sliding will not be seen. This is an issue particularly in patients who are splinting their chest due to pain from rib fractures, because such patients are at risk of PTX.

- False stratosphere sign: if the probe is inadvertently placed over a rib while in M-mode, this will, of course, generate an image that resembles the stratosphere sign (see Figure 3.13).

- False lung point sign: in patients with pauses in ventilation, everywhere the probe is placed can resemble a lung point sign in M-mode. This

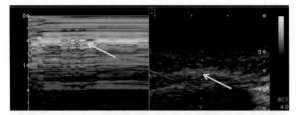

Figure 3.13 M-mode image of *false* 'stratosphere sign' caused by scanning over a rib (arrowed). The horizontal lines seen deep to the leading edge of the rib are simply mirror images of the soft tissue images from above the pleura.

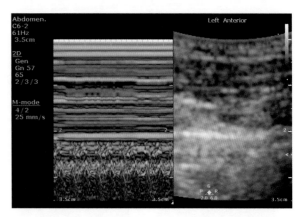

Figure 3.14 M-mode image of cardiac motion. Cardiac motion can be mistaken for lung motion. However, note that cardiac motion has a vertical component, as opposed to lung sliding which is horizontal.

is most apparent in mechanically ventilated patients. The issue can be quickly resolved by scanning elsewhere on the patient and even on the contralateral lung; the same effect will be seen in all lung fields.

- Bulla: this can be difficult to differentiate from PTX. Perhaps the easiest way is to move the patient (e.g. sit the patient up), then to re-scan at the site of the 'PTX'. A true PTX will have moved, but a bulla will remain fixed.

False negatives for pneumothorax

- Cardiac motion: in M-mode, this has a superficial resemblance to lung sliding; however, this motion has a vertical component (as the free wall of the right ventricle moves towards and away from the probe), which does not occur in lung sliding unless there is also a pleural effusion (see Figure 3.14 and Video 3.18 ⬛).

- When PTX causes significant respiratory distress, the entire chest wall moves, and this can generate a false impression of lung sliding under the probe (see Video 3.19 ⬛). Similarly, inadvertent probe movement on the chest wall can also give this impression. This is a problem particularly when using M-mode and can give rise to a 'false seashore sign'. The key is: (a) to ignore all those areas on the image in which grainy movement artefact is seen above the pleural line (grainy 'movement artefact' below the pleura may simply be reflecting this); and (b) to look for *increased* movement below the pleura that is *independent* of chest wall movement (see Figure 3.15).

- Perhaps the most common error is to miss a small PTX that is simply not at the site that was scanned. It may seem obvious, but the lung sliding sign only rules out PTX *at that site*.

Clinical use

In patients presenting with thoracic trauma, the absence of lung slide provides a high degree of sensitivity and specificity for the diagnosis of PTX. Establishing the absence of B-lines, the absence of a lung pulse, or the presence of a lung point increases the diagnostic accuracy but comes at the cost of increasing time and complexity of the examination.

However, if time permits, it is wise to seek the combination of an absent lung slide, absent B-lines, and

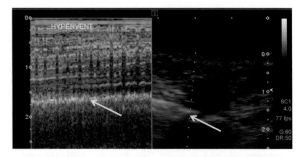

Figure 3.15 M-mode image taken in hyperventilation. Note that there is movement both above and below the pleural line (arrowed), representing movement of the *entire chest* in hyperventilation.

Table 3.4 Ultrasound features of lung versus pneumothorax

Ultrasound feature	Lung	Pneumothorax
Lung sliding	Present	Absent
Lung pulse	Present	Absent
B-lines	Sometimes present	*Never* present
Consolidation	Sometimes present	*Never* present
Lung point	*Never* present	Sometimes present (only if small)

the presence of a lung point before a diagnosis of PTX is made. This is particularly true in critical care, due to the existence of several factors in critically ill patients that can reduce the sensitivity and specificity of the ultrasound examination. See Table 3.4 for a summary.

PoCUS can also help determine the *size* of a PTX. Unlike CXR, ultrasound cannot establish the *depth* of a PTX, but it can establish its *extent*. Simply put, a PTX with loss of sliding that extends throughout the hemithorax indicates collapse of the entire lung, whereas as more lung sliding is seen, then, by definition, the PTX is smaller. For further discussion of this application, readers are directed to the references in 'Further reading', p. 86 for further details.

Pleural fluid

Purpose

PoCUS can be used to detect fluid in the pleural cavity. The nature and significance of the fluid, as with most other PoCUS indications, depend on the clinical scenario.

Perspective

Pathological fluid accumulation in the pleural space occurs in several situations. In thoracic trauma, pleural fluid is taken to represent HTX. The incidence of HTX in this population is between 10% and 20%.

Early detection of pleural fluid can help guide the decision for drainage and further investigation.

Causes of pleural effusion in the non-trauma patient range from heart failure and atelectasis to parapneumonic effusions and empyema. Early detection of pleural fluid can guide the decision for drainage, either for diagnostic or for therapeutic purposes.

Why not use traditional diagnostic modalities?

Clinical studies have shown that supine CXRs cannot detect volumes of <175–525 mL. In ICU patients with coexisting lung pathology (which represents a large proportion of critically ill patients), supine CXRs have a sensitivity of only 39% and a specificity of 85% for the detection of pleural fluid. Placing the patient in the lateral decubitus position, which improves detection of pleural fluid, is often impractical in the critically ill patient.

In thoracic trauma patients, the sensitivity and specificity of supine CXR are greater, with sensitivities of 92–96% and specificities nearing 100%.

How good is ultrasound at detecting pleural fluid, and how does it impact clinical care?

The use of ultrasound for the detection of pleural fluid was first described in 1967. Since that time, ultrasound has been shown to be extremely sensitive for the detection of pleural fluid, with the ability to detect as little as 20 mL.

In the thoracic trauma population, PoCUS has consistently been shown to have a sensitivity of between 92% and 100% and a specificity nearing 100% for HTX. It is worth noting that a single prospective trial of PoCUS in trauma demonstrated a sensitivity of 37% for the detection of HTX. However, all of the missed HTX in this study were 'minimal' and did not require drainage.

In the ICU population, PoCUS has demonstrated a sensitivity of 92% and a specificity of 93% for the detection of pleural fluid, even in the presence of severe pulmonary pathology.

Use of PoCUS drastically reduces the time to clinical diagnosis, when compared to the CXR. In the trauma population, PoCUS has been shown to provide a diagnosis of HTX within 1 minute, compared to 15 minutes by CXR.

PoCUS can also help to quantify the amount of pleural fluid present, to differentiate between transudative and exudative effusions, and to guide thoracocentesis. The use of PoCUS to guide thoracocentesis and chest drain insertion is recommended by the British Thoracic Society.

Use of PoCUS has been shown to increase the success of thoracocentesis, while simultaneously decreasing the complication rate. In a small randomized study, the failure rate in clinically guided thoracocentesis was 33%, compared to 0% with ultrasound guidance. Two large retrospective cohort studies showed that ultrasound guidance reduced the rate of PTX from thoracocentesis by more than half (from 18% to 3%, and from 10.3% to 4.9%, respectively). Further discussion of these applications is continued in Chapter 9.

Image generation

Probe selection, patient position, surface anatomy, and key landmarks

When image interpretation requires deep image penetration, a phased array (cardiac) transducer or a low-frequency (3–5 MHz) curvilinear (abdominal) transducer is preferable. For superficial effusions, a linear (vascular) transducer with a higher frequency (5–10 MHz) is used. The machine can be set to abdominal or lung presets, though as when scanning for consolidation and pleural thickening, pleural fluid is better seen with the 'filters' (tissue harmonics and multibeam) switched on. The examination may be done with the patient in the supine or erect position, as determined by the clinical scenario. In contrast to the examination for PTX, PoCUS for pleural fluid focuses on dependent areas of the chest, as that is where fluid will collect. Greatest success is achieved when the probe is placed just above the diaphragm, on the posterior–lateral chest wall—as was originally described by Lichtenstein's PLAPS point. For clinicians familiar with the FAST scan, this point is similar to the RUQ and LUQ views, in the mid- to posterior axillary zone, level with the xiphisternum. The diaphragm is immediately superior to the spleen or liver and can be found easily using these organs as landmarks.

For thoracocentesis, optimizing the patient position enhances procedural success. Elective thoracocentesis is often performed with the patient in the erect position, leaning forward, with the arms crossed in front. This allows the effusion to collect at the lung bases. The ultrasound probe can then be placed on the back in the posterior axillary line to image the best location for drainage. Critically ill patients are often required to remain in the supine position. A moderate effusion can still be well visualized by scanning the lateral chest wall at the posterior axillary line. The head of the bed may need to be raised, if possible, to visualize smaller effusions. Elevating the patient's arm over the head increases the distance between the ribs, helping to improve image generation. Where this is not practical, the ipsilateral arm can be pulled across the chest to the opposite side.

Image interpretation

Normal appearance

In the *absence* of pleural fluid, air in the lung parenchyma scatters the ultrasound beam and creates a very indistinct image. It is important to note the appearance of the diaphragm when scanning from the trans-hepatic or trans-splenic windows (traditionally used for detecting intra-peritoneal free fluid). On expiration, the diaphragm normally will appear brightly echogenic, as it lies directly adjacent to air-filled lung parenchyma, causing scattered reflection. The diaphragm and intra-peritoneal organs normally will disappear during inspiration, as a 'curtain of air' in the aerated lung moves to lie between them and the probe. This is described as the 'lung curtain' sign (see Video 3.20 🎥). The far-field (medial) vertebral reflections and shadows (seen when scanning in the trans-hepatic or trans-splenic windows) end abruptly at the level of the diaphragm, again as the aerated lung obscures its view. Mirroring of the liver or spleen may be seen at the diaphragm.

Abnormal appearance

Most commonly, pleural fluid is indicated by the appearance of an anechoic area separating the visceral and parietal pleura (representing fluid) just *above* (cephalad to) the diaphragm (see Figure 3.5 and

Video 3.15 📷). This anechoic space varies in size and shape with respiration. When present, this fluid can greatly improve visualization of deeper structures such as the vertebra and the diaphragm, which can be seen almost entirely in larger effusions. The diaphragm will, however, appear less echogenic, when not lying adjacent to aerated lung. In areas where the diaphragm is not present, the fluid is seen between the pleural line and lung parenchyma. The following sonographic signs help to detect effusions more accurately and also help to distinguish fluid from other pathology.

Anechoic/hypoechoic space

An anechoic (or, on occasion, hypoechoic) black space between the pleura that varies in shape with respiration is a key sign for pleural fluid.

Vertebral (V) line/spine sign

As pleural fluid will transmit echoes to the posterior wall of the thorax, these structures, including the vertebrae, will be visualized cephalad to the diaphragm. This is known as the vertebral (V) line or spine sign (see Figure 3.5) and helps to distinguish pleural fluid from the loss of image, or dark lung curtain, seen with normal aerated lung.

Quad sign

The *quad sign* refers to visualization of an effusion between four regular borders: the pleural line, two rib shadows, and the lung line (see Figure 3.16).

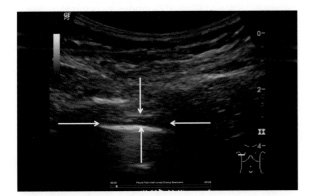

Figure 3.16 The *quad sign*. Arrows indicate the four borders of the effusion: the rib shadows, the parietal pleura, and the visceral pleura.

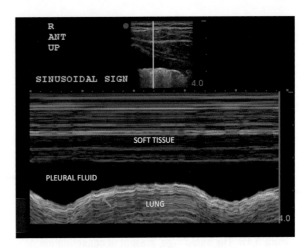

Figure 3.17 M-mode image of the *sinusoid sign* due to the rhythmic to-and-fro motion of the lung within the effusion.

Sinusoid sign

The *sinusoid sign* is seen in M-mode and demonstrates the movement of lung parenchyma in and out of an effusion during inspiration and expiration. This gives the appearance of a sinusoidal wave, as the lung parenchyma moves closer and further away from the pleural line. In B-mode, the lung is seen to 'bob up and down' in the pleural fluid (see Figure 3.17 and Videos 3.10 and 3.14 📷).

Absence of the shred sign

The *shred sign* (see Figure 3.18 and Video 3.14 📷) is seen in consolidation that abuts the pleura (see 'Consolidation or localized effusion?', p. 84) but is absent in simple pleural effusions. This is because it represents pathology that involves the alveoli irregularly, giving an irregular or 'shredded' appearance to the deep border of the area of interest. By contrast, the deep border of a pleural effusion is formed by the visceral pleura and is therefore smooth (see Figure 3.16 and Videos 3.15 and 3.16 📷).

Differentiating transudates from exudates

As the particulate content of pleural fluid increases, it becomes hypoechoic (a few echoes), rather than anechoic (no echoes). As such, if fluid appears to have a homogenously or patchy hypoechoic appearance, or if septae can be seen, it suggests that the

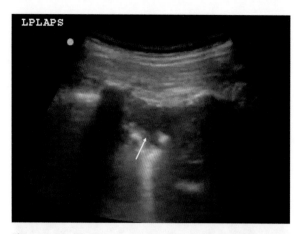

LPLAPS

Figure 3.18 The *shred sign*, present in consolidation that abuts the pleura (arrowed). Note the irregular or 'shredded' appearance of the deep border, representing pathology that involves the alveoli irregularly. By contrast, the deep border of a pleural effusion is formed by the visceral pleura and is smooth. *See Video 3.16* 🎥.

fluid is an exudate or blood. An anechoic appearance can be seen in both transudates and lighter exudates.

Pitfalls—factors that hinder interpretation

Pleural fluid or thickening?

Small effusions may be mistaken for pleural thickening. As seen in 'Abnormal appearance', p. 83, pleural *fluid* is associated with a smooth pleural edge and the quad and sinusoid signs. Pleural *thickening* is often associated with an irregular pleural edge and the absence of the sinusoid sign (see Video 3.11 🎥).

Consolidation or localized effusion?

Interpretation of PoCUS for pleural fluid can be hindered in the presence of alveolar consolidation, which can give the appearance of fluid. However, as noted in 'Absence of the shred sign', p. 83, absence of the *shred sign* assists in differentiating the two conditions. Some authors have suggested the use of colour flow Doppler to differentiate between the two conditions, but the potential for misinterpretation of colour flow Doppler images suggests that further research may be needed before this technique can be recommended.

Interstitial syndrome—cardiogenic pulmonary oedema, ARDS, and pneumonia

Purpose

PoCUS detects interstitial oedema and can differentiate whether the cause is acute cardiogenic pulmonary oedema (APE), ARDS, or pneumonia. Oedematous lung parenchyma has a different echogenicity to 'dry' lung parenchyma, allowing for accurate differentiation between the two.

Perspective

APE and pneumonia can be confused clinically (e.g. both are associated with lung crepitations), and investigations, such as CXR, inflammatory markers, and pro-BNP (prohormone brain natriuretic peptide), can be misleading. Misdiagnosis in an acutely breathless patient can have disastrous consequences.

Why not use traditional diagnostic modalities?

Physical examination and CXR can have poor sensitivities and specificities for the diagnosis of pneumonia, pulmonary oedema, and ARDS.

For community-acquired pneumonia, CXR carries a sensitivity of 69.2% and a specificity of 100%, when compared with high-resolution CT. In pulmonary oedema, the only physical examination findings shown to increase the likelihood of diagnosis—the presence of an S3, jugular venous distension, rales or wheeze, new murmur, and peripheral oedema—have sensitivities of between 13% and 50%. CXR findings shown to increase the likelihood of pulmonary oedema—pulmonary venous congestion, interstitial oedema, cardiomegaly, and pleural effusion— similarly have poor sensitivities of 26–74%. Lastly, a diagnosis of ARDS by auscultation and CXR carries a sensitivity of 34% and 60%, respectively.

How good is ultrasound at diagnosing interstitial syndrome, and how does it impact clinical care?

PoCUS demonstrates a high sensitivity and specificity for the diagnosis of APE, pneumonia, and interstitial syndrome, as listed below:

- APE: sensitivity 97%, specificity 94%;
- Pneumonia: sensitivity 89%, specificity 94%;

- Interstitial syndrome: sensitivity 98%, specificity 88%.

Image generation

As for PTX (see 'Image generation', p. 75).

Image interpretation

The following lung PoCUS findings are used to diagnose and differentiate APE, ARDS, and pneumonia.

1. *Multiple B-lines may be found in diseased lung* (see Figure 3.2 and Videos 3.8 to 3.13 📹): the occasional B-line is a normal finding, as are multiple B-lines in the most dependent portions of the lung in approximately 25% of normal individuals. However, if *three or more* B-lines are seen in a single intercostal space, they are termed *B-pattern* (previously termed 'lung rockets') and the lung is deemed abnormal at that point. *B-pattern* may be found in any condition associated with pulmonary oedema, whether widespread and symmetrical (APE), patchy (ARDS and disseminated pneumonia), or localized (localized inflammation such as lobar pneumonia).

However, pulmonary fibrosis is also associated with B-pattern. Pioneers of lung PoCUS, such as Lichtenstein and Volpicelli, coined the term 'alveolar–interstitial syndrome' (later refined to 'interstitial syndrome'), which is an umbrella term that includes pulmonary oedema and fibrosis.

2. *Distribution of B-pattern differs with the disease process*: any condition which causes interstitial oedema or fibrosis will generate a B-pattern. However, the *distribution* of the B-pattern gives an important clue to the cause:

   - In APE, the B-pattern is widespread and bilateral, and observed throughout the lungs;
   - In ARDS and disseminated pneumonia, it is patchy and alternates with areas of normal lung and even consolidation;
   - In fibrosis, they may be restricted to either the upper or lower lobes, or may be widespread. Furthermore, B-pattern in fibrosis is typically

associated with pleural thickening (see Video 3.11 📹);

   - In localized inflammation, such as lobar pneumonia, they are localized (see Video 3.12 📹).

3. *Interstitial oedema is associated with pleural effusions, which affect lung sliding.* In APE, the effusions are transudative and facilitate lung sliding (see Video 3.10 📹). In inflammatory oedema (pneumonia and ARDS), the effusion is exudative, proteinaceous, and 'sticky'. This sometimes 'glues' the lung to the chest wall, and thus lung sliding may become reduced or even absent (see Video 3.12 📹).

Pitfalls—factors that hinder interpretation

- Occasional B-lines are present in normal lung.
- B-pattern can be present in the lung bases of normal individuals and are seen in pulmonary fibrosis.

Alveolar consolidation

When alveoli fill with fluid (whether pus from pneumonia, blood from pulmonary contusion, areas of malignancy, or even infarcted lung from PE), they transmit sound waves, whereas normal air-filled alveoli scatter sound waves. When areas of fluid-filled alveolar tissue *abut the pleura*, they appear dark and irregular and have a 'liver-like' consistency (*hepatization* or *solidification*; see Figure 3.4) on PoCUS, and they may have an irregular lower border known as the *shred sign*, described in 'Absence of the shred sign', p. 83 (see Figure 3.18 and Video 3.14 📹). Often residual airspaces within consolidation, such as in small airways, appear as bright echogenic points within the solid-appearing zone. These *air bronchograms* may be static (within the consolidation) or sliding, representing movement of fluid and air within the small airways (see Figure 3.4 and Video 3.15 📹).

Note that areas of consolidation may be very small and can give rise simply to a pleural line that appears thickened and 'irregular' (see Video 3.12 📹). Note also that consolidation that is not in contact with the pleura *cannot* be visualized by ultrasound.

What is causing consolidation?

As noted in the previous paragraphs, several conditions can cause consolidation. In most cases, they can be differentiated clinically. However, at times, this can prove difficult, and expert sonologists may choose to employ Doppler sonography to differentiate between them. Subpleural consolidation with a smooth (non-inflammatory) edge may represent infarction, whereas an irregular outline (*shred sign*) implies an inflammatory process such as pneumonia. Using a linear probe with the PRF (scale) reduced as low as possible, scan the consolidated area. If blood flow is present within its substance, the tissue is not infarcted. If blood flow is absent, suspect pulmonary infarction from PE (see Videos 3.21 and 3.22 📹). (*Note that these techniques should be used with caution and only by those experienced in PoCUS, and they always require clinical correlation.*)

What is the overall pattern?

In many cases, this may be the most important question and may be the only way to distinguish between disease processes using PoCUS. The following principles apply:

1. Normal lungs (and those with exacerbation of asthma or COPD) demonstrate predominantly A-lines, or no lines at all, associated with preserved lung sliding.

2. Acute pulmonary oedema is associated with preserved lung sliding and bilateral B-pattern in all lung windows, with smooth pleural surfaces.

3. Pulmonary fibrosis demonstrates some areas of B-pattern (associated with irregular pleural thickening) and some areas of apparently normal lung.

4. ARDS and pneumonia may demonstrate one of the following on PoCUS:
   - Reduced/absent lung sliding associated with widespread, but usually asymmetrical, B-pattern;
   - Patchy B-pattern, alternating with areas of normal lung;
   - Areas of consolidation;
   - Air bronchograms.

Lichtenstein created the 'BLUE protocol' in 2008, which merged the above observations into a single flow sheet. Details of the BLUE protocol (e.g. the 'BLUE' and 'PLAPS' points recommended for probe placement) are beyond this text, and readers are referred to the author's published works on the subject (see Further reading) for a detailed description of the protocol and its limitations.

Two points must be noted at this stage:

1. The BLUE protocol's stated accuracy of 90–95% applies only to patients in extreme respiratory distress. It has not yet been validated in those with mild to moderate illness. For example, although the B-pattern is found throughout the lung fields in APE, the authors observe that they are usually found only in the lower zones in congestive heart failure.

2. The BLUE protocol awaits multicentre validation studies.

That said, the following statements appear to be reasonable in the acutely breathless patient:

- Widespread B-pattern + preserved lung sliding ± bilateral pleural effusions suggests APE (or occasionally interstitial fibrosis);
- B-pattern with reduced lung sliding suggests pneumonia or ARDS;
- Patchy or localized B-pattern suggests a localized disease process (fibrosis, pneumonia, contusion);
- Areas of consolidated lung tissue suggest pneumonia, contusion, or pulmonary infarct;
- Perhaps most importantly for the novice scanner: the above findings should be approached as a 'rule-in', rather than a 'rule-out', guide (i.e. if absent, they may not reliably rule out disease).

📖 Further reading

Additional further reading can be found in the Online appendix at www.oxfordmedicine.com/POCUSemergencymed. Please refer to your access card for further details.

Alrajhi K, Woo MY, Vaillancourt C. Test characteristics of ultrasonography for the detection of pneumothorax: a systematic review and meta-analysis. *Chest* 2012;**141**:703–8.

Alrajab S, Youssef AM, Akkus NI, Caldito G. Pleural ultrasonography versus chest radiography for the diagnosis of pneumothorax: review of the literature and meta-analysis. *Crit Care* 2013;**17**:R208.

Brook OR, Beck-Razi N, Abadi S, *et al.* Sonographic detection of pneumothorax by radiology residents as part of extended focused assessment with sonography for trauma. *J Ultrasound Med* 2009;**28**:749–55.

Ding W, Shen Y, Yang J, He X, Zhang M. Diagnosis of pneumothorax by radiography and ultrasonography: a meta-analysis. *Chest* 2011;**140**:859–66.

Hyacinthe AC, Broux C, Francony G, *et al.* Diagnostic accuracy of ultrasonography in the acute assessment of common thoracic lesions after trauma. *Chest* 2012;**141**:1177–83.

Lichtenstein D. *Whole Body Ultrasonography in the Critically Ill*, 4th ed. Berlin Heidelberg: Springer-Verlag; 2010.

Lichtenstein DA, Mezière GA. Relevance of lung ultrasound in the diagnosis of acute respiratory failure: the BLUE protocol. *Chest* 2008;**134**:117–25.

4

The abdomen

Justin Bowra, Osama Loubani, and Paul Atkinson

Summary

Abdominal PoCUS can be used to answer specific binary questions regarding abdominal pathology.

When to scan (clinical indications):

Core: PoCUS detects *abdominal free fluid*. In the setting of trauma, the presence of free fluid can be diagnostic for haemoperitoneum and is an essential part of the e-FAST examination. PoCUS detects *cholelithiasis, signs of cholecystitis, and CBD dilatation*. This can guide diagnosis and management of the patient presenting with RUQ pain. PoCUS detects *hydronephrosis and absent ureteric jets*. This can assist in the diagnosis of renal colic. PoCUS detects *aortic disease* (see Chapter 6).

Advanced: PoCUS can be used to improve clinical diagnostic accuracy for intestinal pathology, such as small bowel obstruction and appendicitis, in patients with abdominal pain. Because of its variable accuracy in the hands of inexperienced operators, PoCUS is best used to 'rule in', rather than 'rule out', bowel obstruction and appendicitis.

What to scan (PoCUS protocol):

Core: RUQ, LUQ, and pelvis for free fluid; RUQ for the gall bladder and CBD; RUQ and LUQ for the kidneys; aorta for AAA (Chapter 6).

Advanced: as much of the abdomen as possible for bowel obstruction; for appendicitis, begin with the right iliac fossa (RIF).

How to scan (key points on scanning):

Core: curved probe on FAST/lung present, depth 15 cm.

Advanced: after core scan, change to linear probe (on suitable preset such as 'superficial' or 'thyroid') for superficial structures. Consider colour flow Doppler for ureteric jets, renal blood flow, and hyperaemic appendix.

Abdominal free fluid

Purpose

Abdominal free fluid may occur as a result of several disease processes. This chapter will focus in particular on the trauma patient.

PoCUS detects free fluid within the peritoneum. As with all other PoCUS indications, interpretation of the relevance of this finding depends on the clinical scenario and the clinician's index of suspicion. A small amount of intra-peritoneal free fluid in an otherwise well young female, for example, may be normal and clinically insignificant, while free fluid in a patient with severe abdominal trauma suggests intra-abdominal haemorrhage, and in a non-traumatized patient, it can indicate other pathology such as ruptured ectopic pregnancy, intra-abdominal sepsis, and even bowel perforation.

Perspective

Haemoperitoneum occurs in 10–20% of patients suffering from major blunt abdominal trauma and in as many as 50% of patients with penetrating abdominal trauma. Delay in recognition of haemoperitoneum leads to preventable mortality. In one autopsy study of 100 trauma patients, eight of 11 preventable deaths involved intra-abdominal haemorrhage. Of these eight deaths, two were missed entirely, while in six, there were delays in recognition.

Why not use traditional diagnostic modalities?

Physical examination, diagnostic peritoneal lavage (DPL), and CT are traditionally used to detect abdominal free fluid. In trauma, physical examination is notoriously unreliable for the detection of any abdominal injury. As many as one-third of trauma patients with unremarkable physical examinations are later found to have abdominal organ injury. The reliability of the physical examination is further diminished in the context of head injury, polytrauma, intoxication, and lower rib fractures, situations in which detection of major abdominal injury can be of critical importance.

For decades, DPL was the modality of choice for the detection of haemoperitoneum. While DPL is extremely sensitive and specific, it is an invasive test, with reported complication rates of 0.8–9%, including local wound infection, bowel injury, and bladder perforation. Furthermore, the very high sensitivity of DPL has led in the past to a high number of unnecessary operative interventions.

CT is currently the gold standard for identifying intra-abdominal pathology, but it also has its risks. In the very unstable patient, transport to the CT suite can take the patient to a relatively unsafe environment and hinder resuscitation. Conversely, in the entirely stable patient, the risk of ionizing radiation becomes significant, compared with the benefit of the test, especially in younger patients and females of childbearing age.

How good is ultrasound at diagnosing the condition?

In trauma, the PoCUS exam is traditionally known as the FAST exam or 'Focused Assessment with Sonography in Trauma', and more recently known as the *e-FAST or 'Extended FAST'* exam when combined with thoracic scanning. The e-FAST exam combines examination of the peritoneal, pericardial, and pleural cavities for peritoneal fluid, pericardial fluid, PTX, and HTX, respectively. (See Chapters 2 and 3 for detailed descriptions of pericardial and pleural assessment.)

In hypotensive abdominal trauma patients, e-FAST detects haemoperitoneum with great sensitivity and specificity. Over 60 studies, with a combined total of >30,000 patients, have examined the sensitivity and specificity of PoCUS in abdominal trauma. In these papers, PoCUS consistently demonstrated a sensitivity of between 85% and 100% and a specificity of between 95% and 100%. It should be noted that PoCUS is less sensitive in penetrating abdominal trauma (sensitivities for the detection of haemoperitoneum ranging from 50% to 70%) and in those with minor trauma.

How does ultrasound impact clinical care?

In the patient with abdominal trauma, PoCUS enhances the care of the patient in several ways. It has been shown to decrease the time to definitive operative management, the time to disposition, the length of hospital stay, the cost of evaluation by 33–70%, and the overall number of tests (including CT) performed.

Despite these benefits, a Cochrane review of randomized controlled trials of PoCUS in abdominal trauma did not demonstrate a mortality benefit.

Image generation

Probe selection and machine settings

A low-frequency probe (curvilinear or sector) is used to allow for adequate penetration.

Patient position, surface anatomy, and key landmarks

The patient is positioned supine. Trendelenburg (head down) positioning improves the ability to detect free fluid in Morison's pouch but is often impractical. Three main views are used in the detection of intra-peritoneal free fluid (see Figure 4.1):

1. RUQ: perihepatic, including hepatorenal space;
2. LUQ: perisplenic, including splenorenal space;
3. Pelvis: vesicorectal space in men, and vesicouterine and rectouterine spaces in women.

Right upper quadrant

The probe is placed in the coronal plane (marker cephalad). Position the probe approximately at the level of the xiphoid process, in the mid- to anterior axillary line on the right, tilting the probe by about 30° into the bed (see Figures 4.1 and 4.2). The first landmarks

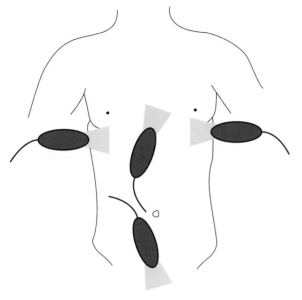

Figure 4.1 **Probe placement for identifying free fluid in trauma. Note that the sub-xiphoid window detects pericardial, rather than peritoneal, free fluid. See Chapter 2 for details.**

sought are the liver and (deeper and more caudal to this) the right kidney, which is darker (less echodense) on ultrasound. Between them, the hepatorenal space, or 'Morison's pouch', can be visualized (see Video 4.1). To find the hepatorenal space, it is often necessary to systematically slide or fan the probe cephalad and caudally, as well as tilting or sliding anteriorly and posteriorly. Once identified, sweep through the hepatorenal and hepatodiaphragmatic spaces, as well as visualizing the tip of the liver (see Video 4.1).

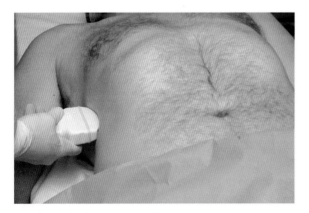

Figure 4.2 **Probe placement for scanning the right upper quadrant.**

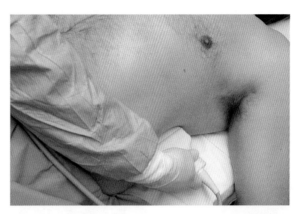

Figure 4.3 **Probe placement for scanning the left upper quadrant.**

Two notes

1. It is advisable to begin e-FAST with the RUQ scan, because in supine patients, fluid is most commonly seen here.

2. However, it is a mistake simply to scan Morison's pouch and ignore the sub-diaphragmatic space and the tip of the liver. It is common for free fluid to be seen in the latter areas, while Morison's pouch itself remains 'clear' of fluid (see Videos 4.2 and 4.3).

Left upper quadrant

The probe position for the LUQ is as for the RUQ, other than beginning more *posteriorly* (in the *posterior* axillary line, rather than the mid-axillary line), with one's hand virtually touching the bed (see Figures 4.1 and 4.3). As with the RUQ, two landmarks are sought—in this case, the spleen and left kidney. From here, the sub-diaphragmatic and splenorenal spaces can be visualized (see Figure 4.4). As with the RUQ, a systematic search superiorly and inferiorly, as well as anteriorly and posteriorly, is required to be certain there is no fluid (see Video 4.4), because fluid often accumulates in the sub-diaphragmatic space first (see Video 4.5). Complete this view by looking for fluid around the tip of the spleen (either by decreasing the depth or zooming in).

For practicality, scan the base of each hemithorax for fluid, while scanning the RUQ and LUQ, as part of the e-FAST scan. (For details on scanning for pleural fluid, see Chapter 3).

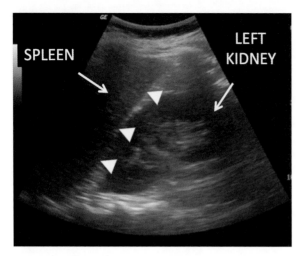

Figure 4.4 Ultrasound image of left upper quadrant: spleen, left kidney, and splenorenal space.

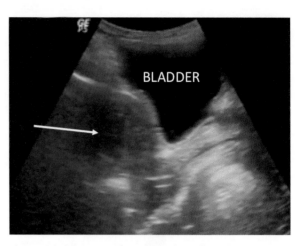

Figure 4.6 Ultrasound image: sagittal view of the female pelvis, negative for free fluid. Note the uterus (arrowed) deep to the bladder.

Pelvis

The bladder is the key landmark in the pelvis. The probe is placed immediately superior to the pubic symphysis, tilting down into the pelvis in the transverse and sagittal (longitudinal) planes and the bladder identified as a walled, anechoic space. Immediately posterior (deep) to the bladder are the prostate and rectum in males (see Figure 4.5) and the uterus in females (see Figure 4.6). Once identified, sweep the space between the bladder and the abdominal organ posterior to it in search of fluid (see Videos 4.6 to 4.9 ▣). Note that the entire bladder should be scanned from the symphysis pubis to past the bladder dome. This will avoid

the pitfall demonstrated in Videos 4.10 and 4.11 ▣. Video 4.10 ▣ demonstrates a false-negative transverse suprapubic view, while in Video 4.11 ▣, a more thorough scan demonstrates that the 'bladder' is, in fact, free fluid delimited by the pelvic brim.

Troubleshooting

In the RUQ and LUQ views, locating the kidney may be difficult initially because of its posterior nature. Often, a more posterior placement of the probe is required. Always 'aim' the probe towards the kidney. If truly unable to find the kidneys in the typical location, check the right and left iliac fossae and pelvis for ectopic pelvic kidneys. Be mindful of other anatomical variants such as horseshoe kidneys.

The next challenge is finding an acceptable image while looking through the intercostal spaces. Ask the patient to inspire and expire to bring desired structures into view, and rotate the probe to align it parallel to the ribs, to scan through the intercostal spaces.

For the pelvic examination, the bladder is best seen when full. An empty bladder can make identification of important structures very difficult, and it can be difficult to locate! With the probe midline in the sagittal plane, fan/slide the probe inferiorly until the symphysis pubis comes into view. With this as a landmark on the right of the screen, the empty bladder typically appears as a small, triangular structure located superiorly.

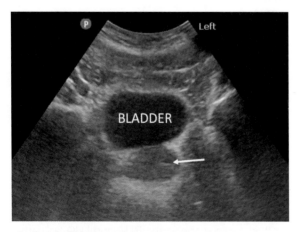

Figure 4.5 Ultrasound image: transverse view of the male pelvis, negative for free fluid. Note the prostate (arrowed) deep to the bladder.

Image interpretation

Normal appearance

Examples of the normal appearance of the different views of the abdomen are shown in Figures 4.4 to 4.6 and Videos 4.1, 4.4, 4.6, and 4.7 🎥.

Abnormal appearance

Fluid will accumulate between the interfaces being scanned. It usually appears as a hypoechoic stripe (unless clotted). Images of fluid in each area are shown in Figure 4.7 and Videos 4.2, 4.3, 4.5, and 4.8 to 4.11 🎥.

Factors that hinder interpretation: 'pitfalls'

Several factors can hinder the interpretation of abdominal PoCUS. If performed too early in the patient's course, PoCUS can be falsely negative because there has not been enough time for sufficient fluid to accumulate. Clinicians should re-scan patients when the clinical situation changes or when suspicion is high.

Some authors advocate scanning only Morison's pouch; however, this decreases the sensitivity of PoCUS. Taking care to systematically examine all three views discussed in 'Patient position, surface anatomy, and key landmarks', p. 105 will improve the sensitivity and specificity of PoCUS.

Intra-abdominal adhesions can localize intra-peritoneal fluid in areas potentially inaccessible to PoCUS, thus causing false-negative results. The presence of abdominal surgical scars or a history of multiple abdominal surgeries should alert the clinician to the possibility of intra-abdominal adhesions.

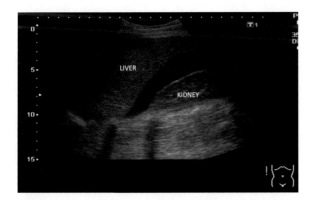

Figure 4.7 Ultrasound image: free fluid in Morison's pouch, seen as a dark stripe between the liver and the kidney.

Clinicians should also consider that PoCUS is not intended to quantify the amount of free intra-peritoneal fluid. PoCUS gives a binary answer—either intra-peritoneal fluid is present or it is not. As with other PoCUS applications, interpretation of this result depends on the clinical scenario and patient condition. While there have been scoring systems developed to help determine the amount and severity of haemoperitoneum in trauma, these scoring systems still require further study.

Clinical use

Interpretation and clinical application of PoCUS results depend on the clinical scenario and patient condition. In the trauma patient, the algorithm for integrating PoCUS into clinical decision-making was clarified by the International Consensus Conference recommendations, as summarized in Figure 4.1s 🖼. In the trauma patient, use of PoCUS for evaluation of haemoperitoneum has become the standard of care, with its use recommended by organizations such as Advanced Trauma Life Support (ATLS), Eastern Association for the Surgery of Trauma (EAST), and the American College of Radiology.

Differentiating between types of peritoneal fluid, and paracentesis

As well as determining whether trauma patients require operative intervention, PoCUS can also help to guide paracentesis of peritoneal fluid, and to differentiate between transudative (anechoic) and exudative (echoic or anechoic) effusions, based on their ultrasound appearance. A discussion of these applications is beyond the scope of this chapter, and interested readers are directed to the references at the end of this chapter (see 'Further reading', p. 105).

Gall bladder disease (focused biliary PoCUS)

Purpose

PoCUS can accurately detect the presence of gallstones, as well as signs suggestive of cholecystitis in patients with suspected biliary pathology. Dilatation of the CBD may also be detected (suggestive of biliary obstruction), though this is technically more difficult.

Perspective

It is estimated that 20 million people in the United States have gall bladder disease, and somewhere between 2.5% and 12% of emergency hospital visits are related to gallstone disease (cholelithiasis). Despite its high prevalence, diagnosis can be difficult and often relies on a formal ultrasound scan performed in the Radiology Department. A systematic review of 61 articles found formal ultrasound to be 97% sensitive and 95% specific for the detection of gallstones. The use of PoCUS to assess for gall bladder disease has been shown to decrease costs, as well as the length of ED stay.

A recent ACEP policy statement on the use of ultrasound states that the primary focus of RUQ PoCUS is to identify or exclude gallstones. A recent systematic review demonstrated that PoCUS detects gallstones in symptomatic ED patients with a sensitivity of 89.8%. This suggests that PoCUS can be used to reliably rule out cholelithiasis in patients presenting with symptoms of suspected biliary origin. Despite this, the presence of gallstones may be an incidental finding in patients with RUQ pain of a different origin.

Image generation

Probe selection and machine settings

Use a curvilinear (abdominal) 2.5–5 MHz probe to allow maximal tissue penetration. Set the image depth initially to 15 cm (to visualize acoustic shadowing from gallstones), and then reduce the depth to more clearly visualize the gall bladder itself. For very superficially placed gall bladders (e.g. in slim patients), increase the frequency and even consider using a linear probe (see also 'Troubleshooting', p. 95).

Patient position, surface anatomy, and key landmarks

The RUQ exam may be performed with the patient in the supine or left lateral position. However, accuracy is improved if both positions are used and, in fact, it is sometimes useful to sit the patient up in order to determine whether a gallstone is impacted. Position the probe initially in the longitudinal (sagittal) plane, just below the xiphoid process in the midline. Angle the probe cephalad, and then sweep it slowly to the right, just below the costal margin (see Figure 4.2s 🎥). The liver should be visible on the screen at this point.

As you slide the probe down to the right (parallel to, and just below, the costal margin) (see Figure 4.2s 🎥), the anechoic gall bladder should come into view. If this does not occur (e.g. in a non-fasted patient with a contracted gall bladder), then reduce the depth and increase the frequency. Ask the patient to take a deep breath in and to hold it—this usually serves to push the liver and gall bladder into view and to push the gas-filled bowel out of view. Or ask the patient to push their abdomen out against the probe—this can remove intervening gas-filled bowel and improve your window.

An alternative approach is to image the gall bladder via the trans-hepatic window; and, in fact, it is good practice to use both windows. The disadvantage of this second window is that the ribs' acoustic shadows can limit the view, but the advantage is that bowel gas does not intervene. For the trans-hepatic window, position the probe over the liver/lower right ribs in the coronal plane, level with the xiphoid process on the anterior to mid-axillary line. This is similar to the RUQ view in the FAST scan (see Figure 4.2), but with the probe placed more anteriorly on the chest wall and aligned between and parallel to the ribs. Fan the probe anteriorly to bring the gall bladder into view.

As with any organ or area of interest, one should image the gall bladder in its entirety, in both planes (transverse and longitudinal), and ideally from both windows described above. Take particular care to carefully assess the area *deep/distal* to the bladder, for acoustic shadowing from gallstones.

The CBD may be visualized as part of *the portal triad*, along with the hepatic artery (HA) and portal vein (PV) at the porta hepatis. The CBD lies anterior to the PV, and the HA may be seen to lie between and alongside the two.

The portal triad and CBD are most easily identified with the patient in the left lateral position. Place the probe at the base of the xiphoid in the transverse oblique position, and angle up towards the liver. Identify the gall bladder, then follow the main lobar fissure from the neck of the gall bladder to the porta hepatis (see Figures 4.8 and 4.9).

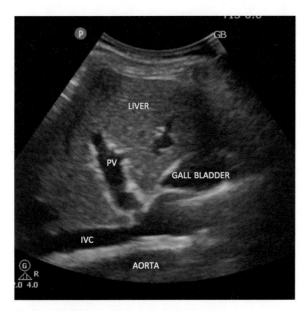

Figure 4.8 Ultrasound image: aorta, inferior vena cava (IVC), portal vein (PV), and gall bladder, visualized from the trans-hepatic (RUQ) window.

Courtesy of Dr Zoltan Galambos.

An alternative approach is to identify the vascular structures from the trans-hepatic coronal plane described above. With the probe in this plane, the liver is imaged from right (top of the screen) to left (bottom of the screen). At the anatomical left (bottom of the on-screen image), first identify the IVC and aorta. Fan the probe anteriorly until the PV comes into view—this is the largest vascular structure that traverses the liver

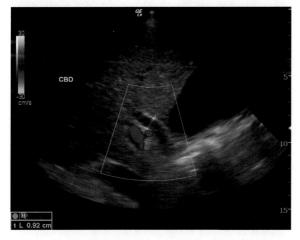

Figure 4.9 Ultrasound image: portal vein, hepatic artery, and dilated common bile duct (CBD) imaged using colour flow Doppler. CBD measured at 0.9 cm (9 mm).

and, unlike the hepatic veins, it does not run into the IVC (see Figure 4.8). Zoom onto the PV, and align the probe parallel to this. A very slight fanning motion will usually reveal the CBD as a very small structure lying anterior to the PV (above the PV on the screen). Usually the HA will also be seen.

To differentiate the CBD from the adjacent PV and HA, ask the patient to hold their breath while the image of the portal triad is zoomed; then scan using colour flow Doppler. With the Doppler scale or 'PRF' set at or below 20 cm/s, flow will be seen in the PV and HA, but not in the CBD (see Figure 4.9). Measure the diameter of the CBD at its widest.

Troubleshooting

Large body habitus, bowel gas, and a recent meal (causing the gall bladder to contract) are the main obstacles to visualization of the gall bladder. In the case of *large body habitus*, increasing the depth and lowering the frequency of the probe can increase the penetration of the beam and aid visualization of deep structures. If *bowel gas* interferes with image acquisition, several techniques can be used to help visualize the gall bladder. A sustained inspiration will lower the gall bladder towards the probe, and placing the patient in the left lateral decubitus position will displace the air-filled bowel to the left, away from the probe. Alternatively, ask the patient to push their abdomen out towards the probe, to remove intervening air-filled bowel.

Paradoxically, the gall bladder can also be difficult to recognize in very thin people because it is so superficial. In this case, change to a linear probe and scan again.

Image interpretation

Normal appearance

The normal, non-contracted gall bladder appears on ultrasound as a fluid-filled (anechoic), thin-walled cystic structure (see Figure 4.10). Wall thickness is measured between the gall bladder lumen and the hepatic parenchyma with a normal thickness of <3 mm. Similarly, the normal CBD will be 6 mm or less in diameter. Older patients may have a normally dilated duct (by approximately 1 mm for every decade past the age of 40), and the CBD may be normally dilated up to 10 mm after cholecystectomy (see Figure 4.9).

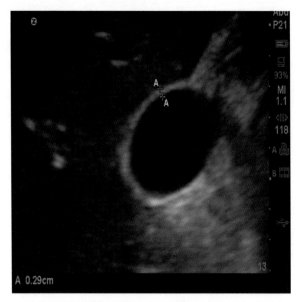

Figure 4.10 **Ultrasound image: normal gall bladder. Gall bladder wall thickness measured at 0.29 cm (2.9 mm).**

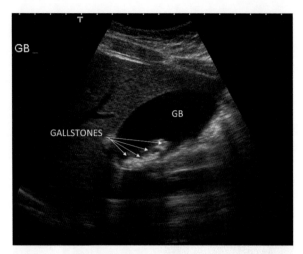

Figure 4.11 **Cholelithiasis. A long-axis view of the gall bladder (GB) showing multiple echogenic gallstones with characteristic acoustic shadowing.**

Abnormal appearance

Particular note should be made of the following findings.

Cholelithiasis (gallstones)

A gallstone appears as a variably sized, rounded echogenic structure, usually with an associated acoustic shadow (see Figure 4.11 and Video 4.12 ▣). Incidental gallstones are usually mobile and will 'roll' to the most dependent portion of the gall bladder. Gallstones impacted in the gall bladder neck cause biliary colic and are the most common cause of cholecystitis.

Sludge will appear as a grey, semi-solid area within the gall bladder, usually without shadowing (see Figure 4.12).

Sonographic Murphy's sign

The sonographic Murphy's sign is positive when the point of maximal tenderness is identified directly under the ultrasound probe in the RUQ, while the gall bladder is identified in the middle of the ultrasound screen.

Thickened gall bladder wall and pericholecystic fluid

(See Figure 4.13.) The most common cause of gall bladder wall thickening is acute cholecystitis. In this condition, the oedematous wall is often visible as two echogenic lines separated by a central echo-poor layer, resembling 'train tracks'. Usually a stone will be seen, impacted in the gall bladder neck. Anechoic fluid may be found around an acutely inflamed gall bladder where it is described as 'pericholecystic fluid'. It is most often seen posterior to the gall bladder and around the neck, but it may also be seen layering on the anterior wall.

Dilated common bile duct

This may indicate biliary obstruction in the appropriate clinical setting (see Figures 4.9 and 4.14 and Videos 4.13 and 4.14 ▣).

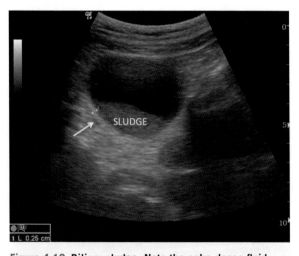

Figure 4.12 **Biliary sludge. Note the echo-dense fluid within the gall bladder and localized free fluid (arrowed) indicating early cholecystitis. Gall bladder wall thickness measured at 0.25 cm (2.5 mm).**

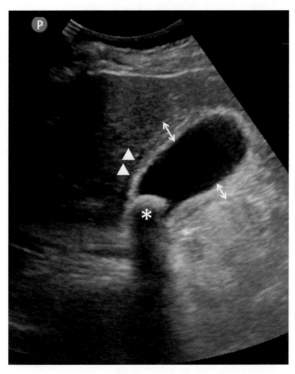

Figure 4.13 **Cholecystitis. In addition to the gallstone (asterisk), note the wall thickening and 'tram tracking' due to wall oedema (bracket), as well as pericholecystic fluid (arrowheads).**

Image courtesy Dr Mo Haywood.

Pitfalls

Polyps may be confused with stones (see Figure 4.3s 🖼). However, polyps will not roll and do not cause shadowing.

False-negative scans can occur with small stones and with impacted stones obscured by overlying bowel

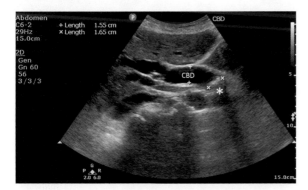

Figure 4.14 **Dilated common bile duct (CBD) measured at 1.55 cm (15 mm), due to impacted stone (asterisk).**

Image courtesy Dr Ahilan Parameswaran.

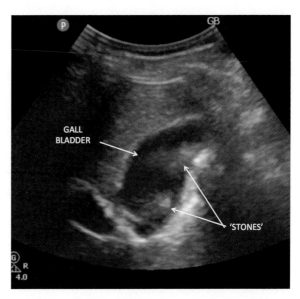

Figure 4.15 **False gallstones (arrowed) due to bowel gas adjacent to the gall bladder, incorporated into the gall bladder image due to artefact.**

gas or a fatty liver. This is why it is important to visualize the neck of the gall bladder. Smaller gallstones may not shadow. To see the smallest gallstones, use the highest available frequency and deactivate compounding or 'multibeam' on the machine.

Another false negative is 'wall echo shadow', wherein a contracted gall bladder containing multiple stones can be mistakenly identified as bowel gas. The echogenic leading edges of the stones obscure the gall bladder itself (see Figure 4.4s 🖼). A clue is that the stones' combined shadow does not move with peristalsis.

False-negative scans for cholecystitis tend to occur early in the disease—most of the gall bladder may appear 'normal', and only a small area of the gall bladder wall will be thickened. Cholecystitis is a dynamic disease process, and repeat scans are sometimes required.

False positives for gallstones include polyps and gall bladder carcinoma. False positives for acoustic shadowing include edge shadowing artefact (seen at the edges of all cystic or rounded structures) and 'dirty' shadowing from bowel gas in the adjacent duodenum (see Videos 4.12 and 4.15 🎬). In fact, slice thickness artefact can cause bowel gas in the duodenum to be 'incorporated' into the image of an otherwise normal gall bladder where it can resemble a gallstone (see Figure 4.15). However, careful fanning will reveal that the 'echogenic stone' is, in fact, air adjacent to the gall bladder. This is one reason why it is important to scan the entire gall bladder very carefully.

Other causes of gall bladder wall thickening and pericholecystic fluid include ascites (see Video 4.16 📹), congestive heart failure, nearby inflammation (such as hepatitis), and gall bladder carcinoma.

CBD dilatation (see Figures 4.9 and 4.14 and Videos 4.13 and 4.14 📹) is a marker of choledocholithiasis and cholangitis, but one should note that these conditions may occur in the presence of a normal-diameter CBD (usually early in the disease process) and that a dilated CBD can be normal in certain patients, as described in 'Normal appearance', p. 95. This is analogous to the fact that hydronephrosis is not identical to ureteric colic.

Clinical use

The results of a PoCUS exam must be interpreted within the context of the clinical and laboratory findings. The presence of gallstones is significant, because it is the primary criterion in diagnosing acute cholecystitis and because 90–95% of patients with acute cholecystitis have gallstones. In the ICU setting, caution is required in patients with burns, severe multisystem trauma, or total parenteral nutrition, as these groups have a higher incidence of acalculous cholecystitis. To establish the sonographic diagnosis of acute cholecystitis, secondary signs, such as pericholecystic fluid, a thickened gall bladder wall, or a sonographic Murphy's sign, must be elicited. CBD dilatation may provide evidence of biliary stasis or obstruction.

Hydronephrosis (focused renal PoCUS)

Purpose

PoCUS can detect the presence of hydronephrosis, which, in turn, may provide evidence of ureteric obstruction. PoCUS can also rule out other important pathology such as an abdominal aortic aneurysm (AAA) in this patient group.

Perspective

PoCUS for hydronephrosis can provide important clinical information in several settings. In the setting of

acute renal failure, PoCUS can rapidly determine if the cause is post-renal, i.e. an obstructive uropathy. Identification of this surgical emergency can expedite specific interventions, such as nephrostomy, or may identify a distal obstruction by demonstrating an enlarged bladder and bilateral hydronephrosis. In the setting of sepsis, evidence of renal obstruction identifies the need for rapid surgical/radiological intervention. In the setting of suspected ureteric colic, the presence of hydronephrosis makes this diagnosis more likely. However, PoCUS alone cannot rule out the presence of renal stones, and CT remains the investigation of choice.

Image generation

Probe selection and machine settings

An abdominal (low-frequency curvilinear) probe should be used to allow maximal tissue penetration. The machine should be initially set to maximum depth and then adjusted as appropriate.

Patient position, surface anatomy, and key landmarks

The renal exam is performed with the patient in the supine or lateral position. The probe is positioned in the longitudinal (coronal) plane, laterally on the posterior axillary line, angled posteriorly by about 30 degrees, similar to the position used for the RUQ and LUQ windows of the FAST scan. The liver/spleen provide the acoustic windows. The probe can then be rotated slightly (aligned with the rib spaces) to obtain a long-axis view of the kidney (see Figure 4.16 and

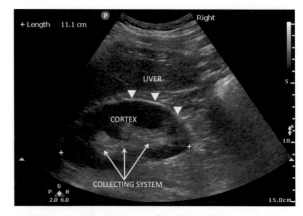

Figure 4.16 Normal right kidney, long axis. Arrowheads indicate an echogenic renal capsule.

Videos 4.1 to 4.3 📷). Each kidney should be visualized entirely by fanning the probe anteroposteriorly and then in short axis by turning the probe 90° and repeating the sweep.

If the patient can be turned, place them in the lateral decubitus position, corresponding to the opposite kidney (i.e. left lateral for the right kidney). The kidney can then be approached directly by placing the probe obliquely in the costovertebral angle or even from an anterior approach. Again, each kidney should be visualized in two planes. Apply colour Doppler across the renal sinus to delineate renal vessels (see Video 4.17 📷). Asking the patient to hold a deep breath (inspiratory hold) can help lower the kidneys towards the probe.

The bladder is an anechoic cystic structure in the pelvis, which expands from a contracted pyramidal shape to a near-spherical shape as it fills. Its volume may be calculated from a simple measurement. Scan the bladder in sagittal and transverse planes, as for the free fluid examination described in 'Abdominal free fluid', p. 92, holding the probe just cephalad to the pubic symphysis and angling the probe caudally into the pelvis (see Videos 4.6 to 4.9 📷). Applying colour Doppler to the base of the bladder will allow visualization of the ureteric jets, which appear as colourful jets shooting into the bladder (see Videos 4.18 and 4.19 📷). Several minutes should be allowed to detect each jet.

For tips on image generation, please refer to Troubleshooting in the 'Abdominal free fluid' section, p. 92.

Image interpretation

Each kidney sits within an echo-bright capsule, surrounded by echo-poor (dark) perinephric fat (see Figures 4.16 to 4.19 and Videos 4.1 to 4.3 📷). The kidney can be divided into the renal cortex and medulla (dark grey on ultrasound) and the central echo-bright renal sinus that contains the normally collapsed pelvicalyceal system, renal vessels, and fibrofatty tissue. Normally, the renal pelvis and calyces cannot be visualized, resulting in the echo-bright renal sinus.

With hydronephrosis, these structures dilate due to obstructed outflow of urine and are seen as an anechoic area in the renal pelvis (see Figures 4.17 and 4.18). There is no absolute threshold for the diagnosis

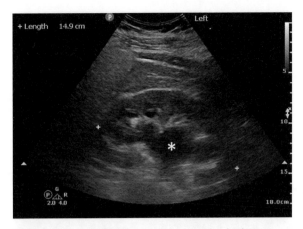

Figure 4.17 Acute hydronephrosis. Asterisk indicates a dilated collecting system.

Image courtesy Dr Jade Knights.

of hydronephrosis; however, the key finding is calyceal dilatation, as renal pelvic dilatation may be normal. Hydronephrosis can be graded as mild, moderate, and severe, depending on the extent of calyceal dilatation. Chronic hydronephrosis will lead to cortical thinning (see Figure 4.18).

If hydronephrosis is due to a stone (calculus) impacted in the ureter, the ureteric jet will be absent on that side. If the ureter is only partly obstructed, there may be a non-pulsatile and constant ureteric jet, which is considered abnormal (see Video 4.20 📷). If the stone is impacted in the vesicoureteric junction (VUJ), a 'twinkling' artefact may be seen with colour Doppler.

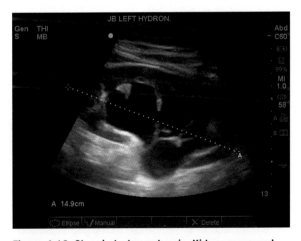

Figure 4.18 Chronic hydronephrosis. Kidney measured at 14.9 cm (enlarged). Note thinning of the capsule, compared to the kidney imaged in Figure 4.22.

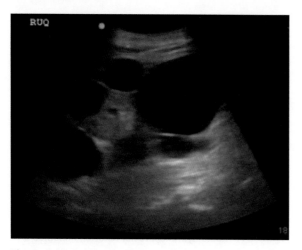

Figure 4.19 Polycystic kidney.

Pitfalls

The medullary pyramids, which are dark grey, should not be confused for dilated calyces. Other pitfalls include mistaking renal cysts for hydronephrosis (see Figure 4.19) or excluding obstructive uropathy in dehydrated patients, when hydronephrosis may not be seen. Dilated calyces should become confluent with the renal pelvis and will not show any flow on colour Doppler imaging.

AAA may mimic renal colic in older patients and should always be considered (and scanned) prior to diagnosing renal colic.

Clinical use

Assessment of the kidneys for hydronephrosis and assessment of the bladder for size and ureteric flow are useful adjuncts to the clinical assessment for patients with suspected renal colic or acute renal failure. Formal sonography or CT scanning should, however, be considered when available.

Bowel obstruction

Purpose

Traditionally, ultrasound is not the first imaging modality of choice in patients with suspected bowel obstruction because: (a) air in the dilated bowel may obscure the ultrasound images and render diagnosis difficult, and (b) ultrasound rarely demonstrates the cause of the obstruction. However, the presence of *fluid-filled* bowel loops can allow ultrasound to make the diagnosis. Ultrasound can even be the preferred modality in some situations, e.g. in the patient whose abdominal X-ray is inconclusive (because the bowel loops are filled with fluid, rather than air) or in the patient for whom one wishes to avoid ionizing radiation (e.g. the pregnant patient). Ultrasound can also differentiate obstruction from paralytic ileus.

Ultrasound can only 'rule in' bowel obstruction. It is unable to rule it out.

Perspective

Why use ultrasound?

Many clinicians have now replaced the abdominal X-ray series with ultrasound when assessing for small bowel obstruction in the acute care setting, because of its advantages described above (see previous section, 'Purpose').

How good is ultrasound at diagnosing the condition?

Studies have shown that ultrasound compares favourably with the abdominal X-ray in the diagnosis of bowel obstruction.

Image generation

Probe selection and machine settings

Begin with a curvilinear probe for the initial 'scout scan', and change to the linear probe when finer detail is required (e.g. when assessing vascularity of the bowel wall).

Patient position, surface anatomy, and key landmarks

Begin with the patient supine, although one may need to roll the patient into the left lateral position if the bowel is difficult to visualize. This manoeuvre will allow gas-filled bowel to 'float up' to the less dependent portion of the abdomen, leaving any fluid-filled bowel easier to interrogate.

Technique

When performing the initial 'scout' scan, be as systematic as possible, ensuring that you scan all quadrants of the anterior abdomen. For example, begin in the RUQ and then proceed to 'mow' the abdomen from cephalad to caudad and from right to left. Once a bowel loop is identified, image it in both its long and transverse axes.

Normal bowel: ultrasound features

Normal *duodenum* is difficult to assess with ultrasound. It lies between the gall bladder and the head of the pancreas. Scatter from air in its lumen can cause 'dirty shadowing' that resembles gallstone shadowing (see Video 4.15). As the gall bladder is often adjacent to the duodenum, this can cause confusion when scanning for gallstones.

The normal *jejunum and ileum* lie more centrally in the abdomen and display the following features on ultrasound:

- Fluid- or air-filled tubular structures;
- Compressible;
- AP diameter of each loop <3 cm;
- Wall thickness ≤3 mm;
- Peristalsis (see Video 4.21);
- Valvulae conniventes: thick and prominent in the jejunum, and nearly absent in the ileum (see Video 4.22).

The normal *caecum and the large intestine* have the following appearance:

- The ascending colon and caecum lie in the right flank. The descending colon lies in the left flank. The transverse colon lies below the liver in the epigastrium;
- Gas and faeces intermingle, generating an appearance of 'dirty scatter' (see Video 4.23);
- No valvulae conniventes. Instead, the colon has *haustra*—folds that do not fully cross the lumen;
- No peristalsis (see Video 4.23).

Bowel obstruction: ultrasound features

- Dilated bowel loops: small intestine ≥3 cm (see Figure 4.20), large intestine ≥6 cm (see Figure 4.21), and caecum >9 cm; initially with vigorous peristalsis proximal to the site of obstruction, often visible as a 'back-and forth' motion on ultrasound (see Videos 4.24 and 4.25)
- The site of obstruction may be seen (also known as the 'transition point').

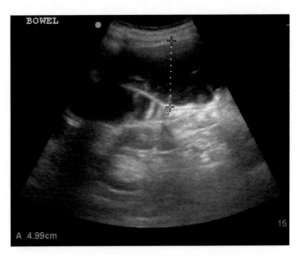

Figure 4.20 Small bowel obstruction (bowel diameter 4.99 cm).

Image courtesy Dr Juan Chiang.

Other findings

- The *cause* of obstruction may be visualized, e.g. intussusception, gallstone, tumour, or bezoar.
- *Complications* of obstruction such as infarction (free fluid surrounding bowel loops and absent blood flow on Doppler assessment).

Pitfalls: factors that hinder interpretation

False negatives

- The most common reason for missing the diagnosis with ultrasound is the presence of intervening air-filled bowel.

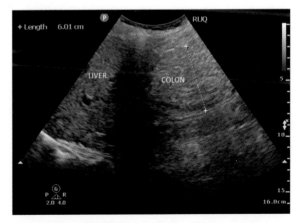

Figure 4.21 Large bowel obstruction (bowel diameter 6.01 cm).

Image courtesy Dr Dirk Bass.

- For this reason, it is imperative to scan the *entire abdomen* before one can rule out bowel obstruction.

Differential diagnosis

- *Paralytic ileus* will also demonstrate dilated, fluid-filled bowel, but peristalsis will be absent.

Appendicitis

Purpose

The role of ultrasound in the patient with suspected appendicitis is to: (a) confirm the diagnosis by identifying a distended, non-compressible appendix at the site of tenderness, or (b) exclude the diagnosis by identifying a normal appendix, or (c) exclude differential diagnoses.

Note that ultrasound can only 'rule out' appendicitis if a normal appendix is visualized, and this is difficult, even for experienced sonographers.

Perspective

The appendix is a blind-ended loop that arises from the caecum (just near the ileocaecal valve) in the RIF. Its length is typically 10 cm, but it may be as long as 20 cm. Although it typically lies medially in the RIF, its location may be quite variable. *Appendicitis* refers to inflammation of the appendix, typically caused by obstruction due to an appendicolith. Other causes include obstruction due to tumour, parasites, and lymphadenopathy. Appendicitis is a surgical emergency. Left untreated, the appendix perforates and the patient may die.

Why use ultrasound?

Traditionally, the diagnosis of appendicitis is made using a combination of clinical features (fever, pain migrating to the RIF, tenderness and peritonism at McBurney's point, and eponymous signs such as Rovsing's, psoas, and obturator) and blood tests (elevated white cell count). Ultrasound has gained in popularity as a non-invasive method of confirming the diagnosis and ruling out differential diagnoses such as a tubo-ovarian abscess. Contrast CT is more accurate but exposes the patient to the risks of ionizing radiation and contrast nephropathy.

How good is ultrasound at diagnosing the condition?

A systematic review of the literature concluded that appendiceal ultrasound had an overall sensitivity of 86% and a specificity of 81%, a positive predictive value of 84%, and a negative predictive value of 85%. However, these figures are extremely dependent on operator experience, as well as patient factors (age, body habitus, and sex), and finally the location of the appendix itself (with the retrocaecal location being the most difficult to image).

Image generation

Probe selection and machine settings

A curvilinear probe is employed for a 'scout scan' (see step 1 in 'Technique', p. 102) and is often required in the obese patient and/or in the case of a retrocaecal appendix.

Although it may seem counterintuitive, the linear probe is often preferred to the curvilinear probe because of its better resolution. Ideally select as wide a linear probe as possible to limit patient discomfort. Consider activating the trapezoid or 'virtual convex' mode, if available, to broaden the field of view. Select a preset with a good dynamic range such as 'thyroid' or 'nerve', and begin with a depth of approximately 5 cm.

Patient position, surface anatomy, and key landmarks

Begin with the patient supine, although one may need to roll the patient into the left lateral position if the appendix is difficult to visualize. Ensure the patient has had adequate analgesia (e.g. with intravenous opiate) prior to scanning (graded compression ultrasound is painful).

Technique

The key to diagnosis is *graded compression ultrasound*, i.e. identifying the appendix and then carefully attempting to compress it. An inflamed, obstructed appendix is *non-compressible*. As described in 'How good is ultrasound at diagnosing the condition', above, the success of graded compression ultrasound in locating the appendix depends on multiple factors—not least of which are time, patience, and a systematic approach. There are many scanning techniques reported. The following technique is typical.

1. The 'scout scan': this is typically performed with a curvilinear probe and is simply a FAST scan limited to a search for free intra-peritoneal fluid.

2. The author (JB) recommends a more focused 'scout' scan (with a curved and also a linear probe) at the site of maximal tenderness. Ask the patient to place a finger on the site of maximal tenderness, and then place the probe there.

3. If the appendix is not seen, the next step is to identify the caecum. Place the probe aligned transversely, just to the right of the umbilicus. The caecum lies caudally and laterally within the abdomen, and it can be identified by the 'dirty scatter' of air in the faeces within its lumen (see Video 4.23 📷).

4. Slide the probe distally, and identify the terminal ileum entering the caecum at the *ileocaecal junction* (see Video 4.23 📷). The ileum lies above the iliac vessels and is recognizably part of the small intestine. By contrast with the caecum, it is smooth-walled, with a smaller diameter of 1–2 cm, demonstrates valvulae conniventes, actively peristalses, and contains fluid—therefore, its posterior wall is often visible (unlike that of the caecum).

5. After identifying the ileocaecal junction (which is about 2 cm above the base of the caecum), scan inferiorly to the base of the caecum. The appendix arises from the posteromedial aspect of the caecum (also check for free fluid around here) (see Video 4.26 📷).

6. If still unable to locate the appendix, continue sliding the probe caudally, *past* the tip of the caecum (see Figure 4.5s 📷).

7. Then turn the probe sagittally, and slide it medially, past the caecum, in order to identify the appendix in cross-section (see Figure 4.6s 📷).

8. Identify the iliac vessels. The appendix may lie draped over these. Turn the probe parallel to these, and look for the appendix in cross-section (see Figure 4.7s 📷).

9. If the appendix has still not been seen, it may be retrocaecal. Roll the patient to the left, and look to the right of, and deep to, the caecum.

10. Use the bladder as a window, and scan deep to this, in case of pelvic lie.

11. If all else fails, consider arranging a trans-vaginal scan in female patients of childbearing age.

Once the appendix is visualized, scan its *entire length* in both longitudinal and transverse planes (important for localized appendicitis).

Troubleshooting

The caecum can often be difficult to locate and identify. This is due to multiple factors:

- A full bladder pushing the caecum higher than expected;
- Patient position can vary the location of the caecum;
- Maldescent of the caecum;
- Situs inversus;
- Other pelvic factors such as fibroids and pregnancy.

For this reason, some sonographers recommend using the *external iliac vessels* as the starting point, as their location is usually consistent. Identify the normal ileum lying anterior to these vessels, then proceed as above.

Normal appendix: ultrasound features

The normal appendix displays the following features on ultrasound:

- Tubular structure arising from the base of the caecum;
- Blind-ended;
- Non-peristaltic;
- AP diameter of 6 mm or less;
- 'Target' sign with alternating anechoic and echogenic layers visible on ultrasound (see Figures 4.8s 📷 and 4.22);
- Compressible (see Figure 4.22).

Appendicitis: ultrasound features

- Point of maximum tenderness with ultrasound probe is over the site of the appendix = analogous to an 'ultrasound McBurney's sign'.

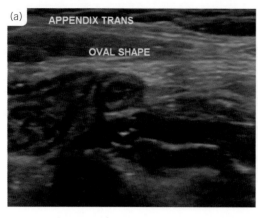
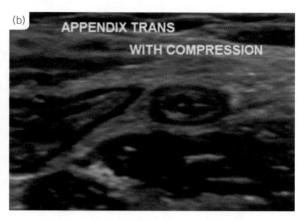

Figure 4.22 Ultrasound image: normal appendix in transverse section. (a) Uncompressed. (b) Compressed.

Image courtesy Rona Girdler, Royal North Shore Hospital Radiology Department.

- AP diameter of >6 mm (see Figure 4.23).

- Non-compressible.

- Appendicolith (see Figure 4.24).

Secondary features

These may be present in appendicitis but do not, in themselves, confirm the diagnosis:

- Echogenic fat surrounding the appendix: inflamed intra-abdominal fat is bright (displays increased echogenicity on ultrasound) and visible in 91% of patients with appendicitis (see Figure 4.25);

- Altered Doppler signal of the appendix (usually increased flow due to hyperaemia but may be decreased, or even absent, if gangrenous);

- No peristalsis of adjacent bowel;

- Surrounding pathological fluid may be present if perforated/localized abscess.

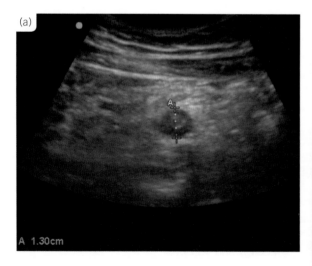
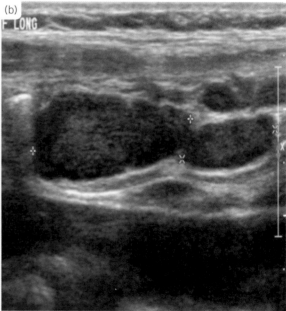

Figure 4.23 Ultrasound images: appendicitis and a mimic. (a) Appendicitis: appendiceal diameter 1.3 cm (imaged in transverse section). (b) Appendix mimic: lymph node.

(a) Image courtesy of Dr Darmas Turner; (b) Image courtesy Rona Girdler, Royal North Shore Hospital Radiology Department.

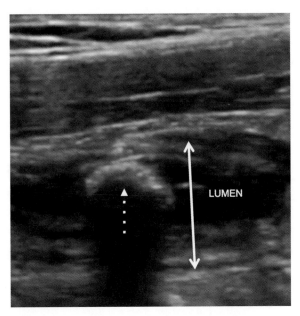

Figure 4.24 Ultrasound image: appendicitis with appendicolith (dotted arrow). Appendix imaged in longitudinal section, diameter indicated by solid arrow.

Pitfalls: factors that hinder interpretation

False negatives

- Possibly the most common pitfall is inadequate compression. The successful operator uses compression first to move intervening bowel 'out of the way' and then to confirm that the appendix cannot be compressed.
- For this reason, it is imperative to scan the *entire length* of the appendix from the base to the tip, in both *longitudinal and transverse planes*, before one can rule out appendicitis.
- Early appendicitis (particularly if the tip of the appendix is not seen on ultrasound).
- If the appendix has already perforated, it may no longer be enlarged.
- Conditions in whom sonography may be technically difficult or non-diagnostic (e.g. obesity, tense ascites, severe pain, retrocaecal appendicitis, and pregnancy).

False positives

False positives (ultrasound mimics of appendicitis) can also occur. For example, a dilated appendix may be seen in Crohn's disease, and a dilated Fallopian tube may resemble an inflamed appendix. However, in neither case will the inflamed tubular structure be obstructed. Another differential diagnosis which can mimic appendicitis is Meckel's diverticulum, which arises from the *ileum* (rather than the caecum). Even a lymph node may be mistaken for a non-compressible appendix, but fanning through the structure will quickly demonstrate that it is not tubular (see Figure 4.23).

Acknowledgement

Thanks to Rona Girdler and her colleagues, General Sonography Department, Royal North Shore Hospital, Sydney, for their advice regarding appendiceal ultrasound.

🗐 Further reading

Additional further reading can be found in the Online appendix at www.oxfordmedicine.com/POCUSemergencymed. Please refer to your access card for further details.

American College of Emergency Physicians. *Policy Statement: Emergency Ultrasound Imaging Criteria Compendium.* Available from: https://www.acep.org/globalassets/new-pdfs/policy-statements/usimagingcriteriacompendium.pdf

Arrillaga A, Graham R, York JW, Miller RS. Increased efficiency and cost-effectiveness in the evaluation of the blunt

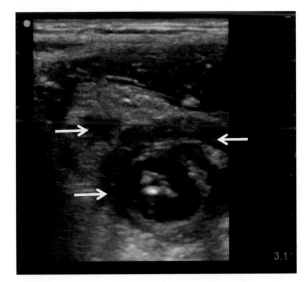

Figure 4.25 Ultrasound image: appendicitis with surrounding fluid (arrowed). Appendix imaged in transverse section.

abdominal trauma patient with the use of ultrasound. *Am Surg* 1999;**65**:31–5.

Melniker LA, Leibner E, McKenney MG, Lopez P, Briggs WM, Mancuso CA. Randomized controlled clinical trial of point-of-care, limited ultrasonography for trauma in the emergency department: the first sonography outcomes assessment program trial. *Ann Emerg Med* 2006;**48**:227–35.

Ross M, Brown M, McLaughlin K, *et al*. Emergency physician-performed ultrasound to diagnose cholelithiasis: a systematic review. *Acad Emerg Med* 2011;**18**:227–35.

Shah K, Wolf RE. Hepatobiliary ultrasound. *Emerg Med Clin North Am* 2004;**22**:661–73, viii.

Shea JA, Berlin JA, Escarce JJ, *et al*. Revised estimates of diagnostic test sensitivity and specificity in suspected biliary tract disease. *Arch Intern Med* 1994;**154**: 2573–81.

Stengel D, Bauwens K, Redemacher G, Ekkernkamp A, Güthoff C. Emergency ultrasound-based algorithms for diagnosing blunt abdominal trauma. *Cochrane Database Syst Rev* 2013;**7**:CD004446.

Teresawa T, Blackmore CC, Bent S, Kohlwes RJ. Systematic review: computed tomography and ultrasonography to detect acute appendicitis in adults and adolescents. *Ann Intern Med* 2004;**141**:537–46.

Zhou J, Huang J, Wu H, *et al*. Screening ultrasonography of 2,204 patients with blunt abdominal trauma in the Wenchuan earthquake. *J Trauma Acute Care Surg* 2012;**73**:890–4.

5

Early pregnancy and pelvic ultrasound

Ryan Henneberry, Chris Cox, Beatrice Hoffmann,
and Paul Atkinson

Summary

When to scan (clinical indications):
 To confirm intrauterine pregnancy (IUP)
 and to help rule out extra-uterine (ectopic)
 pregnancy (EUP).

What to scan (PoCUS protocol):
 Core: Identify the bladder, uterus, endometrial
 stripe, uterine contents, and pelvic free fluid.
 Advanced: Scan the adenexae and for other
 pelvic pathology.

How to scan (key points on scanning):
 Core: Trans-abdominal scanning with a full
 bladder—ensuring that the bladder and uterus
 are juxtaposed, scan through the complete
 uterus in longitudinal and transverse planes.
 Advanced: Trans-vaginal scanning with an
 empty bladder—scan through the complete
 uterus in longitudinal and transverse planes.
 There are no absolute contraindications to
 PoCUS in early pregnancy; however, recent
 gynaecological surgery is considered a relative
 contraindication to trans-vaginal PoCUS.

What PoCUS adds (clinical reasoning—how results
change practice):
 Core: Detect and *rule in* an IUP and exclude
 free fluid.
 Advanced: Ectopic pregnancies and other
 adnexal pathology can often be detected.

Purpose

This chapter will detail how PoCUS, combined with
other clinical parameters, enables the treating physician to accurately confirm the presence of an early
intrauterine pregnancy (IUP). We will provide our suggested approach for the use of bedside ultrasound
and clinical findings to safely assess patients with
first-trimester pregnancy pain or bleeding and rule out
ectopic pregnancy. Common incidental pelvic PoCUS
findings are also covered briefly.

Perspective

Undiagnosed ectopic, or extra-uterine pregnancy
(EUP), is still a major cause of maternal morbidity and
mortality. Up to 13% of pregnant patients presenting
to the ED with abdominal pain or vaginal bleeding
are eventually diagnosed with an ectopic pregnancy.
The physical examination is unreliable and cannot
distinguish between IUP, EUP, or ectopic pregnancy.
In this scenario, imaging with ultrasound and the development of clinical pathways become paramount
to securing the diagnosis and providing guidance for
managing these patients.

The rate of ectopic pregnancy has traditionally been
reported to be 1 in 80, while cases of heterotopic gestation are less frequent. In heterotopic pregnancy,
both IUP and EUP are simultaneously present. While
this event is unlikely, with an incidence of about 1 in

7000 in spontaneous pregnancies, the occurrence jumps to approximately 1% of all assisted reproductive pregnancies.

In a patient with a pregnancy in an unknown location (PUL), the diagnosis of an IUP greatly decreases the likelihood of a simultaneous EUP. Although the risk of a coexisting EUP is not zero and needs to be considered within a rule-out ectopic protocol, PoCUS can provide time and cost savings.

Beta-hCG and serum progesterone testing

The role of quantitative beta-human chorionic gonadotrophin (hCG) levels in diagnosing ectopic pregnancy remains very complex. Levels of the hormone can be quite variable throughout early pregnancy. The levels that determine if an IUP should be visible by means of both trans-abdominal (TA) and trans-vaginal (TV) ultrasound exams (the discriminatory zone) vary considerably. Safe management incorporates the use of beta-hCG discriminatory zones as part of an institution-defined clinical protocol (see Table 5.1). It is important to remember that failure to identify an IUP on PoCUS, with a beta-hCG level above these discriminatory values, does not automatically represent a case of an ectopic pregnancy. Furthermore, a single value of a low or a high beta-hCG level, or a mismatch in expected ultrasound findings, does not automatically define the pregnancy as failed or abnormal. Still, for the emergency physician, the possibility of an EUP should be suspected when no definite IUP can be identified and beta-hCG levels are above the suggested values for each ultrasound modality. Finally, there are also no lower 'cut-offs' for beta-hCG levels at which an EUP is impossible. Specifically, ectopic pregnancies have been confirmed with beta-hCG levels of <10 and also in cases with levels of >100,000. In recent years, the addition of a serum progesterone level has become more prevalent to help facilitate with the diagnosis of an early normal pregnancy. While the serum progesterone level can help distinguish a viable from a failing pregnancy, it cannot distinguish a failing IUP from an ectopic pregnancy and, as a result, is not a significant addition to the rule-out ectopic pregnancy algorithm in the ED.

Identifying intrauterine pregnancy— ultrasound findings

Trans-abdominal approach

Typically, a TA scan is performed using a curved array (curvilinear) transducer with a frequency of usually 3–5 MHz (see Figure 5.1s 🖼). Scanning is conducted in the longitudinal and transverse planes (see Figures 5.2s and 5.3s 🖼). The bladder should be full, in order to create an acoustic window and so that it can push unwanted bowel gas away from the uterus. In the longitudinal plane (see Figure 5.2s 🖼), the probe is placed with the marker pointing to the patient's head, just above the pubis symphysis, and directed caudally. The bladder and uterus should be readily identified on the ultrasound screen (see Figure 5.1). Failure to identify the bladder is often due to not having enough caudal tilt to the probe or not applying enough pressure to disperse unwanted bowel gas (see Figure 5.4s 🖼).

Table 5.1 Beta-hCG levels (mIU/mL) at which an intrauterine pregnancy (IUP) may be expected to be seen with point-of-care ultrasound

Technique	Minimum SI units for IUP by ultrasound
Trans-abdominal (TA) ultrasound	5000–6000 mIU/mL
Trans-vaginal (TV) ultrasound	1500–2000 mIU/mL

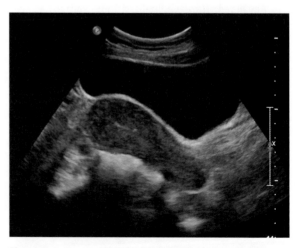

Figure 5.1 Trans-abdominal longitudinal view of the pelvis, demonstrating an anechoic, full bladder (B) in the near field and the uterus in the far field (U).

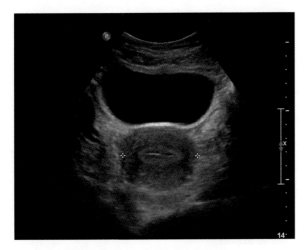

Figure 5.2 Trans-abdominal transverse view, demonstrating an anechoic bladder in the near field and the uterus labelled by calipers in the far field.

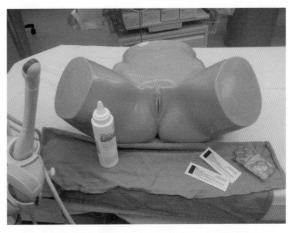

Figure 5.3 Trans-vaginal model. Used to facilitate learning of trans-vaginal approaches to early pregnancy.

Once the bladder is seen on the screen, the uterus can be identified by sliding the probe across the suprapubic region. It should be identified immediately posterior and cephalad to the bladder. The uterus will often be located slightly off midline. It is more difficult to locate when retroverted. Once the uterus is located, it is evaluated from fundus to cervix, looking for the echo-bright endometrial stripe and the subsequent potential signs of an IUP. The uterus is readily identified by its homogenous echogenicity, similar to that of hepatic or splenic tissue. PoCUS images generated in the transverse plane are demonstrated in Figure 5.2.

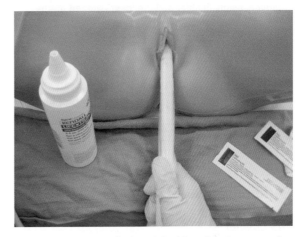

Figure 5.4 Trans-vaginal model with probe, demonstrating probe orientation for trans-vaginal sagittal scanning. Note the probe marker is anterior or on top.

Trans-vaginal approach

TV ultrasound is performed using an endocavitary probe with a frequency of 7.5–10 MHz (see Figure 5.5s 📷). The patient's bladder should be empty. It is typically performed in two planes: the sagittal and coronal plane (see Video 5.11 🎥). Probe position for these two planes are demonstrated in Figures 5.3 to 5.5. The probe handle notch or marker should be kept anterior, while scanning in the sagittal plane. It can be confusing to learn the orientation, while in either plane, and emphasis should be placed on identifying the key anatomical features: the bladder, the uterus, the endometrial stripe, and potential signs of an IUP. Examples of images obtained with TV PoCUS from commercially available models are demonstrated in Figures 5.6 and 5.7.

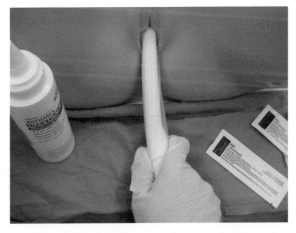

Figure 5.5 Trans-vaginal model with probe, demonstrating the orientation for trans-vaginal coronal scanning. Note the probe marker is located to the right of the mannequin.

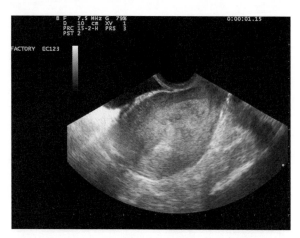

Figure 5.6 Trans-vaginal view of pelvis on the ultrasound screen. This view was obtained from a trans-vaginal model and is taken in the sagittal plane. Note the relatively empty bladder and the 'pear'-shaped uterus.

Use of M-mode

The M-mode is useful for identifying movement and, in particular, fetal cardiac activity. It can be helpful in confirming the presence of the fetal heart rate. A typical M-mode screen is demonstrated in Figure 5.8.

Performing the core scan

The bladder as an anatomical landmark

With the TA approach, transverse or longitudinal views are obtained for evaluation. With TV imaging, the

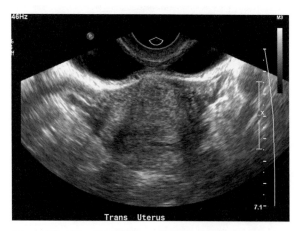

Figure 5.7 Ultrasound image of a trans-vaginal coronal view of the pelvis. Note the relatively empty bladder in the near field and the 'round' shape of the uterus.

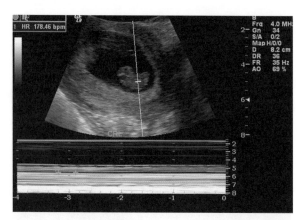

Figure 5.8 M-mode ultrasound image demonstrating fetal cardiac activity.

uterus is typically visualized in the coronal and sagittal planes.

In a standardized approach, one should begin with the TA technique. The bladder is easily identifiable when it is full and thus provides an 'acoustic window' for visualization of the uterus (see Figures 5.1 and 5.2). Once the bladder is identified, the uterus is seen immediately below, and adjacent to, the bladder.

The key point of identifying the juxtaposition of the bladder and uterus cannot be overemphasized, as endometrial-like appearing tissue from the adnexa can often be seen around an EUP, but this type of gestation will be frequently located *remotely* from the bladder.

The same concept also applies to the TV approach whereby the uterus is identified immediately adjacent to an empty bladder. Another key issue is the ability to recognize the borders of *normal* uterine tissue, as the tissue (or ring) around an EUP can be deceiving, but with close examination, it is *unlike* that of '*normal*' endometrial tissue.

Identifying the endometrial stripe

After identifying the bladder and the uterus, the next step would be to identify the endometrial stripe. Within the uterus, the layers of the endometrial wall oppose each other and create a sonographically identifiable, hyperechoic line, referred to as the endometrial stripe (see Figure 5.9). Depending on several factors, including age and timing of the menstrual cycle, the endometrial stripe can be more or less evident.

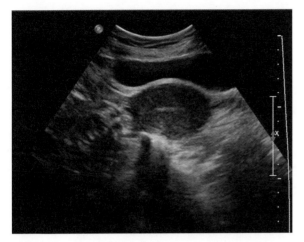

Figure 5.9 Ultrasound image showing a trans-abdominal transverse view of the pelvis. Note the hyperechoic endometrial stripe in the middle of the uterus.

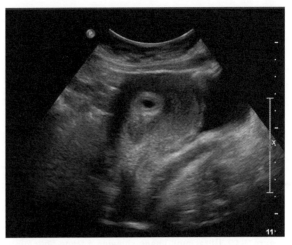

Figure 5.10 Ultrasound image showing a trans-abdominal longitudinal of view of the pelvis. Note the anechoic cavity in the uterus, representative of an early gestational sac.

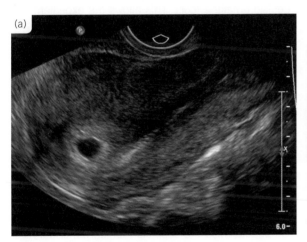

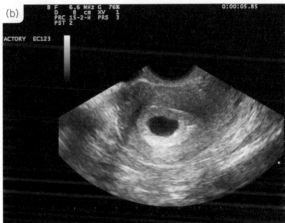

Figure 5.11 Ultrasound image showing a trans-vaginal sagittal view of the pelvis. Note the early gestational sac within the uterus. (a) Early sac transverse view. (b) Trans-vaginal sagittal still of the uterus.

This anatomical area can be visualized by sweeping through the entire uterus.

Identifying the decidual reaction, gestational sac, and yolk sac

Several intrauterine structures must be identified in early pregnancy, in order to confirm an IUP. The first sonographically identifiable finding will form around the normal area of the endometrial stripe and will appear as a hyperechoic 'thickening', called the **de-cidual reaction (DR)**. The DR becomes visible at about 14 days post-fertilization. Eventually, there will be the gradual development of a central cystic area, representing the **gestational sac (GS)**, and becomes visible at around 4.5–5th weeks of gestation. The GS (see Figures 5.10 and 5.11) appears as an anechoic, generally round or oval intrauterine structure. Once the gestational sac is evident, the DR will start to appear as a distinct double layer around the GS, called the double decidual sign (see Videos 5.1 and 5.2). This normal DR is frequently absent when an atypical gestation has developed. However, sometimes a small intrauterine fluid collection can appear as a reaction to

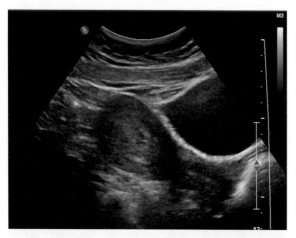

Figure 5.12 Ultrasound image showing a trans-abdominal longitudinal view of the pelvis. Note the irregular anechoic cavity in the uterus, atypical for a normal gestational sac.

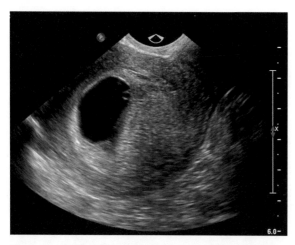

Figure 5.13 Ultrasound image showing a trans-vaginal transverse view of the pelvis. Note the yolk sac within the gestational sac.

increasing pregnancy hormones, triggered by an ectopic pregnancy. This pseudogestational sac is typically also located centrally but can be seen surrounded by only a single decidual layer and does not demonstrate any products of conception (see Figure 5.12).

The **yolk sac (YS)** is the first embryological structure, or product of conception, identifiable by PoCUS. It may be detected around the 4.5–5th week of gestation by TV scanning and around the 5th week of gestation using TA techniques. It is easily identified as a hyperechoic, ring-like structure within the GS (see Figures 5.13 and 5.14, and Video 5.12). Usually,

the YS can be visualized by the time the GS reaches 20 mm with TA ultrasound, and 10 mm with TV ultrasound. Failure to see a yolk sac within a GS of >25 mm will very likely indicate the presence of a blighted ovum or failed development of products of conception (see Figure 5.15).

The presence of a YS within a normal, intrauterine GS is the *minimum* finding required to **confirm** the presence of an IUP (see Videos 5.3 and 5.4). In the absence of risk factors for a heterotopic pregnancy, confirmation of an IUP makes the possibility of an ectopic gestation highly unlikely. Although some guidelines for early pregnancy ultrasound still recommend a comprehensive ultrasound to rule out a heterotopic gestation, identifying an IUP by PoCUS in low-risk patients is a safe approach to excluding an ectopic pregnancy and spontaneous abortion, within the setting of clinical guidelines and using appropriate decision-making tools. This allows the expedient disposition of a stable patient with an IUP, as they are at very low risk for a heterotopic pregnancy. The patient with a confirmed IUP can then wait a certain time for additional first-trimester imaging studies.

Measuring the myometrial mantle

After identifying the intrauterine gestation, it is necessary to confirm that there is an adequate amount of myometrium surrounding it and that the location is indeed central within the uterus. Both a thin endomyometrial mantle or an eccentric location of a GS should raise the suspicion for an abnormally implanted pregnancy (see Figure 5.16). In such cases, an interstitial ectopic pregnancy or a cornual pregnancy, two clinically distinct entities, must be considered. In a cornual pregnancy, the implanted and developing GS is located in one of the upper and lateral portions of the uterus—the 'horn' of the uterus. An interstitial pregnancy is a gestation that implants at the proximal, and still intramural, portion of the Fallopian tube, which is still enveloped by the myometrium of the uterus. Cornual pregnancies are especially potentially devastating, as they tend to rupture late and bleed more. The amount of '*myometrial mantle*' that is regarded acceptable is generally reported to be at least 5 mm. Less than 8 mm as a lower limit of normal is often cited in the emergency medicine literature. This

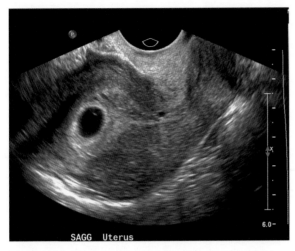

Figure 5.14 Ultrasound image showing a trans-vaginal sagittal view of the pelvis. Note the presence of a yolk sac within the gestational sac.

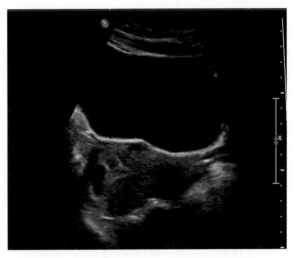

Figure 5.16 Ultrasound image showing a trans-abdominal transverse view of the pelvis. Note the bladder in the near field and the uterus in the far field. There is an eccentrically located gestational sac with a thin myometrial mantle, which should raise suspicion for a cornual or interstitial pregnancy.

more conservative number will increase sensitivity and is more appropriate for point-of-care scanning.

The fetal pole and fetal heart rate

Finally, although not necessary for diagnosing a patient with an IUP, the fetal pole (FP) can often be identified as early as 5.5–6 weeks' gestational age by the TV route, or by 6.5–7 weeks with TA ultrasound (see Figure 5.17). The FP will often be seen initially as a faint echogenic mass of tissue within the GS (see Video 5.5 ▶). Once the FP reaches 5 mm on TV ultrasound (10 mm for TA) the fetal heartbeat (FHB) should be identifiable (see Video 5.6 ▶). Failure to detect the

FHB can mean intrauterine fetal demise. Recent guidelines suggest a cut-off of 7 mm for the crown–rump length (CRL) without a visible FHB, before a non-viable pregnancy should be considered. Although the FHB is often easily seen with bedside ultrasound equipment, the authors caution against labelling an IUP as viable (alive) or not based on identifying the FHB. If there is any indication that the pregnancy might have suffered a demise, comprehensive imaging and consultation with obstetrics services are indicated.

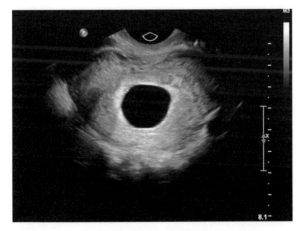

Figure 5.15 Ultrasound image showing a trans-vaginal coronal view of the pelvis. Note the large empty gestational sac, likely representative of a blighted ovum.

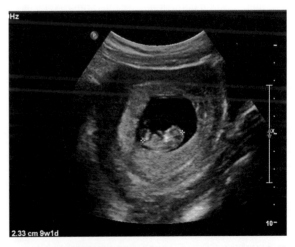

Figure 5.17 Ultrasound image showing a trans-abdominal transverse view of the pelvis. A fetal pole is seen, and the crown–rump length depicted.

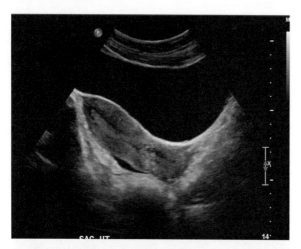

Figure 5.18 Ultrasound image showing a trans-abdominal longitudinal view of the pelvis. Note the anechoic free fluid seen in the retro-uterine space.

Identifying free fluid in the pelvis

The pelvis is the most dependent part of the body in the supine patient. Hence, free fluid can often be found in this location. In some cases, such as trauma, the emergency physician will search for free fluid in the pelvis, which, in the female, is most often seen in the retro-uterine space, also called the 'pouch of Douglas' (Figure 5.18). In the first trimester, a normal amount of free fluid can be encountered in the cul de sac and may be physiological. However, the presence of free fluid may, in fact, be the only detectable finding in a small percentage of ectopic pregnancies. Moreover, haemoperitoneum is found in approximately 40–84% of patients with a complicated ectopic pregnancy, and the greater the quantity of free fluid, the more likely the chance of an ectopic. It is difficult to quantify the amount of free fluid, so the detection of any amount of free fluid (anywhere in the abdomen, including the right or left upper quadrants) in an unstable pregnant patient with an empty uterus should be concerning (see Videos 5.7 and 5.8 📷).

Documentation

The identification of an IUP should be clearly documented in the patient record, as should the lack of an identifiable IUP. Usually the location and measurements of the GS or FP, including the potential detection of an FHB, should be reported, along with copies of representative images or videos.

Other sonographic findings

Identifying a tubal ring

While PoCUS has its goals in ruling in an IUP, some abnormal adnexal findings of ectopics can sometimes be seen. A positive adnexal finding, such as a tubal ring or an adnexal mass, can be present in up to 95% of ectopics. A tubal ring is an extra-uterine, and often hypoechoic, concentric mass, with a thick-walled echogenic ring. It is often found adjacent to the ovary. The ring may appear similar to uterine tissue; however, it will be found far away from the bladder. If seen, it is highly suggestive of an ectopic gestation.

Identifying a potential molar gestation

Again, the goal of PoCUS is to rule in an IUP; however, other abnormal findings may inevitably be encountered within the uterus. Such is the case in molar pregnancies where intrauterine contents will often appear as multiple, cyst-like areas (see Figure 5.19). A normal GS will often be impossible to identify. A comprehensive ultrasound study should be ordered to confirm the diagnosis.

Identifying intrauterine devices

Recognition of an intrauterine device (IUD) may be useful in certain clinical settings. These devices will often appear as a bright, hyperechoic linear object (see Figures 5.20 and 5.21). If positioned correctly, an

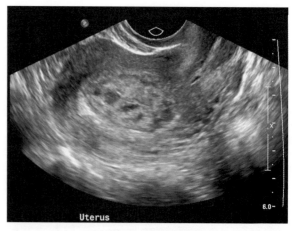

Figure 5.19 Ultrasound image showing a trans-vaginal sagittal view of the pelvis. The intrauterine contents are heterogenous, and no clear gestational sac is identifiable.

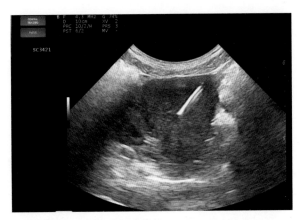

Figure 5.20 Trans-abdominal transverse view showing a copper IUD within the uterus.

IUD can be identified along the location of the endometrial stripe. PoCUS may not be able to identify incorrectly deployed or shifted IUDs at the bedside. If this is a clinical concern in a stable patient, a comprehensive elective ultrasound study should be ordered.

Identifying other pelvic pathology

In female patients with pelvic pain, while performing PoCUS for an IUP or free fluid within the pelvis, the physician may encounter other pelvic pathology. Although the primary goal of pelvic PoCUS should again be to locate an IUP or to detect the presence of free fluid, focused assessment of the adnexa is within the scope of PoCUS.

Each Fallopian tube is approximately 10 cm in length and consists of four segments (from proximal to distal: interstitial cornu, isthmus, ampulla, and

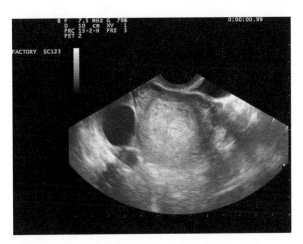

Figure 5.22 Trans-vaginal coronal view of the pelvis, showing a simple cyst in the right adnexa.

infundibulum). Ovaries are elliptical and approximately 4 cm in length, 3 cm in width, and 2 cm in height. Although the location of the ovaries can vary, they are usually anterior to the internal iliac artery.

Pathology that may be seen in the adnexal region includes ovarian cysts, abscesses, and ectopic pregnancies. Such findings become apparent when the clinician sweeps the probe beyond the extremes of the uterus, and the adnexa comes into view. Simple ovarian cysts will generally be thin-walled, round in appearance, with a completely anechoic centre (see Figure 5.22, and Videos 5.9 and 5.10 ⬤). They will also demonstrate acoustic enhancement and will be intimately associated with the ovaries. In women of reproductive age, cysts of up to 3 cm are a normal

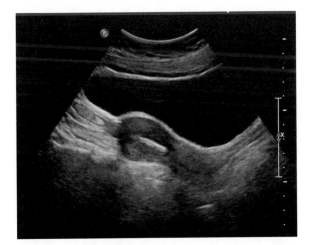

Figure 5.21 Trans-abdominal longitudinal view showing a copper IUD within the uterus.

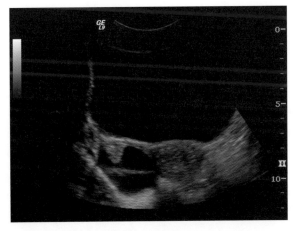

Figure 5.23 Trans-abdominal transverse view of the pelvis, showing a cyst in the right adnexa containing internal echoes and a septation.

physiological finding. These simple physiological cysts do not require follow-up. If a cystic lesion demonstrates internal echoes, or septations (see Figure 5.23), or appears irregular in any manner, then a more prompt follow-up and gynaecological consultation should be obtained in the stable, non-gravid patient. In a patient with a positive hCG, any complex adnexal lesion should be considered as a potential ectopic mass until proven otherwise. Finally, in a febrile patient or one with suggestion of an infectious aetiology, proper gynaecological consultation should again be sought to rule out a pelvic or tubo-ovarian abscess.

Further reading

Adhikari S, *et al.* Diagnosis and management of ectopic pregnancy using bedside transvaginal ultrasonography in evaluation of symptomatic first-trimester pregnancy. *Ann Emerg Med* 1999;**29**:338–47.

Barnhart K, Mennuti MT, Benjamin I, Jacobson S, Goodman D, Coutifaris C. Prompt diagnosis of ectopic pregnancy in an ED setting. *Obstet Gynecol* 1994;**84**:1010–15.

Chetty M, Elson J. Treating non-tubal ectopic pregnancy. *Best Pract Res Clin Obstet Gynaecol* 2009;**23**:529–38.

Condous G, Okaro E, Khalid A, *et al.* The accuracy of transvaginal ultrasonography for the diagnosis of ectopic pregnancy prior to surgery. *Hum Reprod* 2005;**20**:1404–9.

Frates MC, Doubilet PM, Peters HE, Benson CB. Adnexal sonographic findings in ectopic pregnancy and their correlation with tubal rupture and HCG levels. *J Ultrasound Med* 2014;**33**:697–703.

Hu M, Poder L, Filly RA. Impact of new society of radiologists in ultrasound early first trimester diagnostic criteria for nonviable pregnancy. *J Ultrasound Med* 2014;**33**:1585–8.

Kaakaji Y, Nghiem HV, Nodell C, Winter TC. Sonography of obstetric and gynecologic emergencies: Part I, obstetric emergencies. *AJR Am J Roentgenol* 2000;**174**:641–9.

Kaplan BC, Dart RG, Moskos M, *et al.* Ectopic pregnancy: a prospective study with impaired diagnostic accuracy. *Ann Emerg Med* 1996;**28**:10–17.

Moawad NS, Mahajan ST, Moniz MH, Taylor SE, Hurd WW. Current diagnosis and treatment of interstitial pregnancy. *Am J Obstet Gynecol* 2010;**202**:15–29.

Shih C. Effect of emergency physician-performed pelvic sonography on length of stay in the emergency department. *Ann Emerg Med* 1997;**29**:348–52.

6

Vascular ultrasound

Justin Bowra, Osama Loubani, and Paul Atkinson

Summary

When to scan (clinical indications):
   Core: suspected AAA or DVT, and in the shocked patient (IVC).
   Advanced: suspected aortic dissection.

What to scan (PoCUS protocol):
   Core: abdominal aorta and IVC, above-knee DVT (graded compression ultrasound).
   Advanced: above-knee DVT (Doppler ultrasound).

How to scan (key points):
   Abdominal aorta: curvilinear or sector probe, in transverse and sagittal planes.
   IVC: as for the abdominal aorta; the transverse trans-hepatic view from the RUQ window also acceptable (*not* long axis in this window).
   Above-knee DVT: often both linear and curved probe required.

What PoCUS adds (how results change practice):
   AAA can be diagnosed by visualization of an aortic diameter from echogenic wall to echogenic wall of >3 cm, although PoCUS cannot determine rupture.
   Aortic dissection may be diagnosed with the visualization of an aortic flap or suggested by aortic regurgitation and pericardial effusion.
   IVC diameter and respiratory variability can be used to help determine the fluid status of a patient in shock and guide fluid resuscitation (SHoC protocol).

Lack of compressibility of the deep venous system of the leg indicates DVT at or above the knee. Doppler imaging can increase sensitivity.

Introduction

Ultrasound has been a valued modality in the evaluation of vascular pathology since its inception. Vascular PoCUS is one of the earliest, and now most accepted, uses of PoCUS in critical care medicine. PoCUS is used to answer specific binary questions, to assist with diagnosis and resuscitation and to provide guidance for procedures such as vascular access (see Chapter 9).

Abdominal aortic aneurysm

Purpose

PoCUS visualizes the abdominal aorta and can be used to detect AAA. While PoCUS cannot directly diagnose ruptured AAA, the finding of AAA in the proper clinical context can strongly suggest the presence of rupture.

Perspective

AAA is common, and rupture is deadly. AAA is present in 1–8% of those over 60 years of age, with increased frequency in older age, males, and smokers. The risk of rupture varies with the diameter, with an annual risk of rupture of 0.5–5% at diameters of 4–5 cm and as high as 50% annually at diameters of above 8 cm.

The overall mortality of ruptured AAA is 80%, with approximately 10,000 deaths per year attributable to ruptured AAA in the United States. Death from ruptured AAA most commonly occurs prior to arrival in hospital, with 60% dying before reaching medical attention. Of those who survive to reach hospital, only 50% survive to discharge.

Why not use traditional diagnostic modalities?

The modalities most commonly used in the diagnosis of AAA are ultrasound, CT, and physical examination. Physical examination is unreliable for the detection of AAA. The finding of a large pulsatile mass in the abdomen has variable sensitivity and specificity, and these depend on the size of the AAA and whether or not it has ruptured. In unruptured AAA, sensitivity is as poor as 29% for AAA of between 3 and 3.9 cm, and as high as 76% for AAA of above 5 cm. In the case of ruptured AAA, the sensitivity of physical examination ranges from 40% to 90%.

While CT is the gold standard for diagnosing AAA, it presents challenges in both the unstable and the stable patient. In the unstable patient, CT requires transport away from the resuscitation area and can hinder essential patient care. In a stable patient with only a *low* suspicion of AAA, CT can be costly and time-consuming and can expose the patient to a significant radiation dose.

How good is ultrasound at diagnosing the condition?

The ability of non-radiologists, especially emergency physicians, to detect AAA by PoCUS has been extensively studied. Rubano's systematic review of this literature demonstrated a pooled sensitivity and specificity of 99% and 98%, respectively, for the detection of AAA by PoCUS.

How does ultrasound impact clinical care?

Results from several retrospective reviews demonstrate that in cases of *ruptured* AAA, PoCUS decreases the time to diagnosis (5 minutes versus 80 minutes) and the time to the operating room (12 minutes versus 90 minutes) and possibly improves survival—one review demonstrated an improvement in survival, while another showed no improvement in survival between

patients with ruptured AAA who underwent PoCUS and those who did not. There is little evidence on whether detection of *unruptured* AAA by PoCUS has any significant effect on outcomes.

Image generation

Probe selection and machine settings

An abdominal probe should be used to allow maximal tissue penetration. The machine should be set initially to about 15 cm, and the depth altered until the vertebral bodies are identified.

Patient position, surface anatomy, and key landmarks

The examination for AAA is done with the patient in the supine position. The probe is initially positioned in the transverse plane, with the probe marker on the patient's right. The probe is first placed at the level of the xiphoid process in the midline (see Figure 6.1). To ensure that the aorta is visualized as close to its exit from the diaphragm as possible, the heart is first identified in the sub-xiphoid view, and then the probe fanned caudally until it is perpendicular to the patient.

The main landmark for identifying the aorta is the vertebral body beneath. The vertebrae are easily identifiable by their echogenic anterior surfaces and the large shadows they cast (see Videos 6.1 to 6.6 🎦). The aorta and IVC will be immediately anterior to the vertebrae. Care must be taken to properly differentiate the aorta from other vascular structures nearby, especially

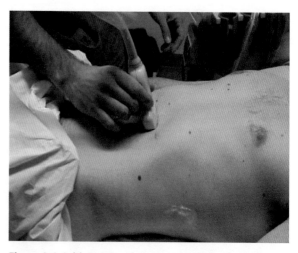

Figure 6.1 Initial probe placement for abdominal aorta scanning.

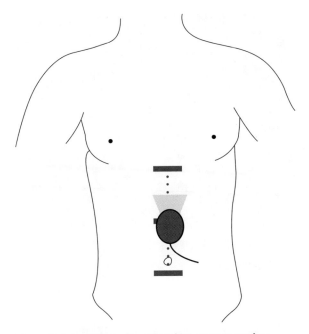

Figure 6.2 Landmarks for abdominal aorta scanning.

the adjacent IVC. The aorta's thick echogenic wall, non-compressibility, and (in older patients) calcification differentiate it from the IVC and other vascular structures. The IVC's oval shape, seen in transverse section (unless distended), change in shape with respiration, and compressibility by the probe itself all help differentiate it from the round, thick-walled aorta (see Videos 6.1 to 6.3 ▢). Pulsatility is not a reliable marker for identifying the aorta, as the IVC can be pulsatile when in close contact with the aorta.

Once the abdominal aorta is identified, scan its entire length from the xiphisternum to the umbilicus (see Figure 6.2), ideally observing its anterior branches—the coeliac trunk (see Video 6.1 ▢) and the superior mesenteric artery (SMA) (see Videos 6.2 and 6.3 ▢). The SMA is a surrogate marker for the

origin of the renal arteries (which are often harder to identify on ultrasound). Then follow the aorta to the level of the bifurcation into the common iliac arteries (see Video 6.4 ▢).

Take care to measure the aorta in true cross-section, because oblique planes will provide diagonal cross-sections of the aorta that will overestimate the apparent size of the aorta (see Figure 6.3). One should scan the aorta in the long axis as well (see Video 6.5 ▢), although one should not measure in this plane because of the risk of underestimating the diameter due to cylinder artefact. Finally, ensure that you measure the true diameter—this is the diameter at the aorta's widest, from *outer wall to outer wall* (see Figure 6.4). Although the difference between this and the luminal diameter may not be great in some cases of AAA (see Video 6.6 ▢), Video 6.7 ▢ demonstrates a case of AAA with true and luminal diameters that were very different—the true diameter was close to 9 cm, whereas the luminal diameter was only 4–5 cm. The difference in this case was very significant in terms of prognosis and likelihood of rupture.

Troubleshooting

Bowel gas and large body habitus are the two greatest obstacles to visualization of the aorta. In the case of large *body habitus*, increasing the depth, decreasing the frequency of the probe, and decreasing the dynamic range can aid visualization of deep structures. Switching off THI may also improve penetration. Finally, asking the patient to bend their knees can also relax the abdominal muscles and make the examination easier.

If *bowel gas* interferes with image acquisition, several techniques may assist. Sliding the probe laterally may evade bowel gas and obtain a clear image. Firm,

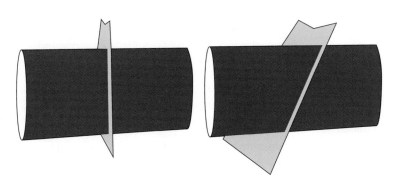

Figure 6.3 The probe angle can affect the apparent diameter of the aorta. Oblique or angled cuts, especially with a tortuous aorta, will exaggerate the true aortic diameter.

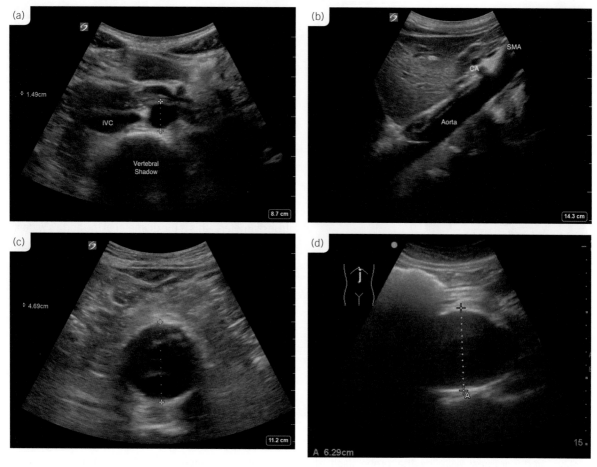

Figure 6.4 Transverse (a) and longitudinal (b) views of a normal abdominal aorta with normal AP diameters of less than 3 cm; and of abdominal aortic aneurysms (c,d) with abnormal AP diameters of almost 5 cm and 7 cm. The aorta lies to patient's left of the IVC, and anterior to the vertebrae.

sustained probe pressure can push the bowel away from the field of view. Asking the patient to take deep breaths in or out may also move the gas-filled intestines out of the way. Placing the patient in the left or right decubitus position can change the position of the bowel gas. At least some of the aorta may be visualized using non-standard windows such as the liver (with the probe in the RUQ, the aorta will be seen deep to the IVC; see Figure 6.1s 🖼) or the spleen.

Image interpretation

Normal and abnormal appearance

The normal diameter of the aorta at the level of the renal arteries is typically 2 cm. An AAA is defined as an aortic diameter at least 1.5 times the normal diameter at the level of renal arteries. Therefore, an aortic

diameter of <3 cm, measured from outer wall to outer wall, is considered to have a normal diameter (see Figure 6.4 and Videos 6.1 to 6.5 🎦). Any diameter of >3 cm provides a diagnosis of AAA (see Figure 6.4, Videos 6.6 and 6.7 🎦). As the diameter increases, so does the likelihood that the AAA is causing the patient's symptoms.

Factors that hinder interpretation: 'pitfalls'

As noted in 'Patient position, surface anatomy, and key landmarks', p. 118:

- Avoid oblique or angled cuts, if possible, which will exaggerate the true aortic diameter (see Figure 6.3) (this can be difficult if the aorta is tortuous);

- Measure the diameter between the *outer* edges of the echogenic walls.

Finally, because the aorta is a retroperitoneal structure, bleeding from an aortic rupture is typically retroperitoneal. As such, PoCUS cannot detect bleeding from ruptured AAA nor can it definitively diagnose ruptured AAA. Rather, ruptured AAA is a clinical diagnosis made when AAA is present in the appropriate clinical context.

Aortic dissection

Purpose

PoCUS cannot exclude an aortic dissection. However, detection of pericardial fluid, aortic regurgitation, a dilated aortic root (see Chapter 2), or an intimal flap in either the thoracic or abdominal aorta (see Videos 6.8 and 6.9 ⬤) may prompt consideration of this diagnosis in the appropriate clinical setting.

Perspective

Aortic dissections form when shearing intravascular forces separate the layers of the aortic wall. If untreated, patients with proximal aorta involvement have a 2-week mortality rate of approximately 80%. Risk factors for aortic dissection include hypertension, Marfan's syndrome, and other connective tissue disorders such as Ehlers–Danlos syndrome.

Why not use traditional diagnostic modalities?

Classic clinical features of aortic dissection include sudden-onset tearing chest pain, differences in blood pressure measurements between the right and left arm, blood pressure or pulse differentials between the arms, neurological deficits, or features of tamponade. However, none of these features is reliable in confirming or excluding aortic dissection.

A plethora of CXR features have been described in aortic dissection. However, these findings are not specific to aortic dissection, and furthermore, CXR may be normal in as many as 10% of patients with aortic dissection.

While the *absence* of the features mentioned above can lower the likelihood of aortic dissection, other tests are often required. Multi-planar TOE/TEE, MRI, and CT are reliable for diagnosing aortic dissection. Unfortunately, in the unstable patient, these tests are usually difficult to obtain and/or unsafe to perform.

How good is ultrasound at diagnosing the condition?

While PoCUS cannot rule out dissection, visualization of an intimal flap by ultrasound may carry a sensitivity of 67–80% and a specificity of 99–100% for dissection.

Image generation and interpretation

Visualization of the heart for pericardial effusion and aortic regurgitation and measurement of the aortic root are covered in Chapter 2. In the setting of typical symptoms or signs, such findings are highly suggestive of an acute aortic dissection.

Visualization of the normal abdominal aorta is described in 'Abdominal aortic aneurysm', p. 117. In the setting of aortic dissection, an echogenic line arising from the vessel wall may be seen within the lumen of the aorta in either longitudinal or transverse views (see Videos 6.8 and 6.9 ⬤). This line represents a flap, resulting from a tear of the intima in the setting of an acute aortic dissection. The flap often moves with flow in the vessel. If colour flow Doppler is used, one may also note flow on only one side of the dissection flap, within the true lumen.

Pitfalls

Visualization of the flap may be difficult in obese patients where the depth settings make the image smaller and where resolution is diminished by using low-frequency settings. It may also be difficult to visualize a flap that is vertically aligned (parallel to the direction of the ultrasound beam), unlike the horizontal flap seen in Videos 6.8 and 6.9 ⬤. A mural thrombus and reverberation artefact may also be mistaken for an intimal flap.

Unlike the above 'mimics', a true intimal flap will demonstrate movement in a different direction from the rest of the aorta.

Clinical use

In a patient with a suspected aortic dissection, detection of the ultrasound findings described in previous section 'Image generation and interpretation', (dilated aortic root with or without aortic regurgitation, intimal flap, and pericardial effusion) should prompt appropriate management of the patient's blood pressure and emergent definitive investigation, according to the stability of the patient.

Inferior vena cava

Purpose

The IVC is a major capacitance vessel, facilitating consistent venous return to the right heart. As such, the diameter of the IVC changes in a non-linear fashion in response to the filling status of the patient, increasing in diameter with increased filling pressure and volume. The IVC also collapses slightly on inspiration in the spontaneously breathing patient (collapsibility). This is reversed in a mechanically ventilated patient, in whom the IVC diameter *increases* during inspiration (distensibility). We will use the term *respiratory variability* to encompass these changes.

PoCUS can visualize the IVC diameter and respiratory variability, and assist the clinician in estimating the patient's fluid status.

Perspective

Hypotension is a predictor of in-hospital mortality, with mortality as high as 25% in those with hypotension in the ED. Identification and rapid correction of hypotension are critical. In the hypotensive patient, one of the first questions a clinician must address is whether the patient requires emergency fluid resuscitation, i.e. is the patient under-filled or overloaded? Or, perhaps more importantly, is the patient likely to be fluid-responsive or not?

Why not use traditional diagnostic modalities?

Clinical assessment often fails to determine the correct cause of hypotension. In one study, the aetiology of undifferentiated hypotension was identified in only 24% of cases. Determining the underlying haemodynamic process in a timely and accurate fashion can allow successful goal-directed therapy. Invasive monitoring techniques can be time-consuming and costly, and they are not always easily performed in the ED or ward setting.

How good is ultrasound at diagnosing the condition?

Ultrasound is rapid and can be performed at the bedside. IVC diameter and respiratory variability have been shown to correlate with CVP, with the strongest correlation seen at extremes of the values (i.e. in low- or high-volume states).

Fluid responsiveness describes a significant increase in CO that results from volume expansion. IVC diameter and respiratory variability have also been shown to be predictive of fluid responsiveness, again at extremes (a large, distended, non variable IVC versus a small, collapsed, variable IVC).

Image generation

Probe selection and machine settings

The IVC can be visualized using either a curvilinear or a phased array probe. Either cardiac or abdominal preset can be used.

Patient position, surface anatomy, and key landmarks

The patient should be in a supine position. Standard measures of IVC diameter assume a supine position, and changes in patient position can greatly affect the IVC diameter. The subcostal, mid-axillary, or transpyloric windows can be used to visualize the IVC (see Figures 6.1s 📷 and 6.5 and Videos 6.1 to 6.3 and 6.10 to 6.15 📹). Longitudinal or transverse planes can provide the needed information on IVC diameter and respiratory variability, although ideally one should image the IVC in both planes to avoid the pitfalls associated with each plane. For example, in the mid-axillary window, the longitudinal plane should be avoided, as discussed in 'Pitfalls', p. 124. Additionally, diaphragmatic movement may cause the IVC to move in and out of the longitudinal plane, leading to a false impression of collapse.

The IVC lies posterior to the liver. It receives the hepatic veins ventrally, before it passes through the diaphragm and into the right atrium (see Figures 6.6 and 6.7). If using the subcostal window, place the probe just caudal to the xiphoid process (see Videos 6.10 to 6.12 📹). If using the mid-axillary window, begin as for the RUQ window for e-FAST; identify the IVC, and then rotate the probe for a transverse view of the IVC (see Videos 6.13 and 6.14 📹). In either window, identify the IVC from its entry into the right atrium and/or its confluence with the hepatic veins. This is to avoid mistaking the aorta for the IVC. If using the transpyloric window, then identify the vertebral artery, IVC, and aorta, as described in the 'Abdominal aortic aneurysm', p. 118 (see Videos 6.1 to 6.3 and 6.15 📹).

Standard sites for IVC assessment are at the confluence with the hepatic veins and at the junction with the left renal vein.

Exercise caution when using M-mode measurements of the minimal and maximal diameter across the proximal IVC, as this is prone to several pitfalls. For example, if the probe is not perpendicular to the IVC, M-mode measurements will overestimate the IVC diameter. Furthermore, the IVC itself moves with respiration, as seen in Video 6.10 📹, and this tends to render inaccurate M-mode measurements of its diameter. Until experienced in IVC assessment, it is wise to avoid M-mode for measuring the IVC diameter.

Image interpretation

Trends of the IVC diameter and respiratory variability in response to fluid resuscitation are better than individual measurements at determining fluid status. However, there is evidence for cut-off values that indicate the under-filled and overfilled extremes of vascular status. In a typical adult, a maximal IVC diameter of <2.1 cm, with collapse of >40–50% with inspiration (in spontaneously breathing individuals), suggests a right atrial pressure (RAP) of <10 mmHg. Conversely, a diameter of >2.1 cm with collapse of <50% suggests an RAP of >10 mmHg. *However, it should be remembered that the RAP and CVP themselves correlate poorly with intravascular volume status and fluid responsiveness.*

In the shocked patient, an initially small IVC diameter with significant or complete collapse suggests a low-volume status that should respond to volume loading (see Videos 6.3, 6.10, 6.13, and 6.15 📹). A large, dilated IVC with no or minimal collapse implies high CVP and a state that would not respond to volume resuscitation alone such as cardiogenic or obstructive shock (see Videos 6.12 and 6.14 📹). Again, these measurements should be repeated during resuscitation to obtain a trend and to guide optimal volumes and rates of intravenous fluid administration.

IVC size and collapse on their own do *not* give a complete picture of fluid status. Other features, such as ventricular size, wall motion, and the presence or absence of pericardial fluid, must be considered to

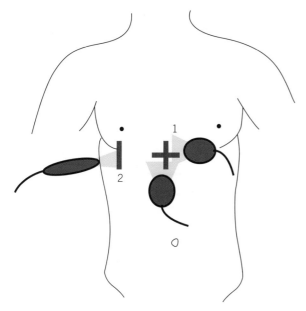

Figure 6.5 Probe positions for subcostal (1) or mid-axillary/RUQ (2) windows used to image the inferior vena cava.

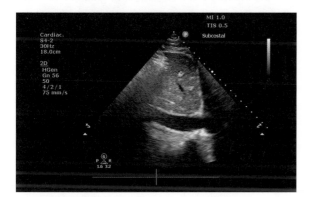

Figure 6.6 Subcostal longitudinal view (general orientation) of the inferior vena cava (IVC) entering the right atrium (RA) in expiration.

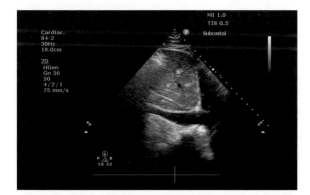

Figure 6.7 Subcostal longitudinal view (general orientation) of the inferior vena cava (IVC) entering the right atrium (RA) in inspiration. Same patient as in Figure 6.6.

gain the clearest picture of the volume status. For example, dry lungs (A profile), a collapsing IVC, and a small, hyperdynamic LV chamber suggest hypovolaemia, while a large pericardial effusion with a distended IVC is consistent with obstructive shock. As such, PoCUS assessment of the IVC is often incorporated into a shock protocol such as ACES, RUSH, or SHoC.

Pitfalls

As noted in 'Image interpretation', p. 123, caution is required when associating PoCUS measurements of the IVC with CVP values, as the CVP itself is an unreliable surrogate marker for volume status. A systematic review of techniques available for the assessment of intravascular volume found that the CVP did not predict fluid responsiveness. As such, it is important to interpret the IVC diameter and respiratory variability within the clinical context they are found, and not as a definitive measure of intravascular volume.

If measuring from the mid-axillary window, the IVC should be imaged in its *transverse*, rather than the longitudinal, axis. This is because the hepatic window visualizes the *coronal* (transverse) plane of the IVC in long axis, whereas in the supine patient, the IVC collapses in the *sagittal* (AP) plane. Therefore, the long-axis IVC view obtained from the hepatic window tends to overestimate the IVC size and to underestimate IVC collapse. This pitfall is overcome by imaging the vessel in its transverse axis, and, in fact, it is good practice to image any structure in two planes (see Figure 6.1s 🖼 and Videos 6.13 and 6.14 📹).

When imaging the IVC in its long axis from the subcostal window, take care to avoid cylinder artefact—if the probe is off-axis, then the IVC will appear smaller and 'under-filled'.

It is also important to be aware of other conditions that affect IVC measurements:

- IVC diameter is decreased in conditions such as raised intra-abdominal pressure or when compressed by external probe pressure. This is a particular issue when imaging the IVC in the transpyloric plane where it is not 'shielded' from the probe by the liver. For example, the IVC in

Video 6.3 📹 may be flattened due to probe pressure, rather than hypovolaemia;

- IVC diameter is increased in athletes and in conditions such as obstructive shock (e.g. tension pneumothorax, massive PE), cor pulmonale, and right heart disease such as moderate/severe tricuspid regurgitation;

- IVC collapse will be exaggerated in respiratory distress;

- IVC compliance decreases with age. Masugata *et al.* showed a decrease in the maximal diameter of the IVC with age and subsequently a greater IVC respiratory variability. However, when analysed, the range was still within normal parameters.

Clinical use

As noted in 'Image interpretation', p. 123, shock protocols incorporate IVC assessment to guide fluid resuscitation. This is discussed in more detail in Chapter 2 on pp. 60–68.

Proximal deep vein thrombosis

Purpose

PoCUS can aid in diagnosing or excluding lower-extremity above-knee or 'proximal' DVT in symptomatic patients by venous compression. The presence of a thrombus within a vein will prevent the vein from compressing completely with probe pressure.

Perspective

DVT is the third most common cardiovascular disease in North America, and in the United Kingdom (UK), its annual incidence is up to 1 per 1000 adults. Untreated, it may progress to PE, which has a high mortality rate (8000 per year in the UK). Patients with lower-extremity DVT typically present with a painful swollen calf, with no history of trauma. DVT is an important diagnosis to consider in any patient with atraumatic unilateral lower leg pain or swelling.

Why not use traditional diagnostic modalities?

The initial approach to the diagnosis of DVT often involves risk stratification using clinical risk scores such as Well's score and D-dimer assays. In the presence of low clinical risk and a negative D-dimer, DVT can be safely ruled out. However, in the large proportion of patients in whom DVT cannot be ruled out in this way, further diagnostic testing is needed.

Ultrasound has become the preferred diagnostic modality for DVT. Venography was once considered the gold standard but has fallen out of favour due to its invasiveness. Other imaging modalities, such as CT and MRI, can also be used to diagnose DVT but are expensive and time-consuming, compared to ultrasound.

How good is ultrasound at diagnosing DVT?

The sensitivity and specificity of *duplex* (combined B-mode and Doppler) ultrasound for proximal DVT have been reported in the 98–100% range. PoCUS for DVT, in the form of a limited 2- or 3-point compression study, has been shown to be reasonably rapid and accurate, with a sensitivity of 93–100% and a specificity of 97–100%, for proximal DVT in ambulatory patients.

Compression ultrasound is not as accurate for below-knee or 'distal' DVT. Because below-knee DVTs rarely embolize without first extending above the knee, the major concern in the ED is proximal DVT. Immobilized patients have a higher risk of having isolated DVTs in the proximal leg veins that may not be detected by the 2-point compression protocol. Also, because of the risk of a distal or isolated DVT extending to become a proximal DVT, repeat ultrasound in 3–7 days is recommended in those with an initially negative ultrasound who have a high pre-test probability of DVT (e.g. high risk by clinical score and positive D-dimer). It should also be noted that patients at risk of pelvic DVT, but with a negative PoCUS study, should have further investigation, such as CT venography, or should have their *iliac vessels and IVC included* in both PoCUS and formal ultrasound studies.

Image generation

Probe selection and machine settings

Traditionally, a linear high-frequency probe is used. A curvilinear low-frequency probe may also be used and is usually required in obese patients.

Patient position, surface anatomy, and key landmarks

The patient can be scanned in virtually any position. Ideally, the leg should be dependent or below the heart, so a seated or semi-recumbent position is preferable. If the veins are difficult to visualize on ultrasound, the patient may also stand and be asked to hum (Valsalva manoeuvre) to increase the venous diameter. The areas to be scanned are the groin, medial thigh, and popliteal fossa.

The technique described below is known most accurately as the *3-point graded compression* technique. Whether two, three, or even four points are used, it should be noted that the 'points' are, in fact, *regions*. At every region described, the probe is, in fact, slid up and down the relevant vein, which is therefore compressed at multiple points. This is to improve the sensitivity of the technique, particularly because thrombi tend to form at areas of venous confluence (which are areas at risk of relatively turbulent flow).

It should also be emphasized that the key is to apply *graded* pressure—to *gradually* increase probe pressure until the artery just begins to indent. This is to prevent dislodgement and embolization of DVT (see 'Pitfalls', p. 127). Hence, the technique is most accurately described as *graded* compression ultrasound.

Inguinal/upper femoral vein

Begin at the level of the inguinal ligament, with the probe in a transverse orientation. The leg should be slightly abducted and externally rotated. Set the depth to at least 4 cm to allow visualization of the vascular structures in the groin. At the saphenofemoral junction [confluence with the great/long saphenous vein (LSV)], gently compress the vascular structures (see Video 6.16 📷). The vein(s) should compress fully and disappear (winking sign), while the artery remains patent (see Figure 6.8 and Video 6.17 📷). Follow the (common) femoral vein distally for several centimetres, compressing and releasing, to the confluence with the profunda femoris vein, and ensure that both the (superficial) femoral and profunda femoris veins are clearly visualized, as well as the proximal LSV.

Some operators choose to enhance their analysis using colour flow and/or PW Doppler augmentation (see Videos 6.18 and 6.19 📷). If Doppler is applied, the femoral artery (which lies lateral to the vein) will demonstrate pulsatile flow, whereas the common femoral

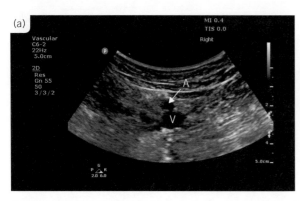
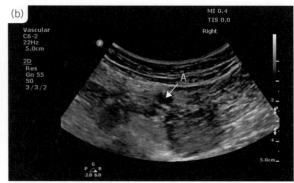

Figure 6.8 Left femoral vein (arrow), uncompressed (a) and compressed (b). Note that, with compression, the femoral vein (V) disappears while the femoral artery (A) is still patent.

vein should demonstrate low or no flow at rest. (See 'Doppler flow augmentation', p. 127.) Some operators also choose to compress and follow the femoral vein distally (see Video 6.20 📷), but this is not essential.

Lower femoral vein

As the femoral vein runs down the thigh, it moves posteriorly before diving through the adductor canal (to become the popliteal vein). Therefore, the vein lies in the *posteromedial* portion of the lower thigh. However, it can be difficult to visualize if the probe is held directly over this area (because of the intervening adipose tissue), and it is more easily visualized with the probe held more anteriorly, over the vastus medialis (medial portion of the quadriceps muscle), and angled directly posteriorly. (Note that a curvilinear probe may be required for this, as the depth may be too great for a linear probe.) In this position, the femoral artery and vein can be seen deep to the muscle and medial to the acoustic shadow of the femur. Once the vessels are seen, the operator should place his or her other hand directly behind the medial thigh and compress the intervening tissue *anteriorly* against the vein (see Figure 6.9 and Video 6.21 📷). If this is difficult, then Doppler should be used instead (see Video 6.22 📷).

Popliteal vein

Finally, move to the popliteal fossa. This is best visualized with the patient seated or erect, but the lateral decubitus position usually suffices. Apply the probe transversely as usual across the popliteal fossa (see Video 6.23 📷). Identify the cortex of the femur and tibia and the deep vessels lying more superficially. The vein is superficial to the artery in this window. Apply

pressure until the vein compresses completely (see Video 6.24 📷). As usual, take care to avoid compressing the artery as well (see Video 6.25 📷). Look carefully for a duplex popliteal vein. Follow the vein proximally and distally, and scan above and the 'trifurcation'.

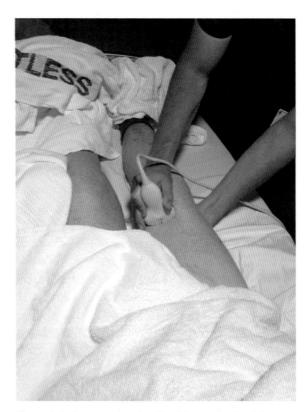

Figure 6.9 Compressing the distal femoral vein. At this level, the vein is fairly distant from the probe, so a curvilinear probe has been used. The operator grasps the patient's posterior thigh and pushes anteriorly against the probe to achieve compression.

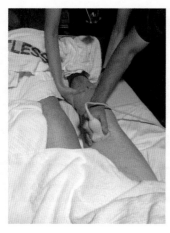

Figure 6.10 If venous compression is difficult, colour or pulsed wave Doppler can be used to detect flow. With the probe held motionless over the vein in question, the calf is gently squeezed more distally (i.e. more caudally). Absence of augmented flow indicates obstruction.

Doppler flow augmentation

If it is difficult to identify or compress veins, turn on colour or PW Doppler and turn down the PRF or 'scale' (e.g. to 5 cm/s) to ensure that you are able to detect any flow in the veins (which are low-flow vessels). With the probe held motionless over the vein in question, gently squeeze the calf distally (see Figure 6.10). Unless the intervening veins are occluded by thrombus, this will augment flow in the veins. On colour Doppler, this appears briefly as a brighter signal. On PW Doppler, this appears as a 'peak' in the venous waveform (see Figure 6.11).

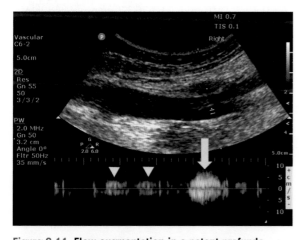

Figure 6.11 Flow augmentation in a patent profunda femoris vein (pulsed wave Doppler). The vein demonstrates respiratory (phasic) flow (arrowheads), with augmented flow when the distal calf is squeezed (arrow).

Image interpretation

Normal veins compress completely, as described. If a vein fails to compress fully (having applied enough pressure to partially compress the artery) or if a clot is visualized within the lumen, then the scan is positive for thrombus (see Figures 6.12 and 6.13, and Videos 6.26 to 6.28). With the addition of Doppler, there will be either no flow or no augmentation (see Videos 6.29 to 6.31).

Pitfalls

False positives for DVT

- *Lymph node* (see Figure 6.14): on ultrasound imaging, lymph nodes usually have a clearly defined structure—notably a dark (echo-poor) cortex and a brighter (echogenic) central area. However, if the overall gain is inadvertently set too low, a lymph node can resemble a non-compressible vessel in cross-section. Fortunately, it is not difficult to confirm that the node 'disappears' when the probe is moved distally or will appear oval (rather than tubular) in longitudinal scanning.

- *Recanalized DVT*: although these may appear identical to a recent DVT on compression ultrasound, old thrombi that have recanalized will demonstrate flow on Doppler imaging.

- *Inadequate probe pressure*: if inadequate pressure is applied, any vein can fail to compress. The key is to apply just enough pressure to begin to indent the accompanying artery.

- *Doppler PRF set too high*: if the Doppler 'scale' or PRF is set too high, no flow will be seen, even in patent veins. This is particularly an issue with colour Doppler. One solution is to decrease the size of the sample volume (the 'Doppler box'), decrease the PRF to the minimum, and increase the colour gain until artefactual flashes of colour appear in the surrounding soft tissue. Another solution is to use PW (spectral) Doppler instead.

False negatives for DVT

- *Non-occlusive DVT*: a small, non-occlusive DVT may *almost completely* compress with probe pressure (see Video 6.26).

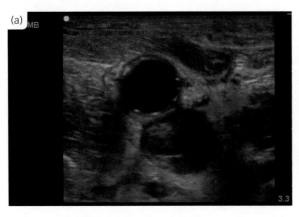
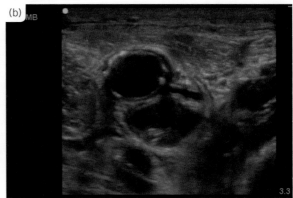

Figure 6.12 DVT. Femoral vein (arrow) is uncompressed in (a) and fails to compress with probe pressure (b).

- *DVT in iliac vessels*: in the presence of a DVT proximal to the common femoral vein (e.g. in the iliac vessels or IVC), the veins of the affected leg are often dilated and more difficult to compress with altered Doppler flow, compared to the unaffected leg. However, they also may appear spuriously normal, particularly on 2D compression ultrasound. One solution is to image the iliac vessels and IVC in the abdomen using the curved transducer, and then to compress them and/or augment them in the same way as the leg veins (see Videos 6.31 and 6.32 ◐).

- *DVT below the knee*: clearly, above-knee compression ultrasound does not interrogate the below-knee veins. However, these tend to propagate above the knee before they embolize. In patients with a high index of suspicion for *below-knee* DVT, some ED operators will extend their scan below the knee (see Video 6.28 ◐); others

will arrange a formal study of the entire limb; others will repeat the above-knee study in a few days. The correct approach is up to the individual clinician and institution.

- *Excessive probe pressure* (see Videos 6.24 and 6.25 ◐): just as inadequate probe pressure is a pitfall, so is excess pressure. If enough probe pressure is applied that the artery is compressed, then even a DVT can be compressed. Worse is the risk that this will dislodge, and even embolize, a DVT. As noted in 'Patient position, surface anatomy, and key landmarks', p. 125, the key is to apply *graded* pressure—to *gradually* increase probe pressure until the artery just begins to indent.

How does ultrasound impact clinical care?

The PoCUS DVT study should be incorporated into a clinical algorithm that considers the patient's risk for

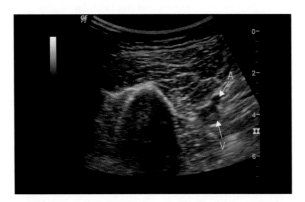

Figure 6.13 Echogenic DVT in the distal femoral vein (V), seen medial to the femur and below the accompanying artery (A).

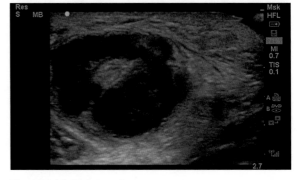

Figure 6.14 Lymph node.

DVT, laboratory tests, and risk factors for pelvic DVT. Negative scans do not rule out DVT in the IVC or iliac vessels, nor below-knee DVT (see 'Pitfalls', p. 128). Therefore, either repeat a negative above-knee scan in a few days, or arrange a formal DVT scan, according to local practice.

Further reading

Additional further reading can be found in the Online appendix at www.oxfordmedicine.com/POCUSemergencymed. Please refer to your access card for further details.

Atkinson PR, McAuley DJ, Kendall RJ, *et al*. Abdominal and Cardiac Evaluation with Sonography in Shock (ACES): an approach by emergency physicians for the use of ultrasound in patients with undifferentiated hypotension. *Emerg Med J* 2009;**26**:87–91.

Marik PE. Techniques for assessment of intravascular volume in critically ill patients. *J Intensive Care Med* 2009;**24**:329–37.

Masugata H, Senda S, Okuyama H, *et al*. Age-related decrease in inferior vena cava diameter measured with echocardiography. *Tohoku J Exp Med* 2010;**222**:141–7.

Plummer D, Clinton J, Matthew B. Emergency department ultrasound improves time to diagnosis and survival in ruptured abdominal aortic aneurysm. *Acad Emer Med* 1998;**5**:417.

Rubano E, Mehta N, Caputo W, Paladino L, Sinert R. Systematic review: emergency department bedside ultrasonography for diagnosing suspected abdominal aortic aneurysm. *Acad Emerg Med* 2013;**20**:128–38.

Sierzenski PR, Leech SJ, Dickman E, Leibrandt PN, Gukhool JA, Bollinger ME. Emergency physician ultrasound decreases time to diagnose, time to CT scan and time to operative repair in patients with ruptured abdominal aortic aneurysm. *Acad Emerg Med* 2004;**11**:580.

7

Musculoskeletal ultrasound

David Lewis

Summary

When to scan (clinical indications):
Musculoskeletal (MSK) PoCUS can enhance diagnostic assessment, trauma care, and procedures. Indications include localized injury, infections, and inflammation.

What to scan (PoCUS protocol):
Core: soft tissue infection/injury/inflammation, joint effusions, fractures, and foreign body (FB). Paediatric applications include assessment for hip joint effusion and toddler's fracture.
Advanced: certain protocols and pathology require greater experience, e.g. rotator cuff assessment, ligamentous injuries, avulsion injuries, neuromas.

How to scan (key points on scanning):
Core: MSK examinations include assessment of the structure in both its long and short axes, using a high-frequency transducer and knowledge of the anatomy and normal ultrasound appearances.
Advanced: advanced MSK applications require detailed knowledge of relative MSK anatomy, specific protocols for joint assessment, and experience.

What PoCUS adds (clinical reasoning—how results change practice):
Core: PoCUS increases diagnostic/prognostic accuracy and guides management, e.g. ruling out FBs, grading muscles injuries, and draining abscesses.

Advanced: PoCUS can become the definitive investigation for MSK pathologies.

Purpose

Physicians with a basic level of experience with PoCUS will already be familiar with the normal ultrasound appearance of the many MSK structures seen while scanning other organs. The concept of visualizing the bone cortex with its associated acoustic shadow is well demonstrated by the vertebral body when visualizing the abdominal aorta and by the ribs when looking for PTX (see Figure 7.1a). Soft tissues, including adipose, fascia, and muscle, are routinely visualized when assessing for DVT or during ultrasound-guided vascular access (see Figure 7.1b). This chapter will outline the key principles of MSK PoCUS and will discuss pathology relevant to emergency and critical care practice.

Perspective

What is the relevance of musculoskeletal PoCUS to a critical care/emergency physician?

Although many MSK PoCUS applications may more appropriately reside within the remit of the sports physician or rheumatologist, there are a number of applications that are frequently used by acute care physicians. Some of these are used during the primary survey of critically ill and injured patients, e.g. triage assessment for long bone fracture, while others

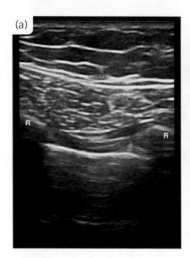
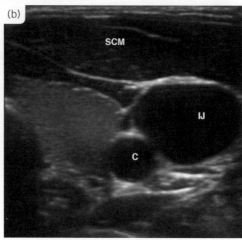

Figure 7.1 **(a) Longitudinal view of the anterior chest wall. R, ribs with posterior acoustic shadow. (b) Transverse view of the anterior neck. SCM, sternocleidomastoid muscle; IJ, internal jugular; C, carotid.**

are used during subsequent workup. For example, is there an MSK cause of this swollen leg in a patient with a negative DVT scan?

Many clinicians will be familiar with the 'dry' abscess tap and the unsatisfactory post-Colles' fracture reduction radiograph. By enhancing clinical assessment with MSK PoCUS, these unwanted outcomes will be less frequent. A radiology ultrasound report identifying the presence of a radiolucent FB is useful but does not help with its removal. Clinician-performed PoCUS-guided FB removal has a high success rate.

Patients' satisfaction is enhanced by incorporating MSK PoCUS into their clinical assessment, often allowing them to immediately see for themselves the cause of their symptoms. This interactivity is to be encouraged, and therefore, consideration of appropriate machine and screen placement should take this into account.

What are the key musculoskeletal PoCUS applications?

1. *Soft tissue infection*: abscess, cellulitis, tendon sheath infection, necrotizing fasciitis;
2. *Soft tissue injury*—subcutaneous haematoma, muscle haematoma, tendon/ligament injury;
3. *Soft tissue inflammation*—bursitis, Baker's cyst, tendonitis;
4. Joint effusions;

5. *Fractures*—diagnosis and manipulation;
6. *FB*—diagnosis and removal.

Principles and general technique for musculoskeletal PoCUS

Machine

For MSK PoCUS, with its focus on finer details and smaller structures, image quality is of paramount importance. Consideration should be given to the quality of the machine and transducers utilized for these applications. While the smaller all-in-one handheld devices with a low-frequency transducer will not generate the resolution required for most MSK PoCUS applications, some of the newer portable devices can provide an acceptable level of quality. For those working in the pre-hospital/austere environment setting, or even in a busy acute care service, there will be a trade-off between machine portability and image quality.

Transducer

The majority of MSK structures of interest to the critical care and emergency physician are relatively superficial. Most MSK PoCUS applications require a high-resolution linear (6–13 MHz) transducer in order to distinguish more subtle pathology. These

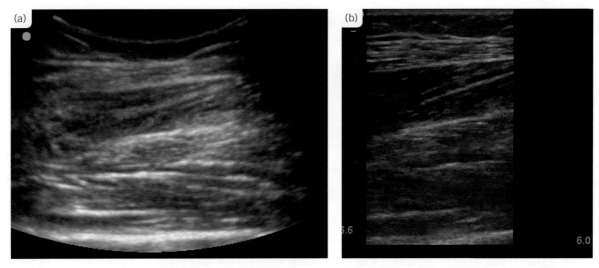

Figure 7.2 Longitudinal view of the anterior thigh, comparing the resolution of a curvilinear transducer (2–5 MHz) (a) and a linear transducer (6–13 MHz) (b).

transducers will generate a high-resolution image but can only achieve a depth of approximately 6–8 cm, which, given the superficial nature of most MSK structures, is usually adequate. One study found that almost all retained FBs were located within 2 cm of the surface.

Deeper structures, such as the adult hip joint, or an athletic thigh can be assessed with a standard curvilinear (2–5 MHz) transducer, although finer pathological detail may not be fully appreciated (see Figure 7.2).

As with any PoCUS application, transducer to body surface contact is of paramount importance. This can be achieved by choosing the correct-sized transducer for the corresponding body part. While the forearm muscles can be readily assessed using a standard-sized linear transducer, a small-footprint hockey stick transducer may be better suited for assessing a digit (see Figure 7.1s 📷).

Stand-off device

Although many modern transducers can provide high-quality images with adjustable focal depth for the most superficial structures, it is sometime advantageous to utilize a stand-off device, such as a fluid-filled surgical glove, to image cutaneous and superficial subcutaneous structures. For the hand

and digits, it is also possible to utilize a water bath, allowing a no-touch technique, which can reduce discomfort when assessing for FB or infection and remove air artefact when assessing wounds (see Figure 7.3).

Doppler

Colour flow can be helpful in MSK PoCUS. Chronic inflammation will often result in localized neovascularization, which can be identified using colour Doppler (see Figure 7.4). Muscle, in particular, is highly vascular, and larger vessels can be confused with small haematomas, especially when viewed in the short axis (transverse plane). Utilizing colour Doppler can help to distinguish small haematomas, cysts, and effusions, which have no flow, from vascular structures. Ensure that Doppler flow velocity/sensitivity and is selected appropriately for the application required. A low-velocity and high-sensitivity setting will be appropriate for most MSK applications.

Transducer orientation and regional survey

PoCUS assessment for soft tissue is performed in conjunction with physical examination. High-frequency linear transducers are used for superficial structures, and lower-frequency curvilinear transducers for deeper structures. While the area of maximal swelling

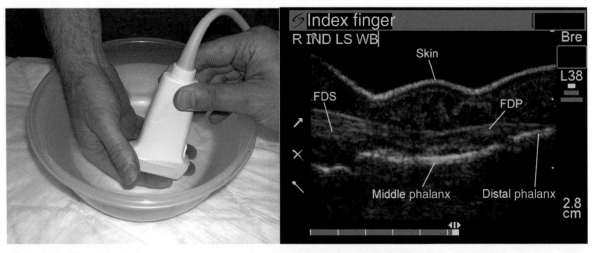

Figure 7.3 Water bath standoff; longitudinal view of the palmar surface of the index finger.

and tenderness should initially be examined, the entire region should be surveyed to ensure all injuries are diagnosed. When considering the orientation of the transducer in relation to the anatomical planes of the body, traditional descriptors, e.g. longitudinal, transverse, and coronal, are not always appropriate for MSK structures. Orientation for MSK structures is better described by the relationship of the transducer to the structure's short and long axes. PoCUS should be performed in both the long and short axes. The long-axis view will generally provide an overview assessment of a structure, while the short-axis view provides a more detailed cross-sectional assessment. It should be appreciated that the echogenicity and sonographic texture of soft tissue structures will vary between the different assessment planes.

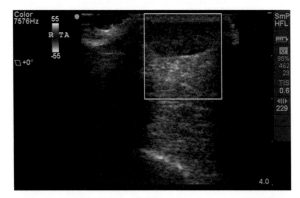

Figure 7.4 Short axis view of the Achilles tendon. Chronic tendinopathy. Thickened tendon with neovascularization demonstrated with colour flow.

Ultrasound artefacts—anisotropy

MSK PoCUS requires an understanding of all the usual ultrasound artefacts, as described in Chapter 1. There is, however, an additional artefact of particular importance to MSK PoCUS that must be appreciated in order to avoid frequent false-positive diagnoses.

Anisotropy describes a property of a material that is *directionally dependent*. In MSK PoCUS, the echogenicity of certain structures is dependent on the direction of the ultrasound beam. When the transducer is perpendicular to a structure, the appearance is echogenic; however, with even small amounts of angulation, the structure can become anechoic (see Figure 7.5). The degree of angulation required to produce this artefact varies for different MSK structures, but it can be seen in muscles, tendons, and ligaments. It is due to the anisotropic reflectivity of fibrous structures within these tissues.

Failure to appreciate this artefact in tendon can result in a false diagnosis of tendon rupture due to the artefactual appearance of an anechoic defect. In muscle, this artefact can mimic free fluid and falsely suggest a haematoma/muscle injury.

With this in mind, when visualizing any area of hypoechogenicity suspected of being pathological, care should be taken to ensure that the transducer is perpendicular to the structure being examined. With curved structures, such as the rotator cuff tendon, it will be necessary to follow the contour of the shoulder with the transducer; focus only on

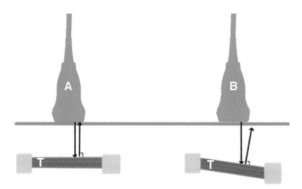

Figure 7.5 Anisotropy. When the ultrasound beam is perpendicular to the tendon (T), reflecting echoes return to the transducer and the structure appears echogenic (A). When there is angulation, the peripheral echoes are reflected away from the transducer and the structure appears anechoic (B).

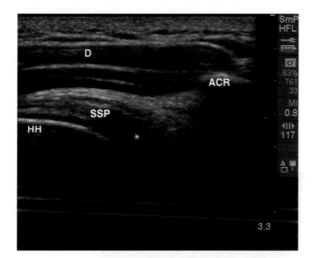

Figure 7.6 Coronal view of the shoulder. Deltoid (D), humeral head (HH), acromion (ACR), supraspinatus tendon (SSP). Anisotropic artefact causing the supraspinatus tendon to appear anechoic (*).

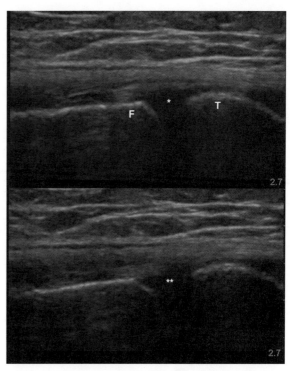

Figure 7.7 Coronal view of medial knee joint. The joint space (*) between the femur (F) and tibia (T) can be seen to widen (**) with a valgus strain. This small amount of opening is normal and can be compared with the contralateral limb, if necessary.

the appearance of the tendon in the centre of the screen, ignoring the anisotropic artefact that interferes with the tendon appearance on either side (see Figure 7.6).

This artefact can also be useful in certain circumstances. When visualized perpendicularly, certain structures can have a similar appearance and echogenicity, e.g. the flexor tendons and median nerve in the wrist. In the transverse plane, gentle angulation of the transducer will result in anisotropy, causing the tendons to become anechoic and highlighting the position of the median nerve (see Figure 7.2s 📷).

Static versus dynamic assessment

Certain structures and pathologies are best assessed without movement. Soft tissue infections, fractures, and retained FBs can be painful, and subtle findings may be missed during active movement. However, other structures and pathologies may only be seen during certain phases of movement. Subtle muscle tears can become apparent during active contraction; ligament integrity can be assessed by stressing a joint, and small joint effusions may only be visible in certain positions (see Figure 7.7).

Atlas of normal ultrasound musculoskeletal anatomy

Becoming familiar with the normal ultrasound appearances of MSK structures can initially seem overwhelming due to the huge variety of structures, views, and orientation. Fortunately, given that almost all MSK structures are bilaterally symmetrical, clinicians can easily access the subject's own 'atlas of normal ultrasound MSK anatomy' by placing the transducer in the same position and orientation on the contralateral side (see Figure 7.3s 📷). Most machines will have a dual-screen function that allows two images to be compared.

Normal ultrasound appearance of musculoskeletal structures

Skin and subcutaneous tissues

Skin (dermis) is hyperechoic and appears as a bright line at the top of the screen. Creases with skin can contain air, causing a shadow artefact. This can be overcome by careful application of ultrasound gel. Subcutaneous tissue comprises adipocytes (hypoechoic), connective tissue (hyperechoic), and superficial vessels (see Figure 7.4s 📷). It can appear hypoechoic or hyperechoic, depending on the size of the adipocytes, but it will always have lower echogenicity than the overlying skin and the underlying fascia.

Muscle

Muscle consists of large hypoechoic bundles, interspersed with hyperechoic strands of connective tissue. Due to the orientation of the muscle fibres and connective tissue, it will generally appear more hypoechoic when viewed in the short axis than in the long axis. Within compartments, surrounded by hyperechoic fascia, individual muscles are also separated by hyperechoic connective tissue layers (see Figure 7.8). It is therefore possible to identify named muscles by their anatomical location, depth, and relations. The thickness of muscle (superficial to deep) can be measured and compared with the contralateral equivalent. Normal muscle is also compressible.

Tendon

Tendon comprises longitudinal parallel collagen bundles. It appears hyperechoic when the transducer is aligned perpendicularly. A typical fibrillar pattern of multiple internal parallel echogenic strands will be apparent in the long-axis view. Multiple scattered internal individual echoes are seen in the short-axis view (see Figure 7.9). However, tendon is particularly

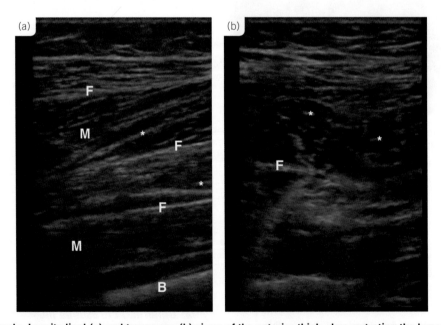

Figure 7.8 Muscle. Longitudinal (a) and transverse (b) views of the anterior thigh, demonstrating the hyperechoic fascia (F), connective tissue (*), and bony cortex (B). The muscle tissue (M) between the fascial layers (F) is relatively hypoechoic.

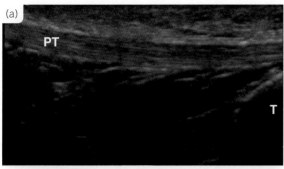

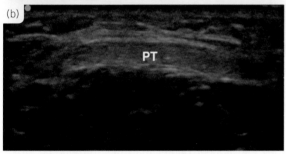

Figure 7.9 Tendon. Longitudinal (a) and transverse (b) views of the anterior knee, demonstrating the typical fibrillar pattern within the patellar tendon (PT).

susceptible to anisotropic artefact and will become more hypoechoic with increasing angulation of the transducer. Tendon often originates within the muscle body, with fibres attaching in a feather-like manner. This is a common site for muscle tears. Thus, internal tendon can be identified and differentiated from a haematoma by gently angling the transducer and utilizing the anisotropic effect.

Tendon changes in structure within the region of bony insertion (the enthesis), becoming more homogenous and hypoechoic, due to an increased proportion of fibrocartilaginous tissue.

Nerves

The ultrasound appearance of nerve tissue varies with location. Large proximal nerve trunks have a short-axis ultrasound appearance, similar to a bundle of vessels, with a hyperechoic circumference and an anechoic centre (see Figure 7.10). Anatomical location and absence of colour flow can help identify these structures.

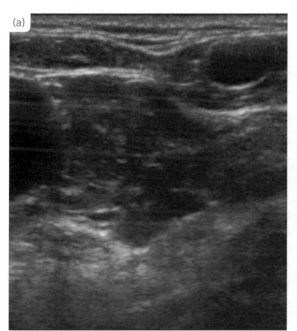

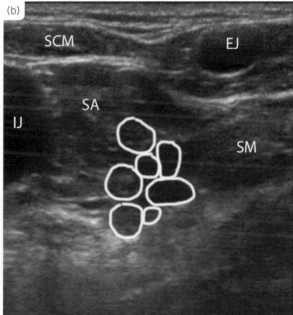

Figure 7.10 Brachial plexus. Transverse view of the right lower neck (a) and labelled (b). The internal jugular (IJ) vein is medial, with the external jugular (EJ) vein lying superficially and lateral to the sternocleidomastoid muscle (SCM). The hypoechoic trunks/divisions of the brachial plexus are seen (white outline) running between the scalenus anterior (SA) and the scalenus medius (SM).

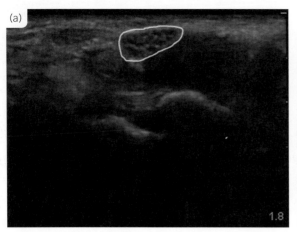
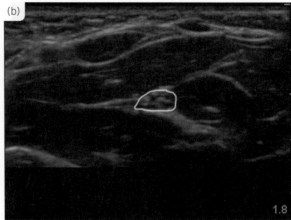

Figure 7.11 Peripheral nerve. Transverse view of the volar wrist (a) and forearm (b). The median nerve is outlined in both images.

In the periphery, individual nerves are more hyperechoic in appearance. They are usually best identified in the short axis (transverse plane) where they appear more hyperechoic that the surrounding muscles. The cross-sectional, honeycombed appearance of peripheral nerves has been compared to a bunch of narrow drinking straws, with multiple anechoic neurons surrounded by hyperechoic fibrous tissue (see Figure 7.11).

Peripheral nerves will usually run in neurovascular bundles between muscle groups. Picking them out on a static image from other hyperechoic, localized fibrous tissue can be difficult. By running the transducer in the short-axis plane, proximally to distally, back and forth, the nerve can often be better perceived, as it maintains a more predictable and slower-changing position than the localized fibrous tissue.

Nerves are non-compressible.

Ligaments

Given the small size and close proximity to bone of many ligaments, it is not surprising that detailed ultrasound visualization can be difficult. Echogenicity can be similar to surrounding tissue, and demarcation therefore difficult. When seen, the hyperechoic collagenous fibrillar structures can have a similar appearance to tendon, although of a much smaller diameter. Although generally hyperechoic, with their

proximity to the bone cortex and surrounding fascia, they can appear darker than the surrounding structures (see Figure 7.12).

Bone and cartilage

Bone cortex has a very high impedance to ultrasound and is highly reflective. The resulting ultrasound appearance is a bright, hyperechoic contour that outlines the bone surface below the transducer. The acoustic shadow deep to this hyperechoic contour is artefactual (see Figure 7.5s ▣). The periosteum is normally closely applied to the bone cortex and will usually be indistinguishable from it on ultrasound. As described later in this chapter, certain pathologies can result in separation of the periosteum from the cortex.

Within the joint capsule, bone is covered in a thin (2–4 mm) layer of hyaline cartilage (see Figure 7.13). The ultrasound appearance of hyaline cartilage changes with the age of the patient. In children and young adults, it is smooth and anechoic, becoming progressively pitted and hyperechoic with advancing years.

Fibrocartilaginous structures, such as the glenoid labrum or meniscal cartilage, are formed by densely packed fibres and have a homogenous hypoechoic appearance, similar in echogenicity to that of the liver (see Figure 7.14).

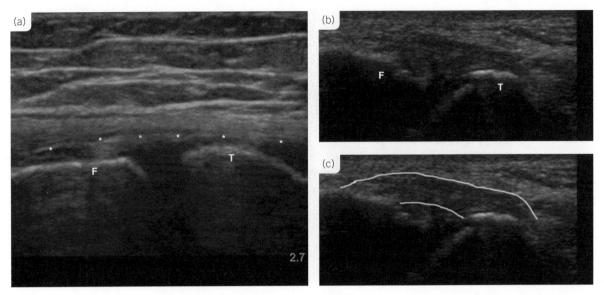

Figure 7.12 Ligaments. Coronal view of the medial knee (a), demonstrating the medial collateral ligament (*) running between the femur (F) and tibia (T). Oblique view of the lateral ankle (b, c), demonstrating the anterior talofibular ligament (outlined in c) running between the fibula (F) and the talus (T).

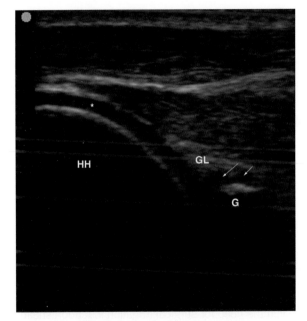

Figure 7.13 Hyaline cartilage. Transverse view from behind the shoulder, demonstrating a posterior dislocation. The hyaline cartilage (*) of the articular surface of the humeral head (HH) has become posterior-facing due to excess internal rotation of the humeral head. A small tear (arrows) between the glenoid labrum (GL) and the posterior glenoid (G) is also demonstrated. See this same view post-reduction in Figure 7.34.

Pathology: soft tissue infection

Cellulitis

Identifying cellulitis with PoCUS can be useful. Consider the following scenarios:

1. Is there an alternative diagnosis for this patient with a red, swollen calf and a negative DVT scan?

2. Is this area of erythema and swelling an abscess that would benefit from incision and drainage, or is it cellulitis?

Cellulitis has a typical appearance on ultrasound. As the pathological process develops, subcutaneous adipocytes become separated and surrounded by inflammatory fluid. This results in an ultrasound appearance of hyperechoic adipocytes surrounded by anechoic fluid, resembling cobblestones (see Figure 7.15 and Video 7.1 ▣).

The cobblestone sign is not specific to cellulitis and can be seen in peripheral oedema due to other causes such as lymphoedema or congestive cardiac failure.

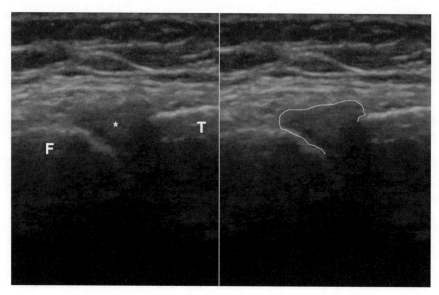

Figure 7.14 **Meniscus. Coronal view of the medial knee. The medial meniscus (*) is outlined in the right panel.**

Abscess

Many subcutaneous abscesses will evolve from an area of cellulitis. Clinical examination will not reliably determine whether an area of erythema and swelling is due to cellulitis or an abscess. Even small collections can appear as if swollen due to a 'ripe' abscess when, in fact, localized oedema is the cause and attempted incision and drainage is unsuccessful (see Video 7.2 ⬛). MSK PoCUS can quickly determine whether there is a drainable collection within the abscess and help guide the procedure. Studies have shown that MSK PoCUS can help clinicians to

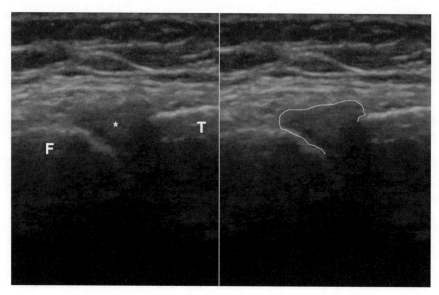

Figure 7.15 **Cobblestone sign. The subcutaneous adipocytes (A) are surrounded by anechoic inflammatory fluid, resulting in a cobblestone appearance.**

more accurately decide when to incise and drain an abscess.

The typical ultrasound appearance of an abscess is an anechoic collection of varying shape, usually containing echogenic debris and surrounded by subcutaneous oedema (see Figure 7.6s ⬛ and Video 7.3 ⬛). Gentle compression of the abscess can result in 'pustalsis', which is the contained debris swirling within the cavity (see Video 7.4 ⬛).

Tendon sheath infection

Tendon sheath infections can be difficult to diagnose clinically. Typically caused by penetrating injuries to the hand, they will normally present as areas of soft tissue infection with associated tenderness on movement. However, in the confined space of the hand, soft tissue infections that have not communicated with the tendon sheath can also be painful on movement. Given the need for surgical irrigation in tendon sheath infections and the potential disability that can result if incorrectly treated, diagnosis is important. The presence of fluid surrounding the tendon within its sheath can be seen on ultrasound (see Figure 7.16).

This appearance, given a typical history and physical examination, would be highly suggestive of tendon sheath infection. While the absence of tendon fluid does not entirely rule out a tendon sheath infection, it would make the diagnosis much less likely and clinical

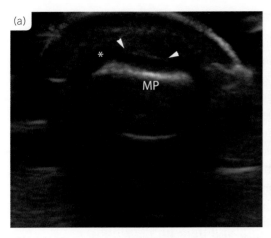

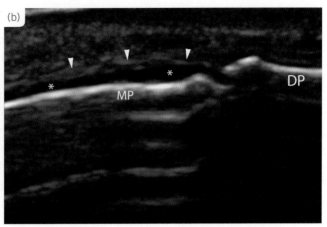

Figure 7.16 Tendon sheath infection. Transverse (a) and longitudinal (b) views of the volar index finger at the level of the middle (MP) and distal phalanges (DP). Anechoic inflammatory fluid (*) is seen between the flexor digitorum profundus (arrowheads) and bone and is within the tendon sheath.

judgement would determine whether further investigations or follow-up are required.

Necrotizing fasciitis

PoCUS has been shown to be potentially useful in the diagnosis of necrotizing fasciitis. This condition is notoriously difficult to diagnose, and any delay in management can have limb- and life-threatening consequences. The ultrasound appearance of necrotizing fasciitis includes subcutaneous tissue and fascial thickening, deep fascial fluid, and, in some cases, subcutaneous air (see Figure 7.17). MSK PoCUS should not be used to rule out necrotizing fasciitis; however, in the correct clinical setting, the above PoCUS findings could be used to fast-track the required surgical management and help to reduce morbidity and mortality.

Pathology: soft tissue injury

The key PoCUS features of any soft tissue injury are:

1. Increased thickness of a structure;
2. The presence of abnormal fluid;
3. A visible defect within the structure;
4. Abnormal movement.

Any or all of these may be visualized following soft tissue injury, although typically, the order presented corresponds with increasing severity of the injury.

Muscle

Closed muscle injury can be caused by blunt contusion or during muscle contraction. Blunt contusion usually results in muscle oedema, which, when compared with the contralateral normal, appears of greater diameter and hyperechoic (see Figure 7.18). Hyperechogenicity of tissue oedema is due to reorientation of connective tissue by increasing interstitial fluid.

Low-grade muscle tears caused by contractive forces will often have a similar appearance to blunt contusion

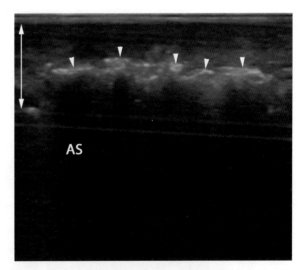

Figure 7.17 Necrotizing fasciitis. Subcutaneous thickening (double-headed arrow), subcutaneous air (arrowheads), and posterior air shadow (AS).

With permission from Vi Dinh MD, RDMS, RDCS.

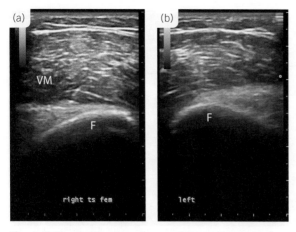

Figure 7.18 Muscle contusion—split-screen comparative. Transverse views of the mid-anterior thigh. The distance from the skin surface down to the femur (F) is greater in the injured leg (a) due to oedema of the vastus medialis (VM). Contused vastus medialis is of greater echogenicity in the injured leg (a) than in the normal leg (b).

injuries, with localized oedema and muscle thickening. Moderate-grade muscle tears will result in the appearance of abnormal fluid, and high-grade tears will result in a visible defect, which changes in size during dynamic examination (see Figure 7.19 and Video 7.5 ⊡).

Differentiating the grade of muscle injury can be important for prognosticating recovery times, especially in the athlete.

Tendon

Injuries to normal tendons are seen following penetrating trauma, especially around the hand, where clinical examination is usually sufficient to make the diagnosis.

Degenerative tendon can tear, or even completely rupture, as a result of muscle contraction or passive stretch. Examples of these injuries that are frequently seen in the acute setting include Achilles tendon and rotator cuff injuries. MSK PoCUS can be very helpful in the assessment of degenerative tendon injuries.

The *Achilles tendon* is formed by fusion of the soleus and gastrocnemius tendons inserting into the calcaneus. The patient is asked to lie prone on the examination couch, with their foot hanging free (see Figure 7.7s ⊡).

The tendon can be well visualized with a high-frequency linear transducer and should be assessed in both the transverse and longitudinal plane. In the transverse plane, the flat posterior margin of the tendon can be seen lying superficially, just deep to the skin, with the curved anterior margin lying deeper, giving this cross-sectional view of the tendon a semicircular appearance (see Figure 7.8s ⊡). In the longitudinal plane, the typical hyperechogenic fibrillar pattern can be appreciated and the diameter can be measured (normal AP diameter = 5–6 mm).

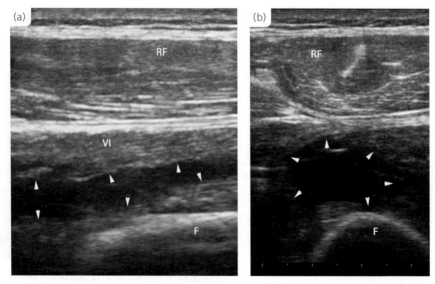

Figure 7.19 Muscle tear. Longitudinal (a) and transverse (b) views of the mid-anterior thigh. A grade 3 muscle tear (anechoic haematoma outlined by arrows) is seen within the body of the vastus intermedius (VI), which lies deep to the rectus femoris (RF) and superficial to the femur (F).

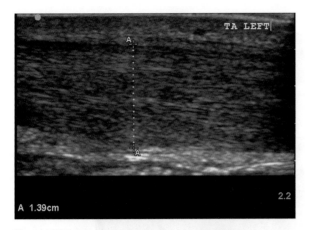

Figure 7.20 Achilles tendonosis. Longitudinal view of the contralateral posterior ankle. Calipers (A) demonstrate the increased anteroposterior diameter of a hypoechogenic tendon.

Localized thickening and hypoechogenicity are suggestive of degenerative Achilles tendonosis, which can be a cause of posterior ankle pain (see Figure 7.20).

With chronic tendinopathy, Achilles tendon rupture usually occurs 5–6 cm proximal to its insertion. Clinicians will be familiar with the typical history and presentation of Achilles tendon rupture (middle aged, male > female, 'it felt like I was kicked in the back of the leg'). Thorough examination, especially the Simmonds test, can be very uncomfortable, and significant swelling can obscure palpation of any palpable tendon defect. PoCUS can enhance the assessment of the Achilles tendon in suspected rupture. In the

longitudinal plane, the tendon will appear thickened and the normal fibrillar pattern will be disrupted. Anechoic haematoma may be visualized around or within the disrupted tendon (see Figure 7.21). Tendon separation may be visualized on dynamic examination during passive ankle dorsiflexion (see Videos 7.6 and 7.7 ⏺).

Diagnostic ultrasound of *rotator cuff* pathology can be challenging, and a detailed guide is beyond the scope of this chapter. However, in acute rotator cuff injuries, utilization of a simplified PoCUS examination can be helpful.

The patient is sat on a stool, facing away from the clinician. The clinician stands behind the patient, with the ultrasound machine in front and visible by both clinician and patient. This allows helpful interaction during the assessment and has been found to improve patient satisfaction. The patient is asked, as pain allows, to place the palm of their hand behind them on their ipsilateral buttock, thus bringing the rotator cuff tendon laterally out from under the acromion. A high-frequency linear transducer is placed in the coronal plane, with the upper end sitting on the tip of the acromion (see Figure 7.9s 🖼). The lower end of the transducer sits over the greater tuberosity (insertion of the supraspinatus tendon).

This view will allow visualization of the deltoid, subacromial bursa, supraspinatus tendon, and head of the humerus cortex. The subacromial bursa is normally empty, and therefore not seen unless pathological

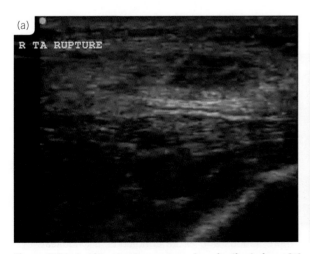
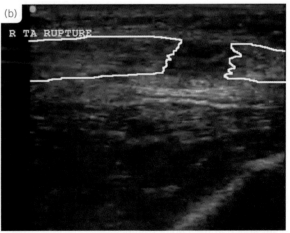

Figure 7.21 Achilles tendon rupture. Longitudinal view of the posterior ankle (a). Same image with the tendon rupture outlined (b).

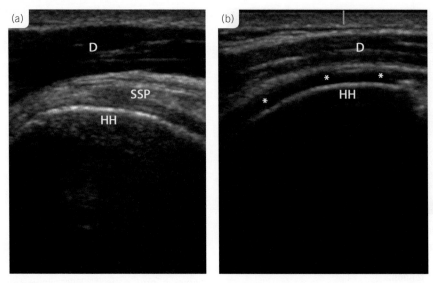

Figure 7.22 Rupture of the supraspinatus tendon (SSP). Coronal view of normal shoulder (a), demonstrating the relationship of a normal supraspinatus tendon (SSP) lying between the deltoid (D) and the humeral head (HH). Coronal view of the shoulder (b), demonstrating the absence of the supraspinatus tendon (*) between the deltoid (D) and the humeral head (HH), indicating a complete rupture of the supraspinatus tendon.

(subacromial bursitis). Care with transducer angulation is required to avoid the pitfall of anisotropic artefact. As with all tendons, chronic tendinopathy of the supraspinatus is visualized with PoCUS as thickening and hypoechogenic. A partial tear of the supraspinatus can be difficult to appreciate, especially when the free edge is involved. It will usually appear on PoCUS as an anechoic defect within the tendon body. A complete rupture of the tendon is demonstrated on PoCUS by the absence of the supraspinatus, and instead the deltoid muscle lies in direct contact with the cortex of the head of the humerus (see Figure 7.22). Calcific tendonitis can be identified as highly echogenic material within the tendon, usually casting an acoustic shadow (see Videos 7.8 to 7.11 ◉).

Ligaments

Ligament injuries can be difficult to directly visualize on PoCUS. They can, however, be inferred by the presence of abnormal fluid (compared with contralateral assessment) and also abnormal bone movement on dynamic examination. Align the high-frequency transducer along the length of the ligament, with the joint space in the centre of the screen and the superficial cortex of the two bones on either side. Assess for joint space opening (abnormal separation of bony cortices), while applying the appropriate stressor force to the joint, e.g. valgus stress for medial collateral ligament of the knee (see Figure 7.7 for normal joint space opening).

The anterior talo-fibular ligament (ATFL) is commonly injured, following an inversion injury to the ankle, although complete rupture is less common. The ligament can be identified by placing the transducer obliquely between the lateral malleolus and the talus. The relatively hypoechoic ligament can be seen extending between the hyperechoic bony cortices (see Figure 7.23). In ATFL rupture, anterior traction results in separation of the bony cortices (see Video 7.12 ◉).

Pathology: soft tissue inflammation

Soft tissue inflammation results in localized oedema (leading to structural thickening) and capillary leak (leading to free fluid generation). Both of these features can be readily appreciated on PoCUS. They can present within the differential diagnosis of some of the more serious and acute conditions, e.g. Baker's cyst and DVT, bursitis, and septic arthritis.

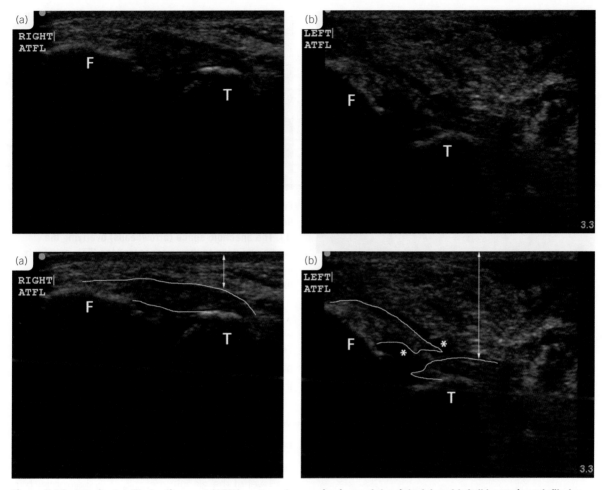

Figure 7.23 Anterior talofibular ligament (ATFL) rupture. Long axis views of the right (a) and left (b) anterior talofibular ligaments. Images are replicated with ligaments outlined below. Fibula (F), talus (T). The ATFL is ruptured on the left, indicated by direct visualization of the defect (outlined), haematoma (*), widened joint space, and soft tissue swelling over the talus (arrowed line).

Baker's cysts are usually formed by an outpouching of the semimembranosus bursa communicating between the tendons of the medial gastrocnemius and the semimembranosus (see Figure 7.24). PoCUS appearance is that of an anechoic cystic structure of varying size and shape, arising medially and lying superficially to the popliteal vascular structures. Absence of Doppler flow can help distinguish it from a popliteal artery aneurysm.

Other bursae can become inflamed, e.g. olecranon bursitis, prepatellar bursitis, and subacromial bursitis. These conditions can present with painful swollen joints that could suggest septic arthritis. PoCUS assessment will demonstrate an anechoic cystic structure in the superficial tissues corresponding to the anatomical location of the bursa (see Figure 7.10s 📷). In addition, PoCUS can demonstrate the absence of a joint effusion, which further lessens the likelihood of a diagnosis of septic arthritis.

Pathology: joint effusions

Joint effusions will appear as protrusions from the joint space of anechoic fluid that displaces but remains constrained by the hyperechoic joint capsule. Small amounts of physiological joint fluid is often apparent, as its anechoic hyaline cartilage.

145

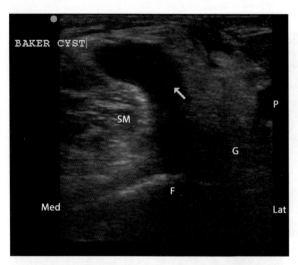

Figure 7.24 Baker's cyst. Transverse view of the posterior knee joint at the level of the medial femoral condyle (F). A Baker's cyst (arrow) is seen emerging between the tendons of the semimembranosus (SM) and the medial head of the gastrocnemius (G), both medial to the popliteal vessels (P).

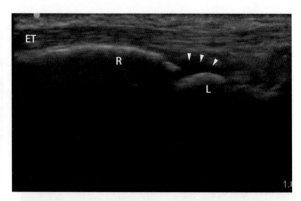

Figure 7.25 Normal wrist joint. Long axis view over the dorsum of the wrist between the radius (R) and the lunate (L). The anechoic space (arrowheads) overlying the lunate and deep to the extensor tendons (ET) represents a small amount of physiological joint fluid and lunate hyaline cartilage.

Contralateral joint assessment and comparison will establish whether the appearances are symmetrical and normal or asymmetrical and abnormal. The nature of the effusion cannot be discerned by PoCUS. Whether an effusion is caused by gout, pseudogout, haemarthrosis, or even sepsis, it will generally have the same anechoic appearance. Once identified, the most superficial and accessible point of the effusion can be determined and, if appropriate, this can guide aspiration, whether for aspirate analysis or simply for symptom relief.

Wrist joint

The transducer is placed over the dorsum of the wrist joint in the longitudinal plane. An effusion is identified by the presence of an anechoic space between the distal radius and the carpus (see Figure 7.25).

Elbow joint

Elbow joint effusions can be detected by placing the transducer in the short axis, posteriorly over the flexed elbow at the level of the olecranon fossa (see Figure 7.26). Larger effusions can be seen in the long axis over the radial head and lateral epicondyle (see Figure 7.11s 🎦) where an effusion, if present, will often be apparent as an anechoic protrusion between these structures.

Shoulder joint

Effusions within the shoulder joint are normally apparent on anterior– and posterior–transverse views at the level of the glenohumeral joint. Subacromial bursitis (see Figure 7.10s 🎦) can occasionally be misinterpreted as a joint effusion, although the latter will normally be seen lying deep to the rotator cuff tendons and extending distally around the long head of the biceps tendon (see Figure 7.27).

Hip joint

The hip joint is best viewed anteriorly along the axis of the femoral neck. This can be found by initially placing the transducer anteriorly, in the short axis, over the proximal femur. The transducer is then moved proximally to the greater trochanter, then rotated along the axis of the femoral neck, before being moved medially until the hip joint is identified (see Figure 7.12s 🎦). In larger adults, a curvilinear 2–4 MHz transducer may be required to achieve the required depth. An effusion will appear as a compressible anechoic space that displaces the joint capsule from the femoral neck.

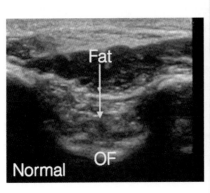
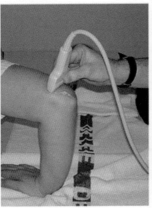
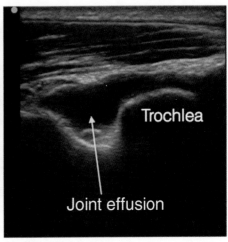

Figure 7.26 Short axis view of the posterior flexed elbow. Compare the normal appearance with joint effusion.

Knee joint

Knee joint effusions are best viewed in the long axis over the medial joint line and the suprapatellar space. As with any joint effusion, they appear anechoic and are compressible (see Figure 7.28).

Ankle joint

Ankle joint effusions are best viewed in the long axis anteriorly between the tibia and the talus (see Figure 7.13s 📷).

Paediatric hip

PoCUS assessment of the paediatric hip joint deserves a special mention. The limping child is a common presentation to the emergency care physician. In the older child, radiography is an appropriate choice of investigation when considering a diagnosis of slipped capital femoral epiphysis (SCFE) or Perthes. In the younger

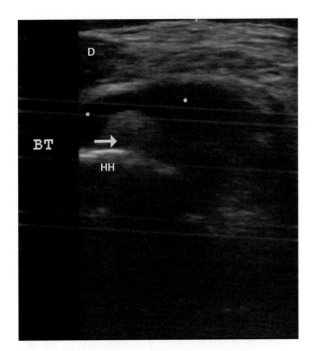

Figure 7.27 Haemarthrosis of the shoulder joint. Transverse view of the anterior shoulder at the level of the mid-humeral head (HH). The intra-articular portion of the long head of the biceps tendon (arrow) is seen in short axis, surrounded by the anechoic haemarthrosis which is distending the capsule deep to the deltoid (D).

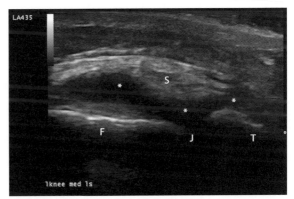

Figure 7.28 Knee joint effusion. A long axis view over the left knee medial joint line (J) between the femur (F) and tibia (T). An anechoic space consistent with a joint effusion (*) is identified. Synovial thickening (S) suggests a chronic condition.

infant, the most common cause of a limp is transient synovitis of the hip (irritable hip). Less common, but potentially devastating if missed, is septic arthritis of the hip. Although widening of the medial joint space on radiographs can occasionally be seen and infers the presence of a large effusion, ultrasound is by far the best modality for imaging paediatric hip joint effusions. Although traditionally performed in diagnostic imaging departments, the technique is straightforward and should be considered an appropriate PoCUS modality to be used as part of the clinical assessment of a limping child.

It is very important to remember that while a hip joint effusion can be diagnosed with PoCUS, the nature of the effusion (septic versus transient synovitis) cannot be determined; in addition, the absence of a visible joint effusion does not rule out septic arthritis. Clinical judgement and, where appropriate, inflammatory markers will be necessary to differentiate these two conditions.

The technique for PoCUS assessment of the paediatric hip is as follows:

- Use a high-frequency linear transduce.

- Spend time explaining the process to ensure a co-operative child and parent. Tips for putting the child at ease include putting the ultrasound gel on the parent's hand first, then asking the parent to apply the gel over the child's hip.

- With one hand holding the transducer and the other holding the leg, and in the absence of an assistant, the parent may even have to be co-opted into pressing the freeze button on the machine.

- The child is asked to lie supine, and appropriate modesty coverings employed.

- Hold the transducer transversely orientated over the proximal femur, and move proximally towards the level of the greater trochanter.

- Rotate the transducer (approximately 45° clockwise) to align along the femoral neck (see Figure 7.14s 🖼).

- Identify the echogenic cortex of the femoral neck and head, with the epiphyseal plate in between.

- Identify the hyperechoic joint capsule and the overlying hypoechoic iliopsoas tendon (see Figure 7.15s 🖼).

- A normal joint may have a small anechoic stripe (normal hypoechoic joint cartilage) between the cortex and the capsule. This will measure <2 mm and will be symmetrical between the hips.

- An effusion will result in a larger anechoic stripe (>2 mm) that takes on a lenticular shape as the capsule distends. Asymmetry between the hips is confirmatory (see Figure 7.29).

- Synovial thickening may also be visualized (see Figure 7.16s 🖼).

Pathology: fractures

PoCUS assessment of bony injury is a relatively new modality. An entry-level PoCUS clinician will be familiar with the complete ultrasound reflectivity of the bone cortex and the posterior acoustic shadow and may wonder how PoCUS can provide any useful information. However, with fractures, it is precisely the alignment of the bone cortex and the overlying periosteum that is of interest. Provided there is an unhindered acoustic window between the skin and the underlying bone, a cortical fracture can be seen with PoCUS (see Figure 7.17s 🖼).

However, with such a narrow field of view, fractures that are not directly below the transducer will be missed. PoCUS will not provide the same quick survey approach of a skeletal radiograph. A detailed PoCUS assessment of the bones in the hand would be extremely time-consuming, when compared with a plain radiograph. The close proximity and shape of the small carpal bones significantly hinder the availability of an acoustic window to each and every cortex. In addition, an appreciation of the degree of angulation and displacement of a long bone fracture may not be readily apparent on PoCUS. Finally, the traditional ability to save a standard-view image to a central repository, both for the medical record and to share with other clinicians (who may not have PoCUS training), continues to favour skeletal radiography as the primary modality for the assessment of the majority of fractures.

There are, however, areas where skeletal radiography is less than satisfactory for both fracture diagnosis and management:

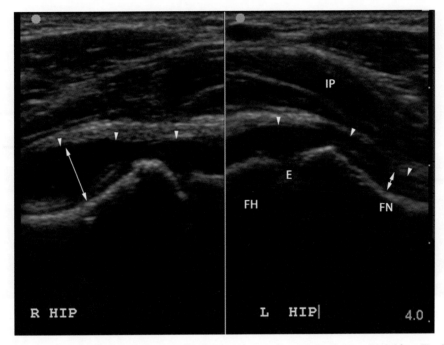

Figure 7.29 Right paediatric hip effusion. Dual-screen view for comparison of the right and left hips. The femoral head (FH), epiphysis (E), femoral neck (FN), and iliopsoas tendon (IP) can be identified on both sides. The capsule (arrowheads) is displaced from the femoral neck by an anechoic stripe on the right hip. There is significant asymmetry between the thickness of the stripe (double-headed arrows) on either side.

1. Chest wall fractures (ribs and sternum);

2. Rapid diagnosis of major long bone fracture in the primary survey;

3. Toddler's fracture and other occult fractures;

4. Pre-hospital and austere environment fracture diagnosis;

5. Inter-reduction fracture imaging (in the absence of fluoroscopy).

It is in these situations that PoCUS can offer advantages over skeletal radiography. These will be described in further detail in the following sections.

General technique

Most bones are well visualized with a high-frequency linear (6–13 MHz) transducer, although a standard curvilinear (2–5 MHz) transducer can be used to visualize the femur, as part of an eFAST scan. The presence of a fracture will be demonstrated by a break in the normally echogenic bony cortex. Displacement and angulation can also be seen. These PoCUS appearances can be correlated with the presence of localized swelling and tenderness. In general, aligning the transducer with the long axis of the bone (usually corresponding to the longitudinal plane) gives the best views. While maintaining this orientation, the transducer can be rotated around the circumference of the limb (in the case of long bones), in order to visualize the anterior, medial, posterior, and lateral surfaces of the cortex (see Figure 7.18s 📷).

The short axis view (transverse) can be used to rapidly screen a length of bone (e.g. tender area overlying a number of ribs) for cortex disruption.

Certain normal structures and artefacts can be misinterpreted on PoCUS as fractures:

- The epiphyseal plate (growth plate);
- Normal cortical surface irregularities;
- Acoustic shadowing from an overlying FB or intra-wound air.

Anatomical knowledge and contralateral comparison will lessen the risk of false-positive PoCUS fracture diagnosis.

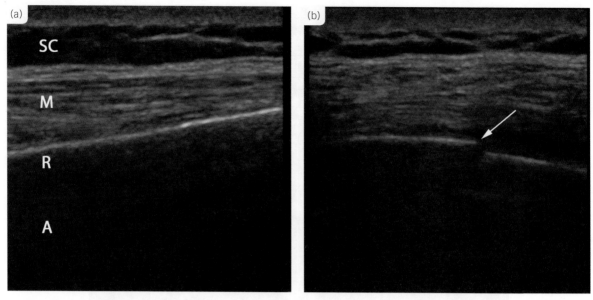

Figure 7.30 Normal rib (a) and rib fracture (b). Long axis view of rib demonstrating subcutaneous tissue (SC), muscle (M), superficial rib cortex (R), and deep acoustic shadow (A). The rib fracture (arrow) can be seen as a step deformity in the cortex.

Chest wall fractures

Rib fractures are notoriously difficult to diagnose on plain chest radiographs, especially fractures of the lower ribs. Clinical assessment of chest wall tenderness following blunt trauma can include PoCUS. Using a high-frequency linear transducer, aligned along the long axis of the ribs in the region of maximal tenderness, a fracture can be diagnosed with a high degree of specificity. The key PoCUS features of a rib fracture are a cortical step deformity, with associated underlying tenderness (see Figure 7.30 and Videos 7.13 and 7.14 ○).

While the majority of rib fractures are benign, occasional associated injuries can be more serious, including PTX, HTX, and liver and splenic injuries. As described earlier in this book, PoCUS can be used with a high degree of accuracy to diagnose PTX and HTX. The haemoperitoneum, which may be associated with abdominal solid organ injury, can also be identified (eFAST). In practice, the presence of a rib fracture overlying the liver or spleen, even in the absence of haemoperitoneum, should raise concerns and would normally warrant further imaging with CT.

Sternal fractures are usually visible on a lateral radiograph; however, rapid diagnosis can be achieved with PoCUS. As with rib fractures, the key features are a cortical step deformity, with associated underlying tenderness. The degree of displacement can be measured easily. In the trauma scenario, the presence of a displaced sternal fracture in a patient with blunt anterior chest trauma and tachyarrhythmia can suggest cardiac injury. Further primary survey cardiac PoCUS assessment for cardiac function and haemopericardium would be warranted.

Long bone fractures

Rapid assessment for long bones fractures is frequently used as part of an eFAST scan. This can be used to assess for other potential sites of blood loss in a patient with shock and also to guide the use of splinting and traction for both haemorrhage control and analgesia.

In the pre-hospital/austere environment, PoCUS may be the only imaging modality available. Patients with a suspected bony injury can be assessed utilizing a thorough PoCUS bone survey, as described in 'General technique', p. 149. This approach can be utilized for the metacarpals, radius, ulna, humerus, clavicle, femur, tibia, fibula, and metatarsals. In these circumstances, confirmed fractures can be splinted and patients can be triaged to the appropriate facility (see Figure 7.31).

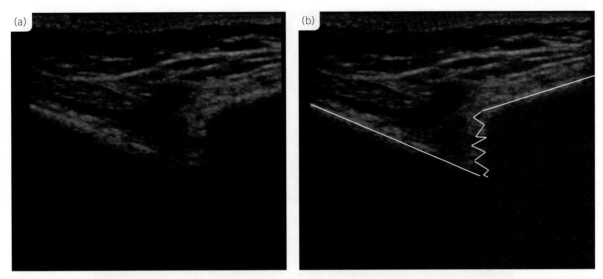

Figure 7.31 Displaced fracture of the distal radius. Long axis view over the distal radius (a) with the bony cortex outlined (b).

Occult fractures

The use of PoCUS to enhance the management of a number of different occult fractures has been described in the medical literature.

A toddler's fracture is an occult fracture of the tibia, which commonly presents in the preschool child after a minor trauma resulting in a torsional injury. The child will be unable to weight-bear, and there may be increased palpable warmth over the shin; however, initial radiographs of the entire lower limb are normal. While an experienced physician may, in these circumstances, suspect a toddler's fracture, they will not be able to confirm the diagnosis until a repeat radiograph in 2 weeks demonstrates the periosteal reaction typical of a toddler's fracture (see Figure 7.19s 📷).

There is a dilemma as to whether to cast all suspected toddler's fractures and accept that, in some cases, this was unnecessary or to cast only in selective cases based on the index of suspicion and parental wishes. PoCUS can help guide this decision. Using a high-frequency transducer on the highest resolution setting and aligned along the long axis of the tibia, a thorough survey can be performed, especially focusing on any areas of increased warmth. A toddler's fracture is confirmed by the presence of an anechoic stripe, superficial to the cortex and consistent with a subperiosteal haematoma (see Figure 7.20s 📷).

Although specific for a toddler's fracture, the absence of a visible periosteal haematoma does not rule out the diagnosis. However, it should guide the clinician to look for other potential causes of a limp/non-weight-bearing. As described in 'Hip joint', p. 147, the hip joint can be assessed with PoCUS for the presence of an effusion.

While the majority of hip fractures in the elderly are apparent on initial radiographs, a small subset will be challenging to diagnose. Disposition may be contentious and result in unnecessary transfer of these frail elderly patients, following a delayed diagnosis with a CT scan. Where there is suspicion of a femoral neck fracture and an inconclusive radiograph, the hip joint can be assessed with PoCUS, in the manner described earlier in this chapter, for the presence of haemarthrosis (see Figure 7.32). In these circumstances, this finding would be diagnostic of an occult hip fracture and should help guide disposition and streamline further imaging.

Fracture manipulation and reduction

It is in this area of fracture management that PoCUS is probably most relevant.

Without access to fluoroscopy, post-reduction alignment can only be surmised clinically and confirmed by transfer to the diagnostic imaging suite. Should the reduction be shown to be unsatisfactory, the cast will

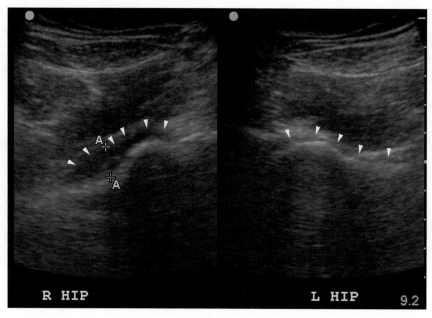

Figure 7.32 Right occult hip fracture. A patient with a history of non-weight-bearing right leg following a fall. Initial plain radiographs were inconclusive. PoCUS assessment demonstrated displacement of the joint capsule (arrowheads) by an anechoic stripe, confirming the presence of a right-sided haemarthrosis and occult fracture.

then have to be removed and the whole process repeated. This can significantly extend the duration of the procedure, consuming personnel resources and complicating the management of conscious sedation or the local anaesthetic block. Even where fluoroscopy is readily available, PoCUS can reduce repeated views and exposure times.

Distal forearm and wrist fractures are common and well suited to the use of PoCUS-assisted manipulation and reduction, although this technique can be used to check alignment of any long bone reduction.

Prior to attempted manipulation and reduction, the fracture should be visualized in the long axis with PoCUS, and the displacement/angulation correlated with the initial radiograph. Should the operator choose a regional nerve block or a haematoma block, then PoCUS should be used to guide the accurate delivery of the local anaesthetic agent (see Chapter 9).

Following attempted manipulation and reduction, repeated PoCUS views can be obtained until the operator is satisfied with the position. Contralateral views can be obtained for comparison and to confirm normal alignment (see Figure 7.33 and Videos 7.15 to 7.18 ▣).

Post-reduction radiographs are still recommended for the following reasons: to confirm maintenance of the fracture position after casting, for medico-legal records, and to assist those involved in the ongoing care of these patients.

Shoulder dislocation

The principles described previously can also be used in difficult cases to check the post-reduction of the glenohumeral joint in patients with shoulder dislocation. A transverse view of the posterior joint space can be used to demonstrate a successful joint reduction (see Figure 7.21s ▣). Both anterior and posterior shoulder dislocations can be diagnosed and reduction confirmed, using this view.

In an anterior shoulder dislocation, the humeral head will appear further away from the transducer than normal (see Figure 7.34).

In a posterior shoulder dislocation, the humeral head will appear closer to the transducer than normal (see Figure 7.22s ▣).

Pathology: foreign bodies

Radio-opaque FBs are easily identified on plain radiographs. However, many retained FBs, such as

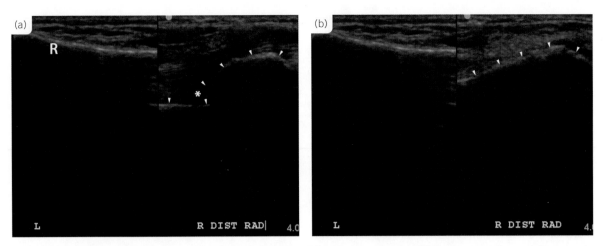

Figure 7.33 PoCUS-guided fracture reduction. Pre-reduction (a) and post-reduction (b) dual-screen views of the normal left and abnormal right distal radius (R). There is significant angulation and some displacement of the distal fragment (arrowheads), which has subsequently been corrected in the post-reduction view. Note the location of the fracture haematoma (*), which can be used to accurately guide a haematoma block.

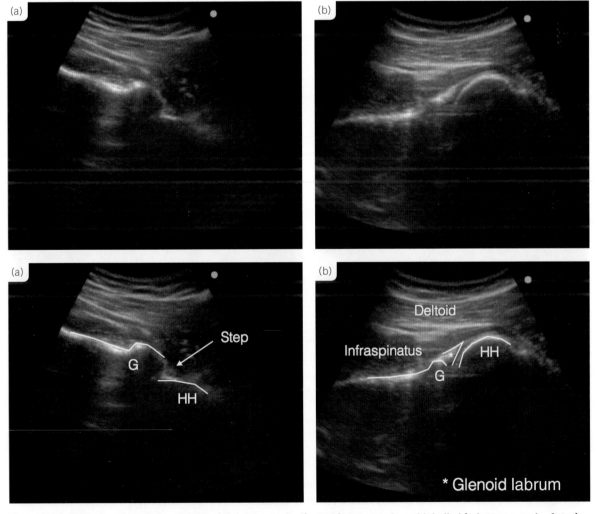

Figure 7.34 Posterior view of the shoulder joint. Images duplicated in top panels and labelled in bottom panels. Anterior shoulder dislocation (a) and post-reduction (b). Note the position of the humeral head appearing deeper (further away from the transducer than normal).

wooden splinters or thorns, are radiolucent and will be missed. This organic material is not only radiolucent, but also most likely to result in infectious complications if retained and missed. Over one-third of retained FBs are missed by plain radiography. While plain radiography can identify the presence of radiolucent FBs, it is of little use in guiding removal. Similarly, diagnostic imaging department ultrasound will identify or rule out radiolucent FBs but will provide little assistance in their removal. The process of identification and guided removal of FBs with PoCUS should be within the skillset of acute care physicians. Many of the associated skills are already learnt and experienced in other applications such as PoCUS-guided vascular access and nerve blocks. Several studies have demonstrated that emergency physicians with standard enhanced PoCUS training (e.g. a short course and limited supervised experience) can identify FBs with high sensitivity and similar accuracy to trained sonographers.

Identification of foreign body

Retained FBs occur as a result of a penetrating injury and while the puncture site will be the initial focus for PoCUS assessment, it should be appreciated that the retained FB may be distant from it. Being a PoCUS assessment, the scan is performed in conjunction with history (nature of material, trajectory of injury) and examination (tenderness, swelling, redness).

A high-frequency transducer, set to maximum resolution on the best-quality machine available, is used. Where the body part is irregular or small, like a digit, or the FB is extremely superficial, a stand-off device (gel pad, water bath) can be used (see Figure 7.35).

The entire region surrounding the puncture should be assessed in at least two planes. The key ultrasound features of most FBs are:

- Hyperechogenicity;
- Posterior acoustic shadow;
- Straight or regular contour.

The degree of hyperechogenicity and acoustic shadowing will depend on the material and duration of retention. Metal and glass are highly echogenic and cast dark acoustic shadows. Wood is less echogenic, becoming hypoechogenic over weeks and months as it denatures *in situ*. Other features that may be seen on ultrasound are:

- Reverberation artefact—this is often associated with metal FBs (see Figure 7.23s 🖼);
- Hypoechoic halo—this develops over days and weeks as a result of localized inflammatory reaction (see Figure 7.36).

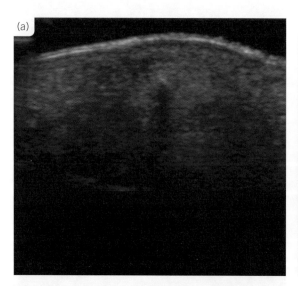
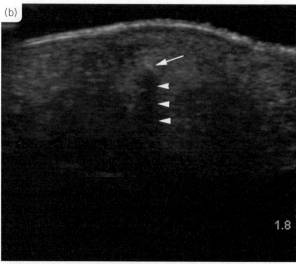

Figure 7.35 Splinter. Water bath, thenar eminence. Short axis view of a wooden splinter. Unlabelled (a) and labelled (b) images. The hyperechoic splinter (arrow) casts a posterior acoustic shadow (arrowheads).

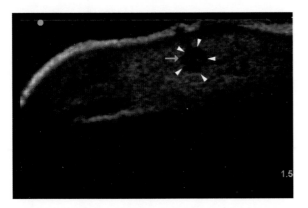

Figure 7.36 Foreign body halo. Water bath, distal thumb, long axis, day 7 post-penetrating thorn injury. A tiny foreign body (green arrow) is seen within the hypoechoic halo (arrowheads).

PoCUS for the assessment of FBs should not be thought of as a quick-look, rapid assessment. Although, when present, the majority of retained FBs are identified within a few minutes of the examination, a thorough survey is required to rule out a retained FB. Clinical judgement, as always, should determine further management, following a negative scan. If a high index of suspicion remains, then referral for a diagnostic imaging assessment may be appropriate. Alternatively, repeating the PoCUS assessment after a few days will give time for a hypoechoic halo to develop, highlighting the enclosed FB.

Once identified, the depth to, and length of, the FB should be measured. This will assist in the extraction and reduce the risk of part removal.

Certain structures can mimic retained FBs. These include small sesamoid bones, calcified scar tissue, and dense fibrous tissue. If the anatomy is unfamiliar, then comparison with the contralateral side may be helpful. One artefact that can be particularly confusing is scatter shadowing caused by traumatic air injection. Penetrating injuries, even when the FB is removed, result in the opening of a false passage through tissue layers, allowing air to enter. The presence of air within the tissues will result in scatter artefact that can mimic the acoustic shadowing caused by an FB. Displacement of this artefact with transducer pressure can help distinguish retained air from a retained FB.

PoCUS-guided foreign body removal

A number of techniques for PoCUS-guided FB removal have been described. One common technique involves localizing the FB with a hollow injection needle. This allows for the local anaesthetic to be infused simultaneously with the localization procedure. PoCUS is used to guide the needle down to the FB in a manner similar to that employed for PoCUS-guided vascular access. Either a short- or long-axis approach can be used, provided the operator is able to precisely localize the needle tip down to the FB. A small incision, along the length of the localizing needle, can then be made and the FB removed with fine forceps.

Alternatively, a real-time ultrasound-guided technique can be utilized. This involves the same needle guidance and local anaesthetic delivery technique described above. However, with this technique, the transducer remains in place, guiding the forceps during the extraction (see Video 7.19 ⬤). Care should be taken to ensure that the incision down to the FB is in line with its long axis to ensure smooth extraction. A pitfall with both techniques is that any injection of air, either during anaesthetic infusion or following the incision, can obscure the ultrasound view of the FB. Copious irrigation with saline during the procedure can help to minimize this risk. High success rates have been reported with the real-time ultrasound-guided extraction technique, which also has the advantage of requiring a potentially smaller incision.

⬢ Further reading

Additional further reading can be found in the Online appendix at www.oxfordmedicine.com/POCUSemergencymed. Please refer to your access card for further details.

Bellah R. Ultrasound in pediatric musculoskeletal disease—techniques and applications. *Radiol Clin North Am* 2001;**39**:597–618.

Cardinal E, Chhem RK, Beauregard CG. Ultrasound-guided interventional procedures in the musculoskeletal system. *Radiol Clin North Am* 1998;**36**:597–604.

Chau CLF, Griffith JF. Musculoskeletal infections: ultrasound appearances. *Clin Radiol* 2005;**60**:149–59.

Dean AJ, Gronczewski CA, Costantino TG. Technique for emergency medicine bedside ultrasound identification of a radiolucent foreign body. *J Emerg Med* 2003;**24**:303–8.

Hashimoto BE, Kramer DJ, Wiitala L. Applications of musculoskeletal sonography. *J Clin Ultrasound* 1999;**27**:293–318.

Klauser AS, Peetrons P. Developments in musculoskeletal ultrasound and clinical applications. *Skeletal Radiol* 2010;**39**:1061–71.

Lewis D, Logan P. Sonographic diagnosis of toddler's fracture in the emergency department. *J Clin Ultrasound* 2006;**34**:190–4.

Martinoli C, Bianchi S, Dahmane M, Pugliese F, Bianchi-Zamorani MP, Valle M. Ultrasound of tendons and nerves. *Eur Radiol* 2002;**12**:44–55.

Mohammadi A, Ghasemi-Rad M, Khodabakhsh M. Non-opaque soft tissue foreign body: sonographic findings. *BMC Med Imaging* 2011;**11**:9.

Woodhouse JB, McNally EG. Ultrasound of skeletal muscle injury: an update. *Semin Ultrasound CT MR* 2011;**32**:91–100.

8

Small parts ultrasound

Michael Rubin, Brandon Ritcey, and Michael Y Woo

Summary

When to scan (clinical indications):

Eyes—to improve sensitivity for underlying conditions [such as retinal detachment (RD)] or when trauma or pain limits the clinician's ability to examine the eye.

Scrotal—to help differentiate the time-sensitive diagnosis of testicular torsion from other causes of testicular pain or swelling.

What to scan (PoCUS protocol):

Eyes—all structures of the globe, from the lids through to the retina, as well as the optic nerve sheath, should be scanned.

Scrotal—scan both testes and other scrotal contents, including colour flow assessment of both sides.

How to scan (key points on scanning):

Eyes—use a high-frequency probe, and ensure use of copious gel or a fluid bag to prevent ocular pressure.

Scrotal—use a high-frequency probe, compare sides, and compare flow.

What PoCUS adds (clinical reasoning—how results change practice):

Eyes—PoCUS provides an additional tool to supplement the evaluation of the eye. Helps diagnose ocular pathologies such as RD and intraocular FB.

Scrotal—although specific for torsion, PoCUS is not 100% sensitive and so should always be interpreted in conjunction with clinical findings and clinical probability.

The eye and orbit

Purpose

Ocular emergencies often present a difficult diagnostic challenge for the clinicians, as the evaluation can be limited by a lack of specialized equipment or consultant support. With the integration of PoCUS as a diagnostic tool, emergency physicians performing ocular PoCUS examinations at the bedside can accurately detect a range of pathological disorders and rule out conditions that would otherwise require immediate ophthalmologic consultation.

Perspective

Ultrasound is non-invasive and enables real-time evaluation of the structures of the eye, even if unable to directly visualize the eye due to trauma. The eye's superficial location and fluid-filled constitution make it ideal for PoCUS evaluation. Ultrasound has been shown to be more effective in the diagnosis of various conditions, such as RD and vitreous haemorrhage (VH), than the conventional static images of CT or MRI. The typical examination time for emergency ocular PoCUS examination can be <60s and can expedite the diagnosis of several ocular emergencies, including RD, retrobulbar haematoma, globe perforation, lens dislocation, VH, and intraocular FB (see Box 8.1).

Box 8.1 Five primary indications to perform ocular ultrasound

- Loss of vision
- Ocular trauma
- Eye pain
- Intraocular FB
- Elevated ICP

Performing the scan

Normal eye anatomy

The normal eye should appear ovoid, with the most anterior portion comprising the anterior chamber. Details within the anterior chamber are not well visualized with ocular PoCUS. The lens appears as a thin, biconvex echogenic structure that, together with the iris, partitions the anterior chamber from the posterior chamber. It is common to see reverberation artefacts caused by the refractive property of the lens. The posterior chamber is filled with gelatinous vitreous humour that appears anechoic on ultrasound. The vitreous is adherent to the retina, choroid, and sclera, which forms the echogenic border of the globe. The optic nerve sheath encases the optic nerve and vessels and appears as a hypoechoic structure at the most posterior aspect of the globe (see Figure 8.1).

Ocular PoCUS examination technique

The eye is a small structure; therefore, the same simple, yet systematic, examination approach can be used to evaluate for all pathology. A high-frequency linear array transducer in the 7.5–15 MHz frequency range is preferred for this examination. The patient should be placed in the supine position. Some providers recommend covering the eye with a clear dressing, such as cling-wrap, Tegaderm™ or OpSite™, prior to applying ultrasound gel; others place the gel directly over the closed eyelid. In either case, a significant amount of gel should be applied to create an adequate acoustic window, to avoid placing unnecessary pressure on a potentially injured eye.

Scanning must be done systematically to ensure that all quadrants of the eye are adequately visualized in both horizontal axial and vertical axial planes. Co-operation is needed from the patient to move their

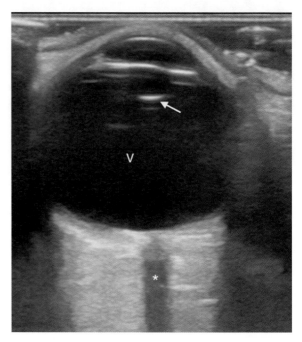

Figure 8.1 Utrasound image of a normal eye. V, vitreous. Arrow indicates the lens. * indicates the optic nerve sheath.

eyes in the horizontal axial and vertical axial planes, to facilitate complete visualization. Ocular PoCUS is a dynamic evaluation, and certain pathology may be best appreciated with kinetic movements of the globe (see Figure 8.2).

Retinal detachment and posterior vitreous detachment

ED ocular PoCUS examination is sensitive for the diagnosis of RD and may have a role in excluding it. A true detachment is an ocular emergency that can often lead to irreversible visual loss without immediate intervention. Classically, patients with RD complain of visual 'flashes' and 'floaters', occasionally with monocular clouding or shadowing in a portion of the visual field. A PVD can present with similar symptoms, and ultrasound may be helpful in distinguishing one from the other but they can also occur concurrently. Definitive diagnosis is made by fundoscopy with dilatation, which can be challenging for an inexperienced ED physician.

In a study of ocular PoCUS by Blavais *et al.*, 60 of 61 intraocular diseases, including nine RDs, were accurately diagnosed in the ED using PoCUS. In a

1. 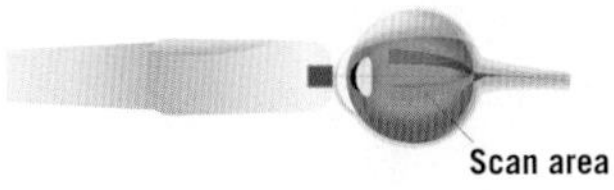 Scan area	Horizontal axial, look straight ahead	7. 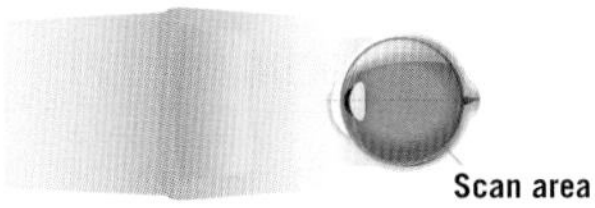 Scan area	Vertical axial, look straight ahead
2. 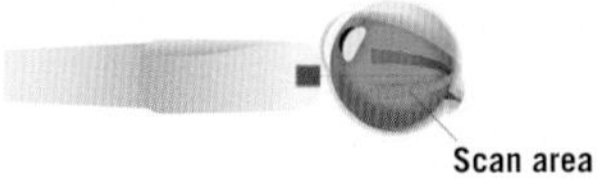 Scan area	Horizontal axial, look up	8. 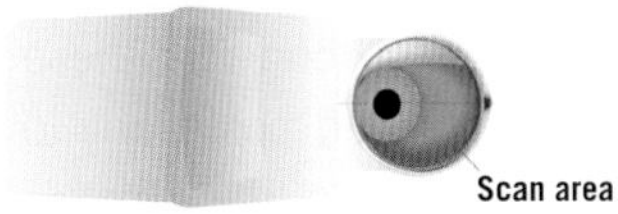 Scan area	Vertical axial, look left
3. 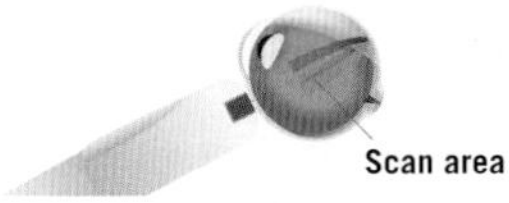 Scan area	Horizontal axial, tilt up, keep looking up	9. 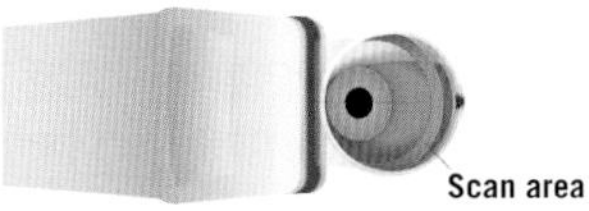 Scan area	Vertical axial, tilt right, keep looking left
4. 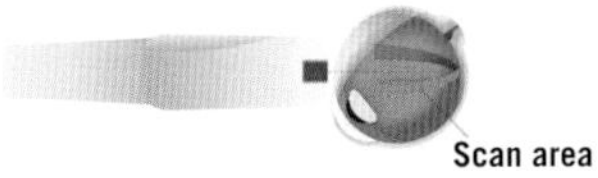 Scan area	Horizontal axial, look down	10. 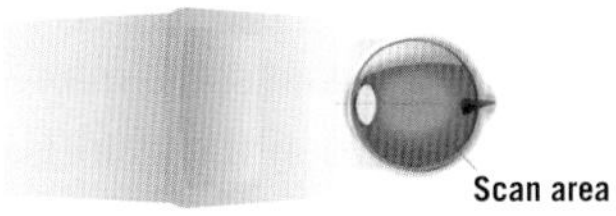 Scan area	Vertical axial, look right
5. 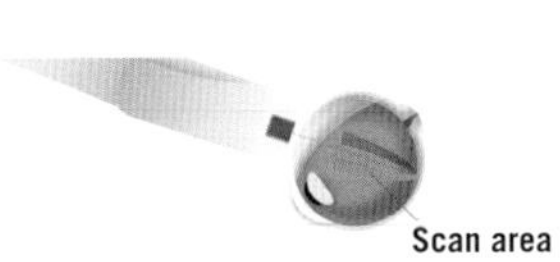 Scan area	Horizontal axial, tilt down, keep looking down	11. 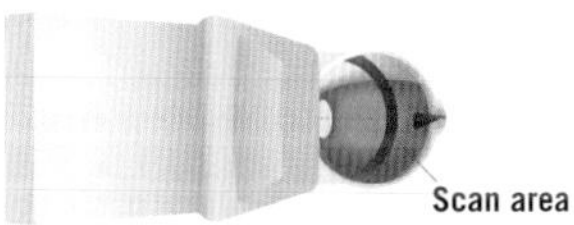 Scan area	Vertical axial, tilt left, keep looking right
6. Keep probe stationary and have patient move eye cephalad-caudal continuously and record 3 second clip of eye movements	Horizontal axial, Look straight ahead	12. Keep probe stationary and have patient move eye nasal-temporal continuously and record 3 second clip of eye movements	Vertical axial, Look straight ahead

Figure 8.2 Protocol for scanning the eye.

Reprinted from *Canadian Journal of Ophthalmology*, 51, 5, Woo MY *et al.*, 'Test characteristics of point-of-care ultrasonography for the diagnosis of acute posterior ocular pathology', pp. 336–41, Copyright 2016, with permission from Elsevier and the Canadian Ophthalmological Society.

prospective observational study, Shinar *et al.* demonstrated that emergency physicians were able to detect RD using ocular ultrasound, with 97% sensitivity and 92% specificity, after a 30-minute training session. Early identification of RD enables the ED physician to appropriately mobilize consultants and facilitate definitive management in a timely fashion. Note that undetached retinal tears may be more difficult to visualize with PoCUS and, as such, cannot be excluded by this technique.

Sonographic appearance of retinal detachment and posterior vitreous detachment

RDs appear as linear echogenic structures tethered within the vitreous. The firm anatomic attachments of the retina, at the ora serrata and optic nerve head, ensure that the detachment does not extend past these sites. As the retina remains suspended posteriorly to the optic nerve, it forms an appreciable 'V' shape on ultrasound. As the eye moves, so too does the tethered echogenic detachment, but it immediately stops once the eye movement ceases (see Figure 8.3).

By contrast, a PVD on ultrasound appears as a thin, less echogenic membrane that may not even be visible, unless the gain is increased. Contrary to an RD, a PVD is rarely attached to the optic disc, and therefore, the detached tissue continues to undulate or float, even after the eye has stopped moving (see Figure 8.4). It is important to have the gain set to maximum, in order to visualize a PVD. When the gain is decreased, the appearance of a PVD may disappear; however, an RD will still be seen.

Vitreous haemorrhage

VH can be spontaneous or associated with trauma. Whether the blood remains liquefied or clots, it can

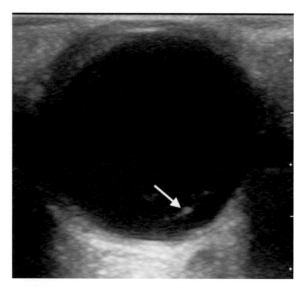

Figure 8.4 Ultrasound image of posterior vitreous detachment (PVD). Arrow indicates PVD.

have deleterious effects on vision. Large clots may appear highly echogenic, whereas small VHs may require an increased gain setting to be identified. VH may be best visualized as the eye is in motion, thereby causing the clots to swirl or bounce around in the vitreous. When the eye is not in motion, the clots tend to layer in the most dependent aspect of the globe (see Figure 8.5).

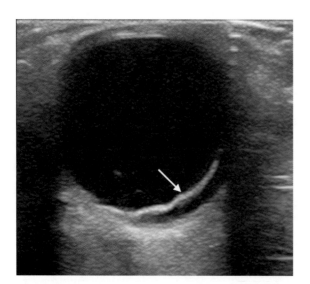

Figure 8.3 Ultrasound image of retinal detachment (RD). Arrow indicates RD.

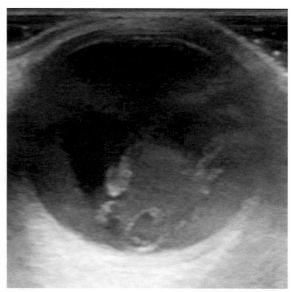

Figure 8.5 Ultrasound image of vitreous haemorrhage (VH). The hyperechoic area represents VH.

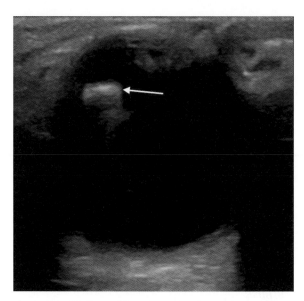

Figure 8.6 Ultrasound image of lens dislocation. Arrow indicates the lens floating in the vitreous.

Lens dislocation

The lens should be clearly visible between the anterior and posterior chambers. It normally remains fixed in position with ocular movements. However, if it subluxes, it may slip behind the iris with movements. Complete lens dislocation may reveal the lens floating within the vitreous, settled in the posterior of the eye or, rarely, in the anterior chamber (see Figure 8.6).

Foreign bodies

Depending on the FB size and consistency, it may present as a hyperechoic mass, often with echogenic reverberation artefact (see Figure 8.7). When colour Doppler is applied over an echogenic FB, it appears as rapidly changing flashes of red and blue, known as the twinkling artefact.

Globe rupture

Globe rupture (GR) may be best diagnosed clinically, but ocular PoCUS can help characterize subtle distortions of the eyeball, identify a perforation, or provide evidence of air or FB inside the vitreous. Ocular PoCUS of the orbit can detect retrobulbar haematomas, which appear as echo-poor areas just posterior to the globe and may distort the posterior aspect of the eye. Ocular PoCUS should not be performed in patients with high clinical probability of GR, as even gentle pressure is dangerous.

Optic disc swelling

A recent study by Teismann *et al.* suggests that emergency physicians may be able to use ocular PoCUS to accurately assess the optic disc for evidence of swelling. Optic disc heights of >1.0 mm were strongly associated with clinically apparent disc swelling, as diagnosed by expert examination (see Figure 8.1s 📷).

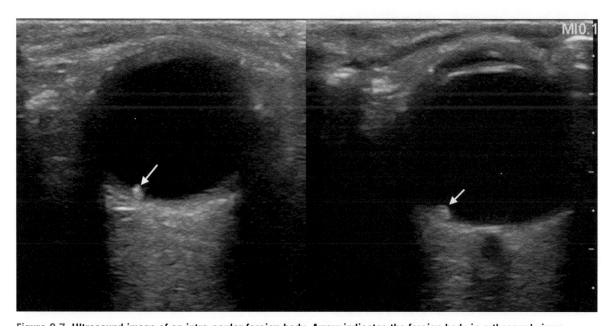

Figure 8.7 Ultrasound image of an intra-ocular foreign body. Arrow indicates the foreign body in orthogonal views.

Optic nerve sheath diameter as an indicator of elevated intracranial pressure

The optic nerve, vessels, and surrounding sheath can be seen at the posterior aspect of the globe. The optic nerve sheath is contiguous with the subarachnoid space, and cerebrospinal fluid flows freely between the cranium and the orbit within the subarachnoid space. The correlation between optic nerve sheath diameter (ONSD) and elevated ICP has been well established. When assessing for ICP, ONSD measurements taken for each eye, 3 mm posterior to the optic disc. Normal ONSD is <5 mm, and anything above 6 mm is considered to reflect clinically significant ICP. Although ocular PoCUS of the ONSD is an indirect method of evaluating ICP, it is non-invasive and quick, can be done at the bedside, and can help establish a diagnosis and guide treatment without delay (see Figure 8.8).

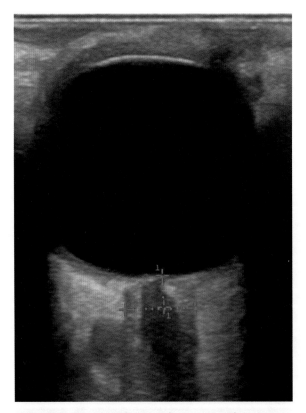

Figure 8.8 Ultrasound image of increased optic nerve sheath diameter (ONSD). Measurement is taken 3 mm back from the retina. The ONSD is increased at 7 mm in this image.

Pitfalls

Always be mindful to avoid placing pressure while scanning the eye, especially if there is suspicion of a GR.

Retinal tears may be small and difficult to appreciate. If suspected clinically, appropriate ophthalmological consultation should be sought, regardless of ocular PoCUS findings.

Ocular PoCUS findings are operator- and patient-dependent and therefore should always be used in conjunction with clinical assessment.

The testicles and scrotum

Purpose

Testicular PoCUS can be utilized to exclude time-sensitive conditions such as testicular torsion, as well as being useful in the assessment of other causes for scrotal pain and swelling.

Perspective

The complaint of a painful and/or swollen testicle is common in the ED, and although frequently due to a benign cause amenable to outpatient treatment, the diagnosis of testicular torsion must be considered, especially for the patient with an abrupt onset of an acutely painful testicle. This time-sensitive, fertility-threatening condition should be foremost in the mind of clinicians. As such, emergency testicular PoCUS examination is largely centred on ruling in or ruling out this high-risk diagnosis. Beyond torsion, PoCUS can also help with other pathology in the differential diagnosis of acute testicular pain (see Table 8.1).

Performing the scan

Patient preparation and positioning

The patient should be supine, with their knees bent in a frog's leg position. A towel should be rolled and placed under the scrotum to keep it elevated. The penis should be directed upwards, pointing towards the umbilicus and covered with a second towel to ensure it stays out of the way during the examination.

Table 8.1 Point-of-care ultrasound (PoCUS) of the painful testicle, with possible diagnoses and findings

Diagnosis	Typical sonographic findings
Testicular torsion	Heterogenous, oedematous, enlarged testicle with reduced flow on colour Doppler. Arterial and venous flows are both usually absent on spectral Doppler
Epididymitis	Normal-appearing testicle with equal flow on colour Doppler. Arterial and venous flows are present to the testicle. The epididymis appears oedematous and has increased flow on colour Doppler
Orchitis	Heterogenous, oedematous, enlarged testicle with increased flow on colour Doppler. Arterial and venous flows are present on spectral Doppler
Hydrocele	Hypo- or anechoic fluid surrounding the free-floating testicle
Varicocele	Anechoic vascular bundle adjacent to the testicle, with internal flow present. More frequently on the left side
Testicular rupture	Irregular testicular border with heterogenous appearance. Possible adjacent traumatic haematocele
Testicular mass	Focal heterogenous or cystic lesion in the testicle

Ultrasound machine initial settings

A high-frequency linear probe (ideally 7.5–10 MHz) is used for scrotal ultrasound. The ultrasound machine should be set to the 'small parts' or 'scrotum' preset, which optimizes the settings for visualizing superficial structures.

Normal sonographic findings of the testicle

The normal B-mode appearance of the testicle should be a homogenous, smooth, rounded structure, with an echogenicity similar to that of the liver (see Figure 8.2s 📷). It is quite easy to compare to the contralateral testicle, even in the same sonographic window, by positioning the probe in a transverse orientation over the central scrotum, so that both testicles can be compared at the same time. Both testicles should be interrogated in transverse and longitudinal planes and compared to the opposite side.

Colour Doppler examination should be performed next, in order to identify the relative amount of blood flow in each testicle. The colour Doppler range setting should be calibrated first on the painless testicle by turning the colour gain to be ultra-sensitive, so that the testicle is washed out by colour artefact. Then colour sensitivity should be turned down until the artefact disappears and there are only small patches of colour flow (see Figure 8.9). The PoCUS sonographer can

then switch to the symptomatic testicle with the same colour settings, and in a normal testicle, they should see approximately the same amount of colour flow. The 'two-testicle view' is also very useful where both testicles are imaged at the same time in a transverse plane, with the colour Doppler activated, so that the amount of flow in each testicle can be directly compared (see Figure 8.10).

Spectral Doppler (also known as PW Doppler) is important to document the presence of both arterial and venous flow. Spectral Doppler is able to identify the presence of arterial and venous flows by producing a

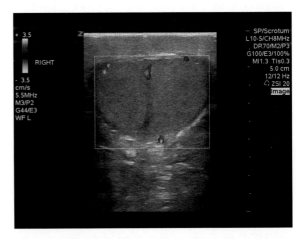

Figure 8.9 Ultrasound image of a normal testicle with colour Doppler.

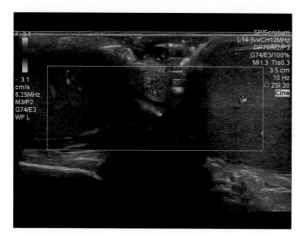

Figure 8.10 Ultrasound image of both normal testicles with colour Doppler.

characteristic waveform, depending on whether the flow is pulsatile or not. With the colour Doppler activated, also turn on the spectral Doppler and place the Doppler gate over an area where there is colour flow seen. The screen will display a waveform representing the velocity of the flow at the location of the Doppler gate. The sonographer may need to adjust the baseline and scale in order to view the whole waveform. Arterial flow will appear like peaks and troughs of flow, representing its pulsatile nature (see Figure 8.3as and bs 🎬). Venous flow will be constant, with only minimal variations in velocity. Several different areas of flow should be interrogated to record both venous and arterial flow in a few areas, to increase the certainty of the findings.

Testicular torsion

Testicular torsion is a time-sensitive emergency condition of the testicle, and PoCUS can be used to help 'rule in' this critical diagnosis. The testicular salvage rate is 90–100% if surgical correction is performed within 6 hours, but drops off to only 10% after 24 hours. The primary use of testicular PoCUS is to rapidly diagnose testicular torsion and minimize delays to surgical intervention.

Ultrasound is considered the first-line investigation for the diagnosis of testicular torsion, although it is important to acknowledge the limitations of this test. The radiology literature cites a range of sensitivities of between 69% and 97% and specificities of between 87% and 100% for Doppler ultrasound of the testicle. The PoCUS literature is still quite sparse for the accuracy

of the emergency clinician in identifying this condition. One small retrospective study found emergency physicians had a sensitivity of 95% and a specificity of 94% for identifying the cause of testicular pain with PoCUS. Most of the PoCUS literature is limited to case reports.

Sonographic findings of testicular torsion

The B-mode findings of testicular torsion evolve, the longer the torsion has been present and depend upon whether the torsion is complete or incomplete. When imaged early, the testicle may appear relatively normal. When torsion is complete and has been present for longer, the testicle becomes hypoechoic and larger, compared to the other side, as oedema develops. Eventually, the testicle becomes necrotic and develops a markedly heterogenous echo texture, which correlates with a lower chance of testicle survival. A twisted spermatic cord may appear as a 'whirlpool sign'.

The colour Doppler findings of testicular torsion depend on the degree of torsion. A high-grade torsion with a complete absence of arterial flow will show no colour flow to the testicle; however, a torsion that is not as severe may simply show reduced flow, compared to the other side (see Figure 8.11). Sometimes the colour flow may even appear equal despite the presence of torsion, or there can actually be increased flow to a testicle that has recently de-torted. Therefore, colour Doppler can be very useful as a 'rule-in' test when colour flow is markedly reduced, but should not be used alone to exclude testicular torsion.

Spectral Doppler findings of testicular torsion may show absent venous and arterial waveforms if the

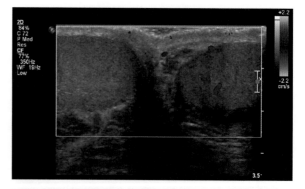

Figure 8.11 Ultrasound image with power Doppler, demonstrating torsion of the right testicle. Note the right testicle has no flow and is larger, when compared with the left testicle, as a result of the torsion.

torsion is complete. However, a partial torsion may only show arterial waveforms, but not venous waveforms if there is only venous obstruction from twisting of the cord. In addition, torsion may cause arterial waveforms to appear similar to venous waveforms, due to lower flow velocity, which is why it is important to attempt to identify both arterial and venous waveforms in every examination.

Until there is further research in the area of PoCUS for the diagnosis of testicular torsion, emergency physicians should use PoCUS as a test to 'rule in' testicular torsion to expedite surgical consultation when they have a positive scan, but should not use PoCUS to 'rule out' testicular torsion in cases where there is remaining clinical suspicion.

Epididymitis

Epididymitis is an infection of the epididymis and is the most common diagnosis in adult patients presenting to the ED with a painful scrotum. In cases where testicular torsion is considered unlikely based on your history and physical examination, it can be helpful to establish epididymitis as an alternate diagnosis.

The epididymis is a slightly heterogenous structure, located adjacent to the testicle, and is often slightly more echogenic than the testicle itself. In epididymitis, the epididymis appears hypoechoic and enlarged due to oedema. Colour Doppler examination shows an increased blood flow to the affected side (see Figure 8.12).

Orchitis

Orchitis is an infection of the testicle that exists along a continuum with epididymitis and, in fact, may coexist

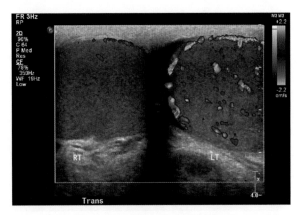

Figure 8.13 Ultrasound image demonstrating increased colour Doppler flow in the symptomatic left testicle, when compared with the right asymptomatic testicle. This is characteristic of left orchitis.

with epididymitis in many cases. In B-mode, the testicle may appear heterogenous and hypoechoic due to oedema. Areas of reduced echogenicity will show an increased flow on colour Doppler examination, due to active inflammation (see Figure 8.13). It is important to note the sonographic appearance of a testicle with orchitis may appear very similar to a recently de-torted testicle with increased vascular flow and areas of heterogeneity. History and physical examination are key to distinguishing between these very different pathologies, and radiology-performed ultrasound and/or consultation should be obtained when the diagnosis is in doubt.

Testicular trauma

Testicular trauma is potentially serious, as testicular rupture can compromise future fertility through disruption of the blood–testicle barrier and the resulting autoimmune reaction. Early exploration can improve outcome in 80% of ruptured testicles, which is where PoCUS can be useful to allow a faster diagnosis.

Findings can be highly variable in testicular trauma. A testicular rupture (see Figure 8.14) will frequently show an irregular testicular border and an associated haematocele (see 'Hydrocele', p. 166). There may be small areas of haemorrhage and oedema, which may appear heterogenous. Any unusual findings on PoCUS after testicular trauma should prompt radiology-performed ultrasound and/or a urologic consultation.

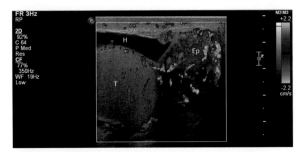

Figure 8.12 Ultrasound image of epididymitis with increased colour flow to the epididymis. H, hydrocele; T, testicle; Ep, epididymis.

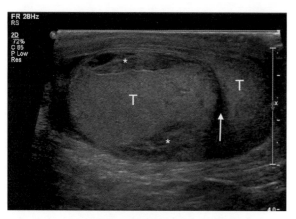

Figure 8.14 Testicular rupture. T indicates a testicle, with the arrow indicating the location of the rupture. * indicates the location of haematomas within the testicle.

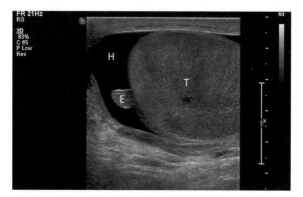

Figure 8.15 Ultrasound image of a hydrocele. H, hydrocele; T, testicle; E, epididymis.

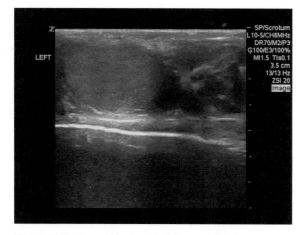

Figure 8.16 Ultrasound image demonstrating a varicocele. V indicates the varicocele. If colour Doppler were to be applied, this area would demonstrate vascular flow. T indicates the testicle.

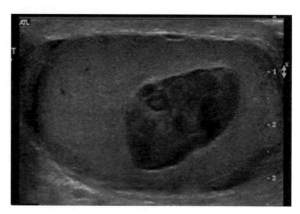

Figure 8.17 Testicular mass.

Hydrocele

A hydrocele appears as anechoic or hypoechoic free fluid surrounding the testicle (see Figure 8.15). It can be due to a primary anatomical defect, or it may be associated with a testicular torsion, orchitis, or testicular rupture.

Varicocele

A varicocele appears as a tortuous, anechoic bundle of vessels that are usually only in the left hemiscrotum (see Figure 8.16). Flow is present within them on colour Doppler and will increase with a Valsalva manoeuvre.

Testicular mass

Any patient presenting with a testicular mass should be referred for urologic follow-up, and identifying a testicular cancer should not be the goal of emergency PoCUS. However, incidental findings do occur. Any focal heterogenous or cystic lesion should be referred for radiology-performed imaging and subsequent consultant follow-up (see Figure 8.17).

Further reading

Additional further reading can be found in the Online appendix at www.oxfordmedicine.com/POCUSemergencymed. Please refer to your access card for further details.

Blaivas M. Bedside emergency department ultrasonography in the evaluation of ocular pathology. *Acad Emerg Med* 2000;**7**:947–50.

Blaivas M, Batts M, Lambert M. Ultrasonographic diagnosis of testicular torsion by emergency physicians. *Am J Emerg Med* 2000;**18**:198–200.

Blaivas M, Sierzenski P, Lambert M. Emergency evaluation of patients presenting with acute scrotum using bedside ultrasonography. *Acad Emerg Med* 2001;**8**:90–3.

Blavais M, Theodoro D, Sierzenski P. A study of bedside ocular ultrasonography in the emergency department. *Acad Emerg Med* 2002;**9**:791–9.

Hassen GW, Bruck I, Donahue J, *et al.* Accuracy of optic nerve sheath diameter measurement by emergency physicians using bedside ultrasound. *J Emerg Med* 2015;**48**:450–7.

Lam WW, Yap TL, Jacobsen AS, Teo HJ. Colour Doppler ultrasonography replacing surgical exploration for acute scrotum: myth or reality? *Pediatr Radiol* 2005;**35**:597–600.

Leo M, Carmody K. Sonography assessment of acute ocular pathology. *Ultrasound Clin* 2011;**6**:227–34.

Roque PJ, Hatch N, Barr L, Wu TS. Bedside ocular ultrasound. *Crit Care Clin* 2014;**30**:227–41.

Sharp VJ, Kieran K, Arlen AM. Testicular torsion: diagnosis, evaluation, and management. *Am Fam Physician* 2013;**88**:835–40.

Shinar Z, Chan L, Orlinsky M. Use of ocular ultrasound for the evaluation of retinal detachment. *J Emerg Med* 2011;**40**:53–7.

Teismann N, Lenaghan P, Nolan R, Stein J, Green A. Point-of-care ocular ultrasound to detect optic disc swelling. *Acad Emerg Med* 2013;**20**:920–5.

Ustymowicz A, Krejza J, Mariak Z. Twinkling artifact in color Doppler imaging of the orbit. *J Ultrasound Med* 2002;**21**:559–63.

Waldert M, Klatte T, Schmidbauer J, Remzi M, Lackner J, Marberger M. Color Doppler sonography reliably identifies testicular torsion in boys. *Urology* 2010;**75**:1170–4.

Wilbert DM, Schaerfe CW, Stern WD, Strohmaier WL, Bichler KH. Evaluation of the acute scrotum by color-coded Doppler ultrasonography. *J Urol* 1993;**149**:1475–7.

Yoonessi R, Hussain A, Jang TB. Bedside ocular ultrasound for the detection of retinal detachment in the emergency department. *Acad Emerg Med* 2010;**17**:913–17.

9

Ultrasound and procedures

Bob Jarman, Beatrice Hoffmann, Miteb Al-Githami,
John Hardin, Elena Skoromovsky, Stuart Durham, David Lewis,
Paul Atkinson, and Justin Bowra

Summary

This chapter covers the principles of how point-of-care ultrasound can be used to augment a range of clinical procedures. Examples of common applications will be discussed; these include:

Ultrasound-guided vascular access: venous and arterial, central and peripheral;

Ultrasound-guided nerve blocks:

> Upper limb—radial nerve, median nerve, and ulnar nerve;
> Lower limb—femoral nerve and the 3-in-1 blocks, fascia iliaca block;
> Haematoma blocks.

Ultrasound-guided aspiration and drainage of fluid:

> Thoracocentesis (thoracentesis); pericardiocentesis; paracentesis; suprapubic catheter insertion; lumbar puncture; abscess drainage.

Miscellaneous:

> Confirmation of endotracheal tube (ETT) placement; confirmation of nasogastric tube (NGT) placement.

The following procedures are described in Chapter 7: aspiration of joint effusions; fracture manipulation and reduction; reduction of shoulder dislocations; and FB identification and removal.

General principles

Introduction

Using point-of-care ultrasound (PoCUS) as an adjunct to a clinical procedure is common. This aspect of PoCUS has allowed clinicians to improve the speed and safety of a wide variety of procedures that are performed at the bedside, as well as in more traditional interventional environments. In the majority of cases, a needle is utilized as part of the procedure, e.g. a simple needle for aspiration of a collection or instillation of local anaesthetic, a cannula-over-needle for peripheral vascular access, or a guide-wire via a needle (Seldinger) technique for placement of a pleural drainage catheter.

This chapter will describe the common principles of how ultrasound can be used as such an adjunct and will describe specific procedures where ultrasound can aid the clinician. Specialist internal cavity ultrasound-guided procedures will not be discussed.

Aims of this section

This chapter will cover the principles of how PoCUS is used to augment a range of diagnostic and procedural procedures. Examples of common applications will be discussed; these include:

- Ultrasound-guided vascular access:
  - Venous and arterial;
  - Central and peripheral.

- Ultrasound-guided nerve blocks:
  - Upper limb:
    - Radial nerve;
    - Median nerve;
    - Ulnar nerve.
  - Lower limb:
    - Femoral nerve and the 3-in-1 blocks;
    - Fascia iliaca block.
  - Haematoma blocks.
- Ultrasound-guided aspiration and drainage of fluid:
  - Thoracocentesis (thoracentesis);
  - Pericardiocentesis;
  - Paracentesis;
  - Suprapubic catheter insertion;
  - Lumbar puncture;
  - Abscess drainage.
- Miscellaneous:
  - Confirmation of ETT placement;
  - Confirmation of NGT placement.

  The following procedures are described in Chapter 7:

- Joint effusions and aspiration;
- Fracture manipulation and reduction;
- Reduction of shoulder dislocations;
- FB identification and removal.

Why use ultrasound to aid procedures?

Safety has been the main driving force for using ultrasound. Ultrasound allows for a visual survey of the anatomy of the region prior to the procedure, so the operator is able to identify potential problems in advance.

Once the anatomy has been surveyed and the operator is aware of potential problems, ultrasound can be used to guide the procedure in real time. The needle can be guided into the right place safely, with minimal damage to adjacent structures. This is often done in a continuous manner, rather than checking the needle position intermittently.

Following delivery of the needle to the area of interest and completion of the procedure, ultrasound can confirm that the procedure has been successful. It can also establish that no complications are evident; examples may include excluding significant haemorrhage or excluding a pneumothorax (PTX).

Evaluating the anatomy

A sonographic survey of the region of interest is important to identify abnormalities or normal variants. It should be undertaken in two planes perpendicular to each other; this is often a longitudinal and transverse window. A key ultrasound skill is being able to rotate the probe between perpendicular planes while keeping the procedure target, e.g. a vessel, in the middle of the screen (see Figure 9.1). This is important, as identifying key adjacent structures is often easier in one plane than both. For example, for internal jugular vascular access, transverse views of the internal jugular vein (IJV) (see Figure 9.2a) clearly show adjacent structures that need to be avoided, especially the carotid artery; however, in a longitudinal view, the IJV may look similar to the carotid (see Figure 9.2b and c). By keeping the target vessel in the centre of the window at all times, 'slipping off' onto an adjacent structure is avoided.

The nature and integrity of the target structure can be evaluated during the survey. If this structure is a vein, looking for the anatomical and physiological features typical of a vein, as well as ensuring that there is no clot in the lumen, is essential. In the latter, simple compression of the vessel, by applying downward pressure to the probe, will cause complete collapse if it is patent. If the target structure is a fluid-filled structure, the user should look for acoustic enhancement below and also identify adjacent structures that may increase the risk of complications if damaged, e.g. concomitant arteries may be injured in venous cannulation, PTX due to a breach of the pleura line in brachial plexus nerve blocks, lung and diaphragm injury in thoracocentesis, and bowel perforation in paracentesis.

Undertaking a survey will also provide an opportunity to optimize the ultrasound image and machine settings, e.g. depth, gain/TGC, dynamic range, etc. Use of other modes, such as Doppler, may aid confirmation of structures, but B-mode should always be used initially.

For some users, ultrasound is used only for surveying the region of interest prior to the procedure. This is called

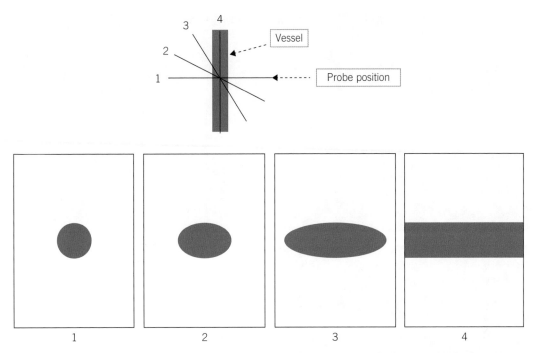

Figure 9.1 Rotating the probe between two planes while keeping the target vessel in the centre of the image.

static ultrasound guidance. In some circumstances, especially when the ultrasonographer is not undertaking the procedure, a skin marker will be used to identify the surface anatomy overlying the procedure target. This has been commonplace for procedures such as thoracocentesis and paracentesis. Complications may arise when the anatomy changes in the interval between the scan and the procedure; this may be due to the patient changing position or changing physiology.

Preparation

For any procedure, preparation is important. This includes consenting the patient, optimizing the environment, getting the patient in position, attaching monitoring, preparing the equipment, establishing a sterile field, and donning personal protective equipment. When using ultrasound as an adjunct, the user also needs to prepare the machine and probe.

Optimizing the environment where the procedure is being undertaken is essential. Sometimes, especially in emergency situations, the user will have to compromise. Try to ensure that the machine's screen is in the line of sight when performing the procedure, so that the user does not need to keep turning around, looking from screen to patient, and vice versa. In addition, there should be task lighting in place over the procedure zone, with the rest of the environment having a lower level of ambient lighting, to enhance the image on the screen.

Orientation

For certain procedures, such as internal jugular cannulation, the operator stands at the head end of the patient, facing caudally, with the machine placed in the line of sight of the operator. This is different to most PoCUS scanning whereby the operator is usually facing rostrally. Therefore, when the operator and machine are in this position, it is recommended that the probe, when transverse, is rotated and aligned to the patient's left, so that its marker remains orientated with the left screen. This will ensure that structures will appear correctly orientated on the screen and procedural guidance will respond appropriately on screen to directional changes of the needle.

In addition, for some applications, the user will need to orientate the probe to the long or short axis of the area of interest, e.g. vessel or nerve, as opposed to the longitudinal or transverse anatomical planes.

Therefore, in procedural ultrasound, the most important principle is that the user is comfortable with

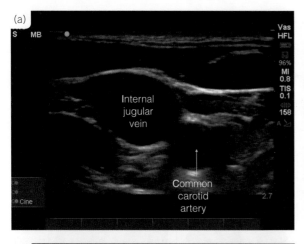

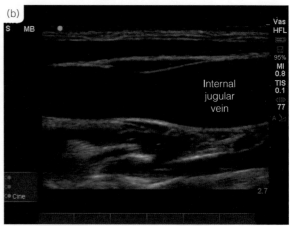

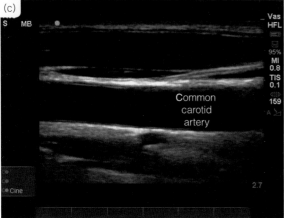

Figure 9.2 (a) B-mode image of transverse internal jugular vein clearly demonstrating the position of the common carotid artery. **(b)** B-mode image of longitudinal internal jugular vein. **(c)** B-mode image of longitudinal common carotid artery.

static (i.e. orientation and anatomical structures) and dynamic (i.e. changes that moving the probe will make and also the direction of needle travel) factors, rather than strict adherence to longitudinal and transverse anatomical orientation protocols.

Which probe?

The depth of the area of interest will determine the type of probe that is used. For applications where the area of interest is within approximately 6 cm of the skin surface, a high-frequency linear probe will be the best choice, especially due to the enhanced axial resolution that will be achieved. Deeper applications will require a lower-frequency probe, such as a curvilinear or phased array, but this will be at the expense of better resolution. Other adjustments, such as time gain compensation (TGC) and focal zone (especially relevant for lateral resolution), will improve the quality of the image.

Keeping clean

For many procedures, a sterile field is required. In addition to the use of an antiseptic cleaner, sterile drapes, a gown, gloves, and other personal protective equipment, the user also needs to ensure that the ultrasound probe does not contaminate the sterile field. The probe and its cord are not sterile (but should be kept regularly clean). In practice, the user can get around this problem by the use of a sterile probe/cord cover (see Figure 9.1s 📷), for which many are commercially available. They are generally packaged folded into a concertina form, with a rigid opening that the scrubbed operator can hold. An assistant then applies some coupling gel inside the area of the cover, adjacent to where the footprint of the probe will sit, before dangling the probe into the cover. The weight of the probe and cord then causes the cover to de-concertina. The final step requires the application of sterile tape or elastic bands to secure the cover to the probe and cord, and especially to ensure that air-filled dead space near the footprint is removed. This results in a probe and a workable length of cord that are now protected by the cover and can be handled by the scrubbed operator. Many probe covers come with a small handle at the opening that can be hung on a conveniently placed drip stand, allowing safe storage of the sterile probe during the procedure.

A cheaper alternative is to use a long, sterile condom or a large, adhesive, transparent wound dressing to cover the probe (with coupling gel on the footprint).

A sterile coupling medium will need to be used between the patient and the covered probe; the user may elect to use a thin layer of sterile gel (usually from a sachet), copious non-alcoholic antiseptic cleaner, or sterile saline.

Once the user, patient, and probe have been prepared, the user will be unable to alter the machine controls, as the console is not sterile. An assistant may be used to adjust the preset, depth, TGC/gain, etc., as required; however, the best practice would be that such settings are adjusted during a preliminary scan prior to establishing a sterile field. Application of a sterile transparent polythene sheet over the console can provide the scrubbed user with some limited ability to operate the machine controls.

Dynamic ultrasound guidance

Once the anatomical survey has been undertaken and the user is aware of potential pitfalls and complications, the next step is to use ultrasound as an adjunct while performing the procedure.

This is called dynamic ultrasound guidance. There are two techniques that are used: out-of-plane or transverse technique and in-plane or longitudinal technique. Both rely on the user being familiar with the plane of the ultrasound beam (see Figure 9.3).

When using the out-of-plane or transverse technique, the user directs the needle towards the plane of the ultrasound beam. At some point, the needle should enter the ultrasound plane (see Video 9.1 📷). However, the B-mode image will not provide information about the location of all the length of the needle, but only the part of the needle in contact with the ultrasound plane (see Figure 9.4). The tip of the needle usually causes a similar reflection to the rest of the shaft, although there are newer specialist needles, which have hyperreflective tips. Only the small part of the needle that is directly within the plane of the ultrasound beam is visible at any one time. Therefore, when using a standard kit, it is not possible to distinguish the shaft from the needle tip by its ultrasound appearance. The reflection seen is bright, or hyperechoic,

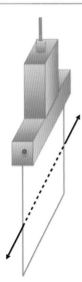
The arrow is traversing within the plane of the ultrasound beam
in-plane or **longitudinal**

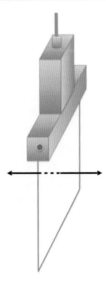
The arrow is not traversing within the plane of the ultrasound beam
out-of-plane or **transverse**

Figure 9.3 **Procedure orientation with regard to the ultrasound beam plane.**

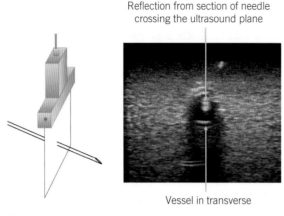

Reflection from section of needle crossing the ultrasound plane

Vessel in transverse

Figure 9.4 Out-of-plane/transverse view of the vessel and needle.

usually with reverberation appearances distally. The reflection is increased, the more the needle is perpendicular to the direction of the ultrasound beam—called parallelism. Therefore, steeply angled approaches to the area of interest will result in less reflection back to the probe.

One way the user can increase the success of the needle tip entering into the area of interest within the beam plane is to use the isosceles triangulation method (see Figure 9.5). The depth of the area of interest is used to guide the distance the needle is introduced from the centreline of the footprint; the user then introduces the needle at a 45° angle.

In addition to utilzing the isosceles triangulation method, the needle can be introduced in stages and further guided towards the area of interest by tilting the

beam plane towards the needle—the so-called 'meet-and-greet' approach (see Figure 9.6 and Video 9.2a and b 🎥). Once the needle is introduced part way, the user tilts the beam plane up towards the needle until the tip of the needle is seen. The user then tilts the beam plane away from the needle by a few degrees; the needle is then advanced until it appears in the beam plane. These steps are repeated until the needle is safely guided down to the area of interest. To the experienced user, this process can be quite fluid and speedy.

The out-of-plane or transverse technique is often used for vascular access techniques at the point of care, as the adjacent structures to be avoided are often in view (i.e. the carotid artery during internal jugular cannulation). It also allows ultrasound to be used when there is limited skin surface access (for the needle and probe)—especially important when the footprint of the probe is large.

When using the in-plane or longitudinal technique, the user directs the needle in a direction where it travels within the ultrasound beam plane. This allows the entire needle residing within the beam plane to be seen at the same time (see Figure 9.7 and Video 9.3a and b 🎥). Keeping the needle within the beam plane requires a degree of practice, skill, and dexterity. The hand holding of the probe needs to be kept still over the area of interest, as it is easy to inadvertently change the beam plane; for example, a slight change in the fanning angle of the beam may move to an adjacent vessel (which may look the same in longitudinal section).

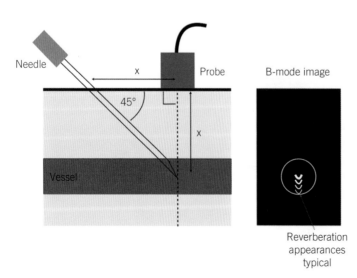

Needle

45°

x

Probe

x

Vessel

B-mode image

Reverberation appearances typical

Figure 9.5 Isosceles triangulation method.

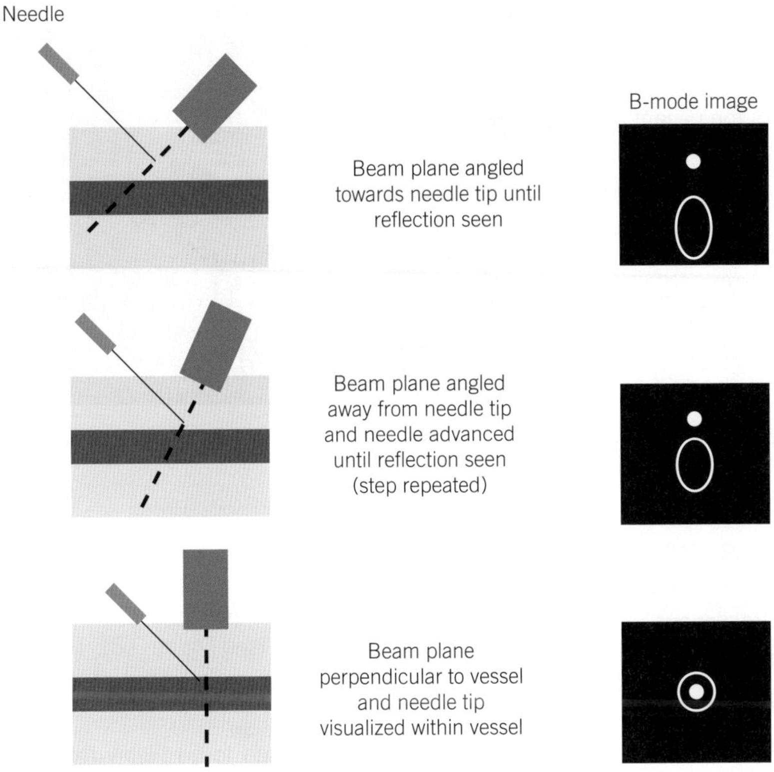

Needle

Beam plane angled towards needle tip until reflection seen

B-mode image

Beam plane angled away from needle tip and needle advanced until reflection seen (step repeated)

Beam plane perpendicular to vessel and needle tip visualized within vessel

Figure 9.6 'Meet and greet' method of guiding the needle.

Similar to the out-of-plane technique, the more perpendicular the needle is to the ultrasound beam, the better the brightness of reflection. In order to achieve this, the needle needs to adopt a shallow angle of approach, and therefore, for most applications, a short needle or minimal surface access is not feasible. This technique is traditionally adopted for procedures such as collection drainage and nerve blocks where greater

surface access can allow this orientation. However, the perception of greater accuracy of needle tip placement with the in-plane technique is being challenged by the newer meet-and-greet approach, as described earlier.

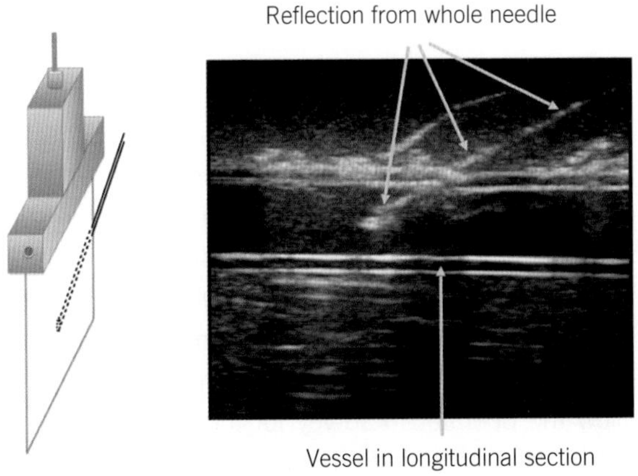

Ensuring the needle tip gets to the right place has been described above using in-plane and out-of-plane techniques. Confirming its location can be checked by using some additional techniques; slight rapid movement of the part of the needle being held by the user will cause the tip to 'vibrate' on the B-mode image; forcefully injecting a small amount of saline, often agitated with air prior to injection to improve reflectivity, will cause an area of transient reflectivity to be seen adjacent to the needle tip. Colour Doppler can be used to visualize a flare at the needle tip when saline is injected. When undertaking a procedure using a Seldinger technique, not only can ultrasound be used to guide the needle into place, but once a guide-wire is inserted, its position can be checked.

After the procedure

The user needs to ensure that following a procedure, appropriate steps are taken to confirm a successful

Reflection from whole needle

Vessel in longitudinal section

Figure 9.7 In-plane/longitudinal view of the vessel and needle.

outcome and no complications. Traditionally, this has been done by clinical reassessment, observations, and adjuncts such as radiological investigations (e.g. CXR). Ultrasound can also be used to reassess the patient in the following ways:

- Local evaluation—e.g. re-evaluating the anatomy and identifying whether there is evidence of local complications such as extravasation;

- Regional evaluation—e.g. in the case of peri-pleural procedures, such as internal jugular cannulation, to ensure that pleural sliding is present to exclude a PTX and that there is no developing pleural fluid collections;

- Systemic evaluation—this may be beneficial, especially in an emergency situation, e.g. fluid responsiveness following peripheral intravenous fluid or cardiac activity following central venous cannulation and inotrope administration.

It is essential to ensure that the machine and probes used are cleaned after each use. Remove and dispose of used probe covers, and clean the probe and cord with a non-abrasive or non-alcohol-based disinfectant.

It is good governance to document the procedure and any complications in the medical record; this should include details about how ultrasound was used. Representative images should be saved, if possible, as this can validate your decision to undertake the procedure, especially if you deviated from the normal protocol, e.g. a particular vessel was not used due to being too small or not patent.

Specific adjuncts

Visualization of the needle by ultrasound is a necessity when performing a procedure. As described previously in 'Dynamic ultrasound guidance', p. 173, the more perpendicular the needle reflective surface is to the direction of the ultrasound beam, the better the reflection seen and the needle representation on the B-mode image. Many machines have probes that allow for ultrasound beams to be sent in a number of directions by electronic beam steering—called compound imaging (manufacturers may use different proprietary terminology). Recently, manufacturers have utilized this principle to direct a greater proportion of beams

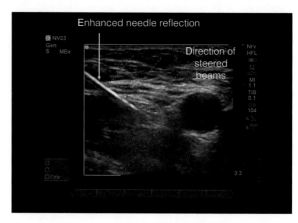

Figure 9.8 Beam-steering technology to enhance needle visualization.
Reproduced with kind permission from Fujifilm Sonosite.

at a predetermined angle that will strike the reflective surface of the needle at 90° (see Figure 9.8). This enhances the reflectivity of the needle due to the dedicated beam steering.

Some needles are designed to be highly reflective and may also incorporate enhanced features like hypo-reflective distance markers and hyperreflective needle tips (see Figure 9.2s 📷).

Many manufacturers supply procedural attachments for their probes, which can act as a guide for the needle during procedures. These attachments usually come with machine software that can be projected on the B-mode image, so the user can estimate the path the needle will follow.

Ultrasound-guided vascular access

Purpose

The use of ultrasound guidance is common to specialties such as anaesthesia, critical care, acute internal medicine, and emergency medicine; all clinicians undertaking central venous access should be suitably trained and expected to use ultrasound guidance.

Using ultrasound can also aid smaller, peripheral venous, and arterial cannulation. In all cases, it will allow the operator to survey for the optimal site and vessel patency to perform cannulation and act as an adjunct during the procedure. Hence, ultrasound can be used as a static and dynamic tool.

Ultrasound-guided peripheral vascular access is of particular benefit in the following groups of patients:

- Obese patients—vessels cannot be palpated within the thick subcutaneous adipose layer;

- Intravenous drug users—vessels are frequently thrombosed due to recurrent use;

- Prolonged illness—vessels are frequently thrombosed due to recurrent use;

- Shock—superficial peripheral vessels are collapsed and cannot be palpated.

Ultimately, the patient will benefit from efficient and effective cannulation using a portable ultrasound system as an adjunct.

Perspective

In 1993, Denys *et al.* published a prospective series of using ultrasound-guided internal jugular cannulation in 928 patients versus a landmark technique only in 302 patients. They described a significant improvement in first and overall success rates, time taken to perform the procedure, and carotid puncture rate. This was further supported when the National Institute for Health and Care Excellence (NICE) in the UK published guidance advocating the use of ultrasound for central venous access. They performed a meta-analysis and described a reduction in the relative risk of failed first and overall attempts and also complications associated with the procedure. NICE recommended that ultrasound should be used for all elective central lines and considered for emergency ones.

Performing the scan

Where?

For central venous access, the common sites used in clinical practice are:

- The internal jugular vein (IJV);

- The femoral vein;

- The subclavian/axillary vein.

The IJV lies in close proximity to the common carotid artery (CCA) on the right and left sides of the neck, before joining the subclavian veins (SCVs) on each side to form the right and left brachiocephalic veins, respectively (see Figure 9.9). The typical site of cannulation is within a triangle formed by the two heads

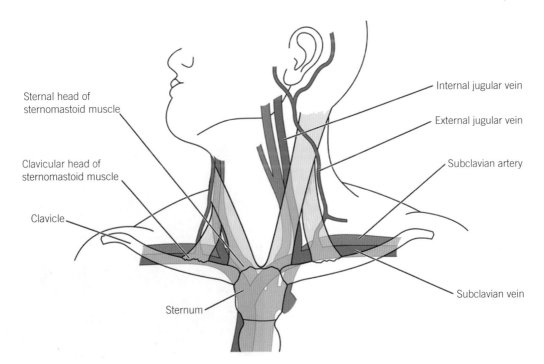

Figure 9.9 Vascular anatomy of the neck.

Peter Lamb, Slovenia © 123rf.com

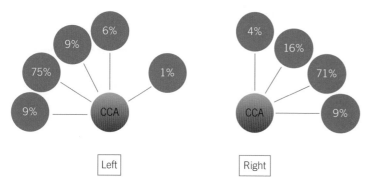

Left   Right

View from head end (i.e. looking towards to feet)

Figure 9.10 Variation of the internal jugular vein position in relation to the common carotid artery (CCA).

Reprinted by permission from Springer Nature: Springer Nature, *Cardiovascular and Interventional Radiology*, Anatomic relationship of the internal jugular vein and the common carotid artery applied to percutaneous transjugular procedures, Turba UC *et al.*, 28, 3, pp. 303–306. © Springer Science+Business Media, Inc. 2005.

of the sternocleidomastoid muscle. The IJV tends to lie anterolaterally to the CCA in most cases (see Figure 9.10 and Video 9.4). However, the location of the IJV in relation to the CCA at this level is variable and also influenced by excessive head rotation. Maecken *et al.* (2011) described a study of 600 patients placed in the supine position, with the probe placed at the level of the cricoid, scanning at an angle of 45° to the vertical (i.e. flush with the contour of the patient's neck). They found that the IJV, in relation to the CCA, is anterior or anteromedial in 49% on the right and in 59% on the left, and only lateral in 3–3.3%. In a minority of patients, the IJV was medial to the CCA (0.7–2.0%). Therefore, in a significant number of cases and dependent on probe angulation, the IJV will be overlying the CCA, increasing the risk of inadvertent arterial puncture if the IJV is traversed. The likelihood of traversing the IJV is greater in a shocked patient when hypovolaemia results in poor venous filling. Ultrasound guidance can clearly highlight such potential dangers to the operator. Changing the position or angulation of the probe may reduce the risk of CCA puncture by moving the artery out of the path of the needle. Head tilt away from the site of interrogation should be kept to <40° to avoid changing the relationship of the IJV to the CCA. The right side is often preferred over the left side due to the presence of the thoracic duct joining the left IJV and the increased risk of a chylothorax if injured.

The femoral vein may be found by locating the inguinal ligament—from the anterior superior iliac spine to the pubic tubercle. This is more proximal than the groin crease. The clinician should put the probe in a transverse position, approximately 1 cm distal to the inguinal ligament. At this level, the common femoral vein,

artery, and nerve are adjacent to each other. The vein is the most medial and the nerve is the most lateral, although not easily identifiable on B-mode (see Figure 9.11). If the clinician chooses a site more distal, the vascular anatomy does change; confluence with the femoral vein and the great saphenous and profunda femoris veins occurs (see Figure 9.12), and the femoral artery bifurcates to superficial and deep branches.

A less commonly used option for central access is the axillary vein. The basilic vein becomes the axillary vein, and medial to the lateral border of the first rib, the axillary vein becomes the SCV. The latter is not amenable to ultrasound evaluation due to its position behind the medial clavicle. Hence, subclavian cannulation is undertaken as a landmark-guided technique. However, the axillary vein can be used and can be found inferior to the lateral half of the clavicle (see Figure 9.13). It lies slightly deeper and lateral to

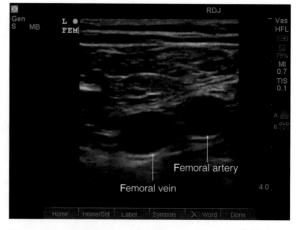

Figure 9.11 B-mode image of the transverse femoral vein just below the inguinal ligament.

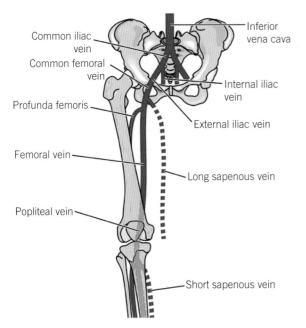

Figure 9.12 Venous anatomy of the pelvis and lower limb.

Peter Lamb, Slovenia © 123rf.com

the vein. The brachial plexus is at the most lateral aspect of the infraclavicular region, and thus the clinician may want to avoid cannulation in this area; in addition, the brachial plexus is not easily identified by B-mode. Galloway *et al.* (2003) found significant

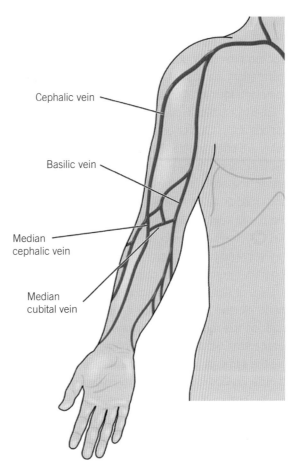

Figure 9.14 Venous anatomy of the upper limb.

Peter Lamb, Slovenia © 123rf.com

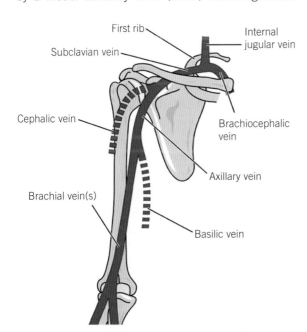

Figure 9.13 Venous anatomy of the shoulder and upper limb.

Peter Lamb, Slovenia © 123rf.com

variability in the position of the axillary vein on ultrasound that would not have been appreciated by landmark techniques. They also noted more vessel overlap medially; however, the vein was deeper, the more lateral the probe is placed, and may not be seen with a high-frequency linear probe.

For peripheral venous access, any identifiable vein is potentially suitable. In patients who are hypovolaemic or have multiple thrombosed veins, often secondary to multiple cannulations or intravenous drug use, a good place to start is the antecubital fossa (see Figure 9.14 and Video 9.5). A minimum depth of only 2–3 cm is required on the B-mode settings using a high-frequency linear probe. A good habit for the clinician to develop is to initially identify structures that need to be avoided such as the brachial artery. Using a tourniquet, as would be the norm for a traditional cannulation, will allow the vein to be as distended as possible.

Once a vein has been identified, and its patency confirmed by simple probe compression, it should be tracked proximally and distally to enable the clinician to ascertain the path of the vein. The number of viable veins and their location are extremely variable.

Often in difficult circumstances where peripheral venous access is challenging, the proximal upper limb veins are often usable. There are two main veins: the cephalic and the basilic. The former lies anterolateral in the arm, and the latter can be found deeper and medial—a transverse B-mode appearance of the basilic vein is shown in Figure 9.3s 📷 and Video 9.6 🎥. The basilic vein ultimately becomes the axillary vein and has traditionally been a choice for a peripherally inserted central catheter (PICC).

Uses of ultrasound-guided vascular access also include elective or emergency cannulation of arteries, such as the radial artery, for non-invasive BP measurements in a critical care environment. The principles are the same as for venous cannulation, although the clinician needs to be aware of the different ultrasound characteristics of arteries and veins; Table 9.1 shows a summary of the main differences.

When ultrasound has been used to facilitate vascular access to enable insertion of a temporary pacemaker wire, ultrasound can also be used to confirm placement of the pacing wire (usually in the apex of the right ventricle) via TTE windows.

How?

Prior to undertaking the procedure, informed consent should be obtained, if possible. The clinician should be competent to perform this procedure or be supervised as part of a training programme. The clinician should ensure that they adhere to good aseptic practice during the procedure, including establishing a sterile field and using a sterile probe cover. For larger cannulae and central access, local anaesthetic should be injected under the skin at the needle insertion site. Generally, a high-frequency linear probe should be used and the ultrasound machine optimized—utilization of vascular access preset, correct depth, and the highest frequency setting that will allow the best resolution of the area being interrogated.

The clinician can utilize in-plane and out-of-plane techniques for this procedure—this is often based on clinician preference, size of probe used, and surface space available. A preliminary scan should be undertaken to identify a suitable location, and the chosen vessel should be evaluated in transverse and longitudinal views.

For IJV cannulation, it is preferable to have the patient supine, with the trolley/gurney tilted head down (approximately 30°); this reduces the risk of air embolism and ensures optimal filling of the vessel. For femoral cannulation, the patient should be tilted head up (approximately 5°). Peripheral cannulation is aided by the application of a tourniquet and positioning the limb in an optimal position to improve ergonomic considerations.

The ultrasound machine should be in the clinician's line of sight to reduce head-turning during the procedure. In IJV cannulation, the clinician may be placed at the head of the patient, looking caudally; in such cases, reversing of the standard probe/B-mode image orientation is adopted, so that lateral movements of the probe correspond to movements in the same direction on the B-mode image.

As previously discussed, patency of the vessel should be confirmed by performing a proximal and distal sweep of the vessel to look for potential problems such as thrombus, aberrant vessels, branches, and valves, etc. However, too much operator pressure may compress and hide the vessel sought, so the amount of probe pressure applied should be minimal. Colour Doppler may be used to confirm the presence of flow (important for small radial arteries prior to cannulation); although colour Doppler should not be activated while searching for a vessel, due to degradation of the B-mode image.

Table 9.1 Differences between arteries and veins

Characteristic	Veins	Arteries
Shape	Variable, often oval	Round
Wall	Thin, poorly echogenic	Thick, echogenic
Compressibility	Easily compressible	Not easily compressible
Pulsatility	Double pulsed waveform	Single pulsed waveform
Anatomy	Often variable	Less variable

Complications include haemorrhage, damage to adjacent structures, false aneurysms, and fistulae. PTXs are more common when cannulation is undertaken near the thorax, e.g. the IJV. Haemothorax and chylothorax are also possible. Infection may be a consequence of poor technique or where lines are inserted in the groin region, e.g. femoral veins. In cases where the patient is hypovolaemic or no attempt was made to tilt the trolley/gurney, air embolism is possible.

Ultrasound can be used to confirm the presence of the guide-wire in the lumen when undertaking Seldinger cannulation. It can also be used to evaluate for complications such as those described in the previous paragraph.

Ultrasound-guided nerve blocks

The practice of regional anaesthesia has continued to gain popularity, as has the scope of what types of nerve blocks are undertaken. The main reasons are:

- The target area, i.e. nerve(s), is directly visible in real time;

- Adjacent structures that should be avoided are seen in real time, especially relevant when there is dynamic movement, e.g. the diaphragm in respiration;

- The needle can be visualized along its whole pathway (if in-plane technique adopted);

- Smaller volumes of local anaesthetic may be used, as it is delivered closer to the target; this reduces the risk of local anaesthetic toxicity.

A 2015 Cochrane database systematic review, which included 18 trials (ten upper limb and eight lower limb), concluded the following:

- Improved sensory and motor blocks by using ultrasound alone or in combination with peripheral nerve stimulation (PNS);

- Reduced need for supplementation;

- Fewer minor complications;

- Using ultrasound alone shortens performance time, compared to PNS (however, increases performance time when used with PNS).

This systematic review was not able to ascertain whether its conclusions were influenced by studies utilizing more experienced operators or ascertain the learning curve considerations, compared to other techniques.

It is unfeasible for this chapter to include all nerve blocks currently undertaken; however, we have provided several examples of the ones commonly undertaken. More advanced users are advised to refer to specialized literature.

A safe and aseptic approach to regional anaesthesia needs to be maintained, with particular attention to monitoring, needling techniques, and a local protocol to recognize and manage local anaesthetic toxicity. Users should be familiar with the pharmacology of the most common agents lignocaine/lidocaine (they are the same drug) and bupivacaine (or the newer S-isomer levobupivacaine). Use of adrenaline (epinephrine) is associated with less vasodilatation and a longer duration of action. Typical doses are shown in Table 9.2.

In the case of local anaesthetic severe toxicity (LAST), there should be clear departmental guidance on recognition and management. It is recommended that lipid emulsion should be available, along with a rapid treatment protocol, within areas where regional anaesthesia is undertaken.

Care has to be taken that the use of regional analgesia does not mask the symptoms of compartment syndrome. A high index of suspicion, frequent patient assessment, and compartment pressure monitoring are essential for early detection of compartment syndrome.

Careful documentation of pre-procedural sensory and motor examination is imperative. Also, detailed

Table 9.2 Typical doses and formulations of common local anaesthetic agents

Local anaesthetic	Maximum dose recommended	Formulation
Lignocaine/lidocaine	3 mg/kg without adrenaline 6 mg/kg with adrenaline	1% = 10 mg/mL 2% = 20 mg/mL
Bupivacaine	2 mg/kg	0.25% = 2.5 mg/mL 0.5% = 5 mg/mL

patient instruction about the duration of anaesthesia and post-block care should be given.

Ultrasound-guided radial nerve block

Purpose

Ultrasound-guided radial nerve block allows for the treatment of small hand lesions or injuries in the ED without the use of procedural sedation or multiple local anaesthetic injections. The use of ultrasound guidance has several advantages over landmark-based techniques, such as avoidance of vascular structures and direct visualization of the nerves, with improved success rates of the block.

Perspective

Radial nerve block provides effective analgesia for different hand procedures such as reduction of fractures, exploration and treatment of hand wounds, and evacuation of abscesses. The supracondylar radial nerve block can be used for analgesia in the treatment of distal radius fractures. A block of the radial nerve, performed under ultrasound guidance above the elbow, is effective for analgesia for reduction of this type of fracture.

The radial nerve runs in the spiral groove of the humerus and descends anterior to the lateral epicondyle in the elbow. At the elbow, it divides into the superficial branch, which provides sensory innervation to part of the hand (see Figure 9.15), and the deep branch, which innervates the dorsal compartment of the forearm. The superficial branch travels with the radial artery in the mid forearm but divides away from the artery in the distal forearm.

Performing the nerve block

Using a high-frequency (9–18 MHz) linear probe, the nerve is found by tracing the radial artery from distal to proximal. It can be blocked at the upper arm and mid forearm. An in-plane approach is preferable for greater control of the needle tip; an out-of-plane approach is also possible but requires advanced spatial skill for localizing and aligning the needle tip with the target tissue. Typical block volumes are 3–5 mL and should achieve anaesthesia within 15 minutes.

Upper arm

The nerve can be visualized and blocked at the level of the upper third of the humerus. The probe is placed over the triceps muscle in transverse orientation, localizing the brachial artery. Lateral to it, the radial nerve can be found crossing over the humeral shaft in the mid upper arm (see Figure 9.16). The needle is inserted from the lateral side of the arm.

Forearm

At the level of the mid forearm, the cutaneous branches will reform the radial nerve, lateral to the artery. The nerve may appear triangular or oval. Colour Doppler

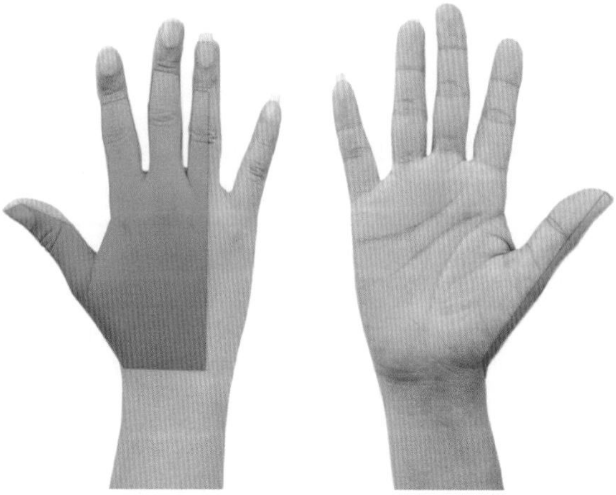

Figure 9.15 Radial nerve sensory distribution to the hand.

Sommai Larkjit, Thailand © 123rf.com. Augmented by Bob Jarman.

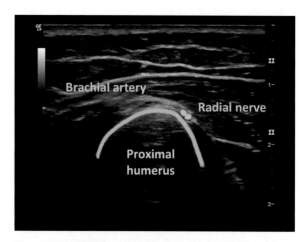

Figure 9.16 Radial nerve at the upper arm, adjacent to the humerus, in close proximity to the brachial artery.

Reproduced with kind permission from Matt Nixon.

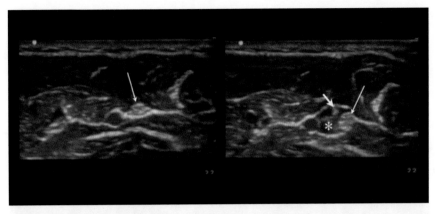

Figure 9.17 Left image: out-of-plane approach for the radial nerve (long arrow) at the level of the mid forearm, close to the brachial artery (red). Right image: the needle tip (short arrow) and the injected anaesthetic (*) surounding the nerve.

Reproduced with kind permission from Matt Nixon.

can assist in identification of the vessel. The needle is held in the dominant hand and carefully inserted from the radial side of the forearm. After identifying the needle tip, the needle is advanced slowly towards the base of the radial nerve. Local anaesthetic is injected to surround the nerve. Readjustment of the needle to the superficial border of the nerve is often necessary to fully surround the nerve. An out-of-plane or in-plane approach is possible (see Figure 9.17).

Ultrasound-guided median nerve block

Purpose

Ultrasound-guided median nerve block allows for the treatment of small hand lesions and injuries. There has been increasing popularity for ultrasound use, as it provides effective analgesia without the use of procedural sedation or multiple local anaesthetic injections.

Perspective

Ultrasound-guided median nerve block can be used for several hand procedures such as reduction of fractures, exploration and treatment of hand wounds, and evacuation of abscesses.

After it is formed from the medial and lateral cords of the brachial plexus, the median nerve runs very closely to the brachial artery until it passes through the cubital fossa into the elbow where it gives off the

anterior interosseous nerve. This nerve supplies the deep volar muscles of the forearm. Distal to the elbow, the median nerve is found between the muscle of the flexor digitorum superficialis and the flexor digitorum profundus, before passing through the carpal tunnel into the wrist. It supplies radial sensation of the palm (see Figure 9.18).

Performing the block

Using a high-frequency (7–15 MHz) linear probe, the nerve can be blocked at three levels: the elbow, the forearm, and the wrist. An in-plane approach is preferable for greater control of the needle tip. An

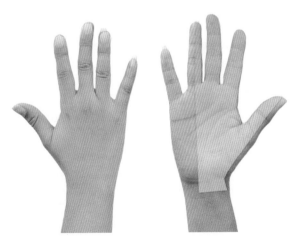

Figure 9.18 Median nerve sensory distribution to the hand.

Sommai Larkjit, Thailand © 123rf.com. Augmented by Bob Jarman.

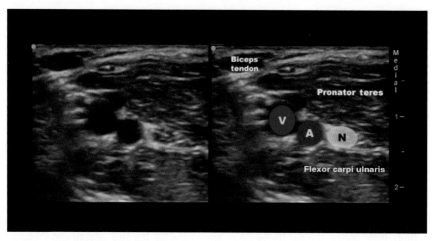

Figure 9.19 The median nerve at the antecubital fossa.
Reproduced with kind permission from Matt Nixon.

out-of-plane approach is possible and may aid in separating the nerve from the artery, but it usually requires significant spatial skill and experience. Typical block volumes are 5–7 mL of anaesthetic.

Elbow

In the antecubital fossa, the median nerve lies medial to the brachial artery. With the arm extended and externally rotated, a high-frequency (8–18 MHz) probe is placed transversely over the brachial artery pulse (see Figure 9.4s 🔲). Medial to the artery, the median nerve will have a classic honeycomb appearance (see Figure 9.19). For an in-plane approach, the needle is held in the dominant hand and carefully inserted medial to the probe. After identifying the needle tip, the needle is slowly advanced towards the base of the median nerve. Local anaesthetic is injected and should surround the nerve. Readjustment is often necessary.

Forearm

At the mid forearm, the median nerve is found deeper between the muscles of the volar compartment. The probe is placed transverse over the flexor aspect of the mid forearm (see Figure 9.5s 🔲). Its honeycomb appearance should stand out against the surrounding hypoechoic muscle (see Figure 9.20). It can be traced from distal to proximal, if needed, starting at the carpal tunnel (see Figure 9.21). In a similar fashion to its block at the elbow, local anaesthetic is injected to surround the nerve.

Wrist

Scanning starts on the volar wrist, transversely at the first carpal crease. Several round, fibrinous structures are identified, including the tendons and median nerve in the carpal tunnel. Fanning or rocking the probe will change the appearance of these structures from hypoechoic to hyperechoic. This is called anisotropy and is more obvious with tendons than nerves. The median nerve has less anisotropy and lack of movement on flexion and extension of the digits. An out-of-plane approach is generally preferred (see Figure 9.6s 🔲). The needle is inserted perpendicular to the ultrasound plane. Once the needle tip is identified, it is slowly directed to one side of the median nerve. Anaesthetic is injected until the entire nerve is surrounded. Both sides of the injection will ensure full anaesthetic surrounding the nerve (see Figure 9.22).

Ultrasound-guided ulnar nerve block

Purpose

The hand can be especially problematic when providing anaesthesia, given the difficulty of anaesthetizing through tough and painful palmar skin. Thus, blocks of the ulnar nerve are excellent for complex laceration repairs and painful lesions (i.e. burns) in this area. Fortunately, both pain and the amount of local anaesthesia can be reduced, utilizing regional nerve blocks.

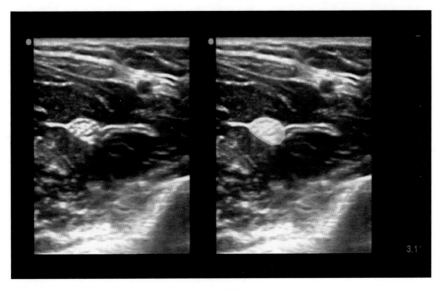

Figure 9.20 The median nerve (yellow) at the level of the mid forearm.

Reproduced with kind permission from Matt Nixon.

Perspective

The use of ulnar nerve block is for sensory anaesthesia of the supplied portion of the hand—namely the fifth digit and the ulnar half of the fourth digit and palm of similar distribution (see Figure 9.23). The ulnar nerve does not provide any sensory innervation to the forearm.

The ulnar nerve begins at the medial cord of the brachial plexus (C8, T1 roots) and is a combined motor and sensory nerve. The nerve courses along the medial aspect of the humerus before coursing posterior to the medial epicondyle of the humerus

in the cubital fossa where it is at its most superficial and is prone to injury. It continues its course near the ulnar artery in the forearm, passing into the palm, superficial to the flexor retinaculum through Guyan's canal; thus, it is not spared in carpal tunnel syndrome. The sensory distribution is described in the previous paragraph, and the nerve (through muscular, superficial, and deep branches) innervates the flexor carpi ulnaris, the ulnar portion of the flexor digitorum profundus, the hypothenar muscles, the interosseus and lumbrical muscles, and the flexor (brevis) and adductor pollicis.

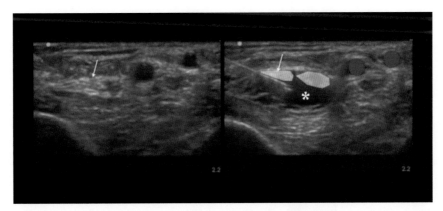

Figure 9.21 Left image: the median nerve (arrow) further distally. Right image: the median nerve (yellow) and duplicated brachial arteries (red), demonstrating injected anaesthetic (*) surrounding the nerve.

Reproduced with kind permission from Matt Nixon.

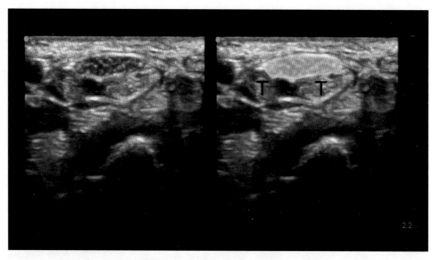

Figure 9.22 The median nerve (yellow) with tendons (T) at the level of the wrist.

Reproduced with kind permission from Matt Nixon.

Performing the scan

Although the ulnar nerve can be successfully located and blocked at any level distal to the brachial plexus, in the ED, we recommend utilizing the mid forearm as the location for a block for regional anaesthesia of appropriate hand injuries (see Figure 9.7s 📷). This approach has two main advantages—firstly, the ulnar nerve has anatomical separation from the ulnar artery at this point in its course, and secondly, the potential risk of cubital compartment syndrome from injections in the cubital fossa can be avoided.

At this location, the ulnar artery can still be utilized as a landmark, and the ulnar nerve will be ulnar to its corresponding artery (see Figure 9.24) The nerve should be localized in axial view and the artery identified, and needle insertion should be performed in an 'in-plane' orientation, with direct visualization of the needle tip at all times. During injection of the anaesthetic, the operator can now observe how the nerve is separating from its surrounding connective tissue and is now clearly visible and surrounded and 'floating' in anaesthetic fluid (see Figure 9.25); a total of 3–5 mL of anaesthetic is injected.

An alternative anatomical approach is to inject the anaesthetic several centimetres above the elbow (see Figures 9.26, 9.27, and 9.8s 📷). This approach will also avoid the risk of potential compressive injury in the cubital fossa.

Ultrasound-guided femoral nerve block

Purpose

Ultrasound-guided femoral nerve block (FNB) has been established as an option for regional pain management at the anterior thigh in patients with femur and patella fractures and those requiring extensive laceration repairs or abscess drainage in this region. The so-called '3-in-1' modification of the block gives additional peripheral blockade to the hip area, since it provides regional anaesthesia to the femoral, obturator, and lateral cutaneous nerves.

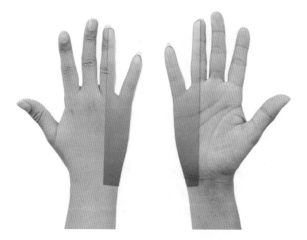

Figure 9.23 Ulnar nerve sensory distribution to the hand.

Sommai Larkjit, Thailand © 123rf.com. Augmented by Bob Jarman.

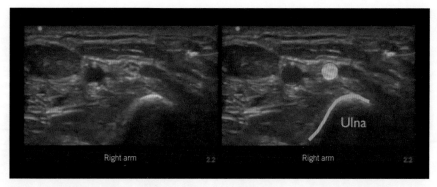

Figure 9.24 The ulnar nerve (yellow) with the ulnar artery (red) at the level of the mid forearm.

Reproduced with kind permission from Matt Nixon.

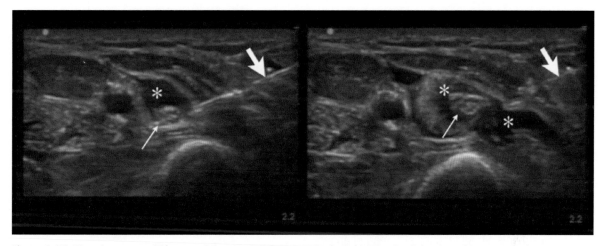

Figure 9.25 The ulnar nerve (thin arrow) surrounded by anaesthetic fluid (*), after injection with anaesthetic, and visualized needle (thick arrow).

Reproduced with kind permission from Matt Nixon.

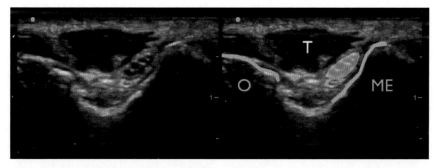

Figure 9.26 The ulnar nerve (yellow) can be easily identified in the posterior view of the elbow, adjacent to the medial epicondyle (ME), olecranon (O), and triceps tendon (T).

Reproduced with kind permission from Matt Nixon.

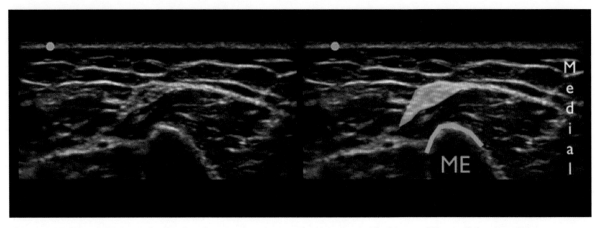

Figure 9.27 The ulnar nerve (yellow), a few centimetres proximal to the cubital fossa. ME, medial epicondyle.

Reproduced with kind permission from Matt Nixon.

Perspective

The anatomy of the femoral nerve compartment at the inguinal region makes the FNB ideal for ultrasound guidance. The femoral nerve is large, superficial, and easily located adjacent to the femoral vessels. Fletcher *et al.* found that ultrasound guidance for FNBs resulted in a significantly higher success rate versus a blind technique. Visualization with ultrasound also helps the practitioner monitor needle placement and the spread of local anaesthetic and facilitates appropriate adjustments, should the initial spread of anaesthetic fluid be deemed inadequate. Moreover, because of the proximity to the relatively large femoral artery, ultrasound may reduce the risk of arterial puncture, as it is performed under visual guidance. This would be particularly beneficial in obese patients, in whom a femoral pulse can be difficult to detect.

The femoral verve, the largest branch of the lumbar plexus, derives from the ventral rami of the L2–L4 nerves. It provides sensory innervation to the femur periosteum, anterior thigh, and knee, as well as the medial knee and lower extremities. It also gives off motor fibres to the quadriceps muscle. The femoral nerve enters the thigh under the inguinal ligament, between the psoas and iliacus muscle, and is located below the fascia iliaca. The lateral cutaneous femoral nerve originates from the L2 and L4 roots and is located proximally and laterally to the femoral nerve, providing sensory innervation to the lateral thigh. The obturator verve also arises from L2 and L4 and is located medially to the femoral nerve, providing sensory innervation to the medial thigh. Figure 9.9s shows the branches of the lumbar plexus.

The femoral nerve is easily recognizable by its 'honeycombing' appearance bounded by the:

- Femoral artery—medially;
- Iliopsoas muscle—infero-laterally;
- Fascia iliaca—superiorly.

(See Figure 9.28.)

Performing the procedure

The patient is placed in the supine position, with the probe positioned at the level of the groin crease in a transverse orientation. Firstly, the femoral artery is identified, and then the highly echogenic area lateral to the artery is located, which is the femoral nerve. Then the needle is inserted through the skin at an approximate 45° angle and is advanced under direct vision through the ilio-pectinal fascia into the immediate proximity of the nerve. The anaesthetic should be instilled after initial aspiration attempts are made. If blood is aspirated, the needle should be repositioned and the needle tip location should be re-verified under visual guidance. Once the optimal position for injection is attained, local anaesthetic is infiltrated under visual guidance at the 12 o'clock position just above the nerve, and then towards the 6 o'clock position just underneath the nerve. The goal should be to reach full bathing of the nerve in anaesthetic fluid (see Figure 9.29).

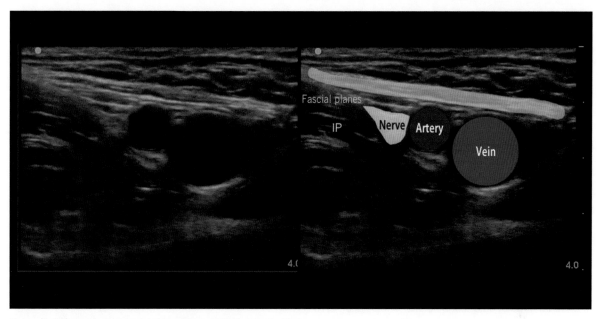

Figure 9.28 The femoral nerve bounded medially by the femoral artery (red), the iliopsoas (IP) inferomedially, and the fascia iliaca superiorly—right side shown.

Reproduced with kind permission from Matt Nixon.

The technique for the 3-in-1 block is similar to that described previously for the FNB, with two differences:

- A larger volume of local anaesthetic is used to aid spread. The minimum volume of 20 mL is recommended, but up to 30 mL may be necessary.

- Pressure is applied 2–4 cm distal to the needle site and held for 30 s by an assistant. This encourages the necessary spread of anaesthetic agent.

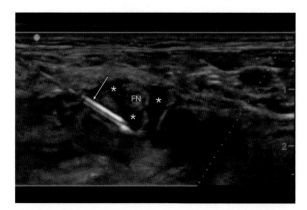

Figure 9.29 In-plane needle (arrow) injecting local anaesthetic (*) around the femoral nerve (FN)—right side shown.

Reproduced with kind permission from Matt Nixon.

Ultrasound-guided fascia iliaca compartment block

Purpose

Fascia iliaca compartment block (FICB) is an anaesthetic technique designed to provide effective pain relief to patients with lower limb injury, especially for femoral fractures.

Perspective

Optimal analgesia management for fractured neck of the femur (FNOF) includes avoidance of delirium. Under-managed pain, an over-reliance on opiates, and anticholinergic anti-emetics can all contribute to delirium in this vulnerable group. Timely FICB should become part of a package of care for FNOF, as well as for femoral shaft fractures.

Ultrasound-guided FICB is more efficient than a landmark technique and superior to traditional approaches to FNOF pain management. There is also evidence that this block is superior to the 3-in-1 block described previously.

The lumbar plexus gives origin to the peripheral nerves that provide sensory and motor supply to the hip joint

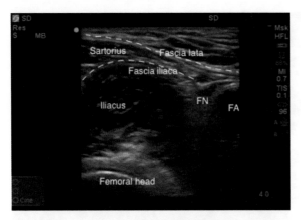

Figure 9.30 Ultrasound image of the anatomy for fascia iliaca nerve block. FN, femoral nerve; FA, femoral artery.

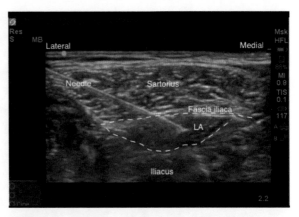

Figure 9.31 Ultrasound image of the in-plane needle position and local anaesthetic (LA) injection under the fascia iliaca.

and lower limb, namely the sciatic, obturator, femoral, and lateral femoral cutaneous nerves. The sciatic nerve lies posteriorly and the obturator nerve lies medially, neither being easily accessible, particularly in an elderly patient in pain with a hip fracture. The femoral and lateral femoral cutaneous nerves, however, both lie in the same fascial compartment under the fascia iliaca, which covers the iliacus muscle and is bounded superiorly by the iliac crest and inferiorly blends with the psoas fascia. MRI and ultrasound images demonstrating the anatomy are shown in Figures 9.10s 📷 and 9.30, respectively.

Performing the scan

The simplest technique for the FICB is to obtain a transverse view of the femoral neurovascular bundle orientated close and parallel to the femoral crease identifying all the structures. Infero-laterally lies the iliacus muscle, and more superficially and laterally lies the sartorius muscle, which crosses the field laterally to medial, as we descend down the neurovascular bundle. The aim is to deliver a block as cranial as possible, certainly above the level of the bifurcation of the common femoral artery.

Concentrate on the dome of the iliacus muscle lying somewhere lateral to the femoral nerve, yet medial to the sartorius. Reduce the scan depth to put the plane of the fascia iliaca in the centre, with the femoral artery just visible medially.

The needling technique should be using an in-plane approach from the lateral aspect, maintaining constant visualization of the moving needle tip (see

Figure 9.11s 📷). Insert the needle tip at the lateral border of the transducer, descending medially through a portion of the sartorius, aiming for the top of the dome of the iliacus (see Figure 9.31). There is both a visual and tactile confirmation of penetration of the fascia iliaca, with a sudden increase, then loss, of resistance. Test aspiration, followed by delivery of a small amount of local anaesthetic, will delineate the undersurface of the fascia iliaca; failure to do so should prompt repositioning. The remainder of the local anaesthetic (typically up to 40 mL of 0.25% levobupivacaine) can now be delivered and will be seen to spread medially and laterally under the overlying fascia iliaca. A long-acting local anaesthetic should be used, taking into consideration that this is a compartment block, so the volume and distribution are paramount, i.e. 20 mL of 0.5% or 40 mL of 0.25% levobupivacaine.

Ultrasound-guided haematoma block

Purpose

The haematoma block involves infiltration of local anaesthetic to the peri-fracture haematoma, thus enabling an effective blockade of adjacent nerves (e.g. periosteal branches).

Perspective

This block is commonly undertaken in many EDs for analgesia prior to reduction of displaced distal radial fractures. Using ultrasound can aid in locating the haematoma—which will be adjacent to the fracture line. In many cases, this is palpable; however, when there is significant swelling or large patient body habitus, this may prove difficult. Additionally, the patient may not tolerate palpation of a painful site. Hence, ultrasound allows locating the haematoma area and also guides placement of the needle.

Other sites have been described, e.g. the humeral shaft and sternal fractures. However, in many cases, the haematoma block has been superseded by more nerve-specific regional blockade, which may utilize less local anaesthetic agent and produce more effective analgesia.

The procedure is considered safe; however, the operator should avoid higher concentrations of local anaesthetic. A study by Quinton took arterial samples at predefined intervals on nine patients receiving haematoma blocks for severely displaced and comminuted Colles' fractures. The author found plasma concentrations of lidocaine were potentially toxic when 10 mL of 2% lidocaine was used versus similar doses of 1%; the peak concentrations were noted after manipulation was undertaken. No patients displayed any signs of toxicity, and all received satisfactory blocks.

Performing the block

The fracture area is evaluated using a high-frequency probe, e.g. linear or hockey stick. Plenty of couplant gel should be used in this initial evaluation to avoid unnecessary probe pressure and patient discomfort. The bony cortical reflection should be identified and followed in a longitudinal direction towards the fracture site until a step is seen. Excess couplant gel is then removed, and the skin cleaned. A liberal spray of chlorhexidine will act as a skin cleaner and couplant. A 20G or 22G needle and a 10-mL syringe with 10 mL of 1% lidocaine (lignocaine) should be introduced under ultrasound guidance towards the fracture area (often from a proximal direction in the case of distal radial fractures). An in-plane technique is best for this procedure, as the entire needle is seen. Once the needle tip has reached the optimal site, aspiration may draw back some blood. Five to 10 mL of local anaesthetic can then be introduced slowly. Adequate analgesia is normally achieved within 10–15 minutes.

In cases where there is more than one fracture site, e.g. associated ulnar styloid fracture, the procedure can be repeated. However, the operator needs to ensure the amount of local anaesthetic used does not exceed safe doses.

Technically, the operator is creating an open fracture. However, the reported incidence of subsequent infection is very low. This block should not be undertaken in the presence of an adjacent infection (e.g. cellulitis).

Ultrasound-guided aspiration and drainage of fluid

Ultrasound-guided thoracocentesis

Purpose

Pleural effusions are clinically common and may be a result of many local and systemic problems. This is covered in more detail in Chapter 3. The purpose of thoracocentesis (also known as thoracentesis or pleural aspiration) is to remove air or pleural fluid (effusion or blood).

Perspective

Ultrasound can increase the success rate and safety of this procedure, compared to traditional non-ultrasound-guided practice. Ultrasound may also contribute to establishing the presence of pleural fluid; it also will guide the clinician in determining an optimal site to perform the thoracocentesis and as an adjunct during the procedure. As described earlier in this chapter, ultrasound guidance can be static or dynamic, depending on whether it is used to simply identify an optimal site or whether the procedure will be guided by ultrasound in real time. Static ultrasound-guided thoracocentesis is not recommended, unless the pleural effusion is large, because the anatomy can change, depending on patient positioning and physiological considerations. Using ultrasound to guide the needle is the next step—dynamic guidance.

In the emergency setting, this may be performed for diagnostic or therapeutic purposes. Diagnostic samples may be obtained with a simple needle and syringe and sent for cytology, protein, lactate dehydrogenase, pH,

Gram stain, and culture and sensitivity. Therapeutic thoracocentesis may be undertaken to relieve symptoms of respiratory distress or guide the introduction of a chest drain. Removal of large volumes is thought to increase the risk of re-expansion pulmonary oedema. Therefore, a maximum volume of 1.5 L in one attempt is recommended.

Performing the scan

Where?

Thoracocentesis can be performed from the anterior, lateral, or posterior approach. However, to reduce iatrogenic injury, the preferred site of pleural drainage in the supine patient (especially relevant when inserting a Seldinger drain) should be within the triangle of safety (see Figure 9.12s ⬛). This is bordered anteriorly by the lateral border of the pectoralis major muscle, posteriorly by the lateral border of the latissimus dorsi, inferiorly by the line of the fifth intercostal space, and superiorly by the base of the axilla.

Commonly, with the patient sat upright, sites lower down and posterior to the mid-axillary line are used and are safe (e.g. seventh to ninth intercostal spaces posterior to the mid- and/or posterior axillary lines). When draining fluid, the operator needs to ensure that the site chosen allows direct access to the pleural fluid and that adjacent structures (e.g. liver and spleen) will be away from the trajectory path throughout the respiratory cycle. In addition, procedural safety can be maximized by considering the size of the underlying fluid collection. Preference should be given to the site where the collection is the largest, as this reduces the risk of damaging lung tissue. When choosing a site to drain air, the only consideration is avoidance of underlying structures (e.g. collapsed lung, liver, and spleen).

How?

The patient should be sitting, either supine or in the lateral decubitus position, depending on what is achievable, given the clinical scenario. The ultrasound machine is positioned adjacent to the patient and within reach for the operator to comfortably adjust the settings and apply the probe to the patient's thorax. The patient should be encouraged to raise their arms in order to increase the intercostal space. Due to the depth required to evaluate the pleural space and adjacent structures (up to 15 cm), a low-frequency probe, such as

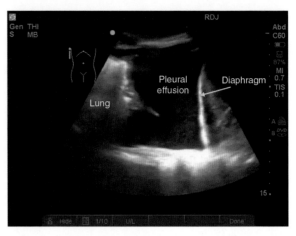

Figure 9.32 Identifying a potential site for needle insertion in thoracocentesis.

a curvilinear or phased array probe, is used. Once the site is identified, the clinician may change to a high-frequency linear probe, but this is not essential. The clinician should perform a preliminary scan of the chest to confirm the diagnosis and the potential site of safe needle insertion (see Figure 9.32 for an example). Use of the quad and sinusoidal signs may aid in the diagnosis of pleural fluid (see Chapter 3). It is imperative that the diaphragm is identified; starting at the bases easily identifies the diaphragm initially. In the majority of cases, the B-mode appearances of pleural fluid will be hypoechoic. Pleural exudates or HTX may show up as mixed echogenicity on B-mode. In some cases, there will be loculated pockets of fluid, which require skill and experience to drain—these should be referred for specialist intervention. The clinician should ensure that there is a minimum of 10 mm depth of pleural fluid, no intervening lung at maximal inspiration (i.e. when the lung moves closest to the chest wall), and a minimum risk of injury to adjacent structures such as the diaphragm, liver, spleen, and kidneys. Lower margins of the rib (i.e. the upper intercostal space) should be avoided due to the presence of the adjacent intercostal neurovascular bundle; ultrasound has not been shown to reduce inadvertent injury to these intercostal vessels.

Local anaesthetic is not always required for simple needle aspiration for diagnostic purposes. However, when used, local anaesthetic should be injected under the skin at the needle insertion. The local anaesthetic should be then infiltrated down to the adjacent rib periosteum and parietal pleura—this can be facilitated using ultrasound. Ensuring the length of the needle is adequate for the patient's body habitus is essential.

The clinician can utilize in-plane and out-of-plane techniques for this procedure, although the former is preferable as the needle is visualized throughout its length. Some clinicians rotate from an initial longitudinal orientation to one in alignment with the intercostal space—this is not always transverse as the rib orientation is variable, depending on the site chosen on the thorax.

For diagnostic thoracocentesis, the clinician may elect to use a needle and syringe, to obtain 20–50 mL of fluid (depending on the laboratory samples required). A small-bore needle is recommended, if possible, to reduce the risk of post-procedure PTX.

Non-urgent pleural aspirations and drainage should be avoided in coagulopathic or anticoagulated patients. The most common complications from pleural aspiration are PTX, procedure failure, pain, and haemorrhage. There is also a risk of visceral injury. Evidence suggests that ultrasound can reduce these complications.

The clinician should not choose a site where infection, such as cellulitis, is present.

Re-expansion pulmonary oedema is a complication of large-volume pleural fluid drainage.

Ultrasound-guided pericardiocentesis

Purpose

The purpose of pericardiocentesis is to remove pericardial fluid for diagnostic or therapeutic purposes, which includes for palliative reasons. The causes and features of pericardial effusions and cardiac tamponade are covered in more detail in Chapter 2; however, one of the primary causes is malignancy, and a high index of suspicion should be assumed for haemodynamically compromised oncology patients.

Perspective

Ultrasound can increase the success rate and safety of this procedure, compared to traditional non-ultrasound-guided practice; it will guide the clinician in determining an optimal site to perform the pericardiocentesis and as an adjunct during the procedure. Hence, ultrasound can be used as a static and dynamic tool.

In the emergency setting, pericardiocentesis is undertaken for therapeutic indications in patients who are *in extremis* due to pericardial effusion resulting in cardiac tamponade and/or cardiac arrest (PEA). Drainage of relatively small volumes can improve the patient's haemodynamic status significantly (as little as 50 mL). In the non-emergency setting, patients requiring diagnostic and non-urgent pericardiocentesis would normally be referred to interventional cardiologists.

Performing the scan
Where?

The established site for traditional pericardiocentesis is the subcostal approach; this involves traversing the left lobe of the liver (see Figure 9.33) and may be complicated by a distended stomach. However, with increasing use of PoCUS, an approach via the anterior chest wall has also been advocated; parasternal to apical windows have been described (see Figure 9.13s 🖻).

When using anterior chest wall sites, the clinician should be aware of, and avoid, the left internal mammary vessels (artery and vein), which run at the left lateral edge of the sternum. The left internal mammary vessels can be identified as vascular structures parallel to the sternum and under the costal cartilages at a depth of approximately 2 cm (see Figure 9.34). These can be identified using a high-frequency probe, and their position indicated with a surgical marker pen.

Avoid the lower border of the ribs, if using an anterior chest wall approach, to reduce the risk of inadvertent injury to the neurovascular bundle.

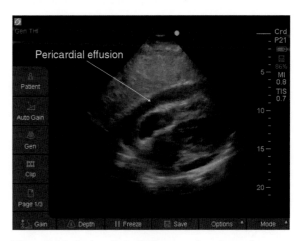

Figure 9.33 Pericardial effusion seen in subcostal window.

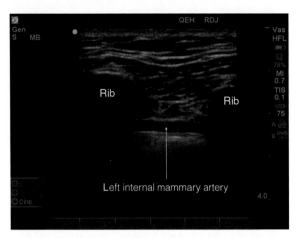

Figure 9.34 B-mode image of the left internal mammary artery (longitudinal orientation).

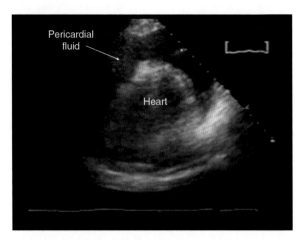

Figure 9.35 B-mode visualization of the needle (*) during pericardiocentesis.

How?

The patient should be positioned 30–45° head up or in the left lateral decubitus position to pool the pericardial fluid in the inferior pericardium/apex (especially in smaller collections), but in a cardiac arrest situation, only the supine position is feasible. The ultrasound machine should be positioned adjacent to the patient and within reach for the operator to comfortably adjust the settings and apply the probe to the patient's abdomen. Due to the depth required to evaluate the echocardiographic windows and navigate the thoracic cage, a low-frequency probe, such as a phased array or small curvilinear probe, is used. The clinician should perform a preliminary scan of the heart to confirm the diagnosis of pericardial fluid and the potential site of insertion of the needle. In many of the cases, the B-mode appearances of pericardial fluid will be hypoechoic. Exudates or aged haemorrhagic effusions may show up as mixed echogenicity on B-mode. Where the largest pericardial collection is seen, with minimal intervening structures, should be considered as the preferred site. The clinician should be aware of heart movements during the cardiac cycle and respiratory cycle. Ultrasound will allow the depth to the effusion to be assessed—either using the depth graduations on the side of the B-mode or by using calipers. A surgical skin marker may then be used to mark this spot.

Local anaesthetic would ideally be used at the needle insertion site (skin and along the needle tract); however, in emergency cases, this may not be feasible. There are dedicated pericardiocentesis kits available (see Figure 9.14s). These often include catheters that can be inserted for repeated or continuous drainage—utilizing the Seldinger technique. Anterior chest wall approaches do not need long needles, as the depth to effusion is minimal; subcostal approaches require longer needles.

The clinician can utilize in-plane and out-of-plane techniques for this procedure, although the former is preferable as the needle is visualized throughout its length. The in-plane B-mode visualization of the needle is shown in Figure 9.35.

Once in the pericardial sac, confirmation that the needle tip is in the right place may be demonstrated by injection of a small volume (1–2 mL) of agitated saline. This will result in a transient reflective flush being seen.

ECG monitoring may be adopted as a further safeguard against inadvertent myocardial injury—most pericardiocentesis kits will have a crocodile clip lead to attach to the needle for ECG monitoring during the procedure.

Coagulopathy is a relative contraindication to performing pericardiocentesis. In cardiac tamponade secondary to dissection of the aorta, pericardiocentesis should be considered as contraindicated.

Complications include damage to structures such the liver, diaphragm, gastrointestinal tract, heart chambers, coronary vessels, lung, and vessels. A PTX or pneumopericardium is also possible. Later complications include infection. However, as this will only be performed in an emergency scenario in a moribund patient, the benefits will often outweigh the risks.

In cases where there is clotted blood or pus in the pericardium, i.e. in trauma and infection, respectively, pericardiocentesis may not be able to drain the collection and a surgical option will need to be undertaken.

Ultrasound-guided paracentesis

Purpose

Paracentesis is used to remove ascitic fluid for diagnostic or therapeutic purposes. Ultrasound can increase the success rate and safety of this procedure, compared to traditional non-ultrasound-guided practice.

Perspective

Ultrasound may also have contributed to establishing the presence of ascites; it also will guide the clinician in determining an optimal site to perform the paracentesis and as an adjunct during the procedure. Hence, ultrasound can be used as a static and dynamic tool.

In the emergency setting, diagnostic samples may be sought. Often this sample is tested for cell counts (white, neutrophils, and red), glucose, albumin, protein, amylase, lactate dehydrogenase, cytology, tumour markers, Gram staining, and culture. This may be to ascertain whether there is an infection in suspected spontaneous bacterial peritonitis (SBP). Patients should be screened for the development of SBP, which is present in approximately 15% of patients admitted with cirrhosis and ascites. Evaluation for other potential causative conditions, such as malignancy or pancreatitis, may also be required.

Therapeutic paracentesis may be undertaken to relieve pain or reduce diaphragmatic splinting and respiratory distress; however, removal of large volumes can increase the risk of electrolyte disturbance, renal impairment, and encephalopathy. This procedure is often undertaken in an inpatient setting by specialty teams.

Performing the scan
Where?

The established sites for paracentesis are the lower abdominal quadrants. The left side is usually preferred in order to avoid the liver and caecum. The clinician should be aware of, and avoid, the inferior epigastric artery, which runs from the mid-inguinal point to lateral to the umbilicus. Therefore, the surface landmark approximately 15 cm lateral to the umbilicus or 4–5 cm superior and medial to the anterior superior iliac spine is generally used (see Figure 9.15s 📷). Sites where there are scars or a previous stoma should be avoided.

The location of the fluid, its proximity to the abdominal wall, and the maximal depth will also influence positioning (often >3 cm depth would be expected). This reduces the risk of iatrogenic injury, especially to the bowel.

How?

The patient should be supine, and the ultrasound machine positioned adjacent to the patient and within reach for the operator to comfortably adjust the settings and apply the probe to the patient's abdomen. Due to the depth required to evaluate the peritoneal space and adjacent structures, a low-frequency probe, such as a curvilinear or phased array probe, is used. The clinician should perform a preliminary scan of the abdomen to confirm the diagnosis of ascites and the potential site of insertion of the needle (see Figure 9.16s 📷 for the typical appearance of ascites in B-mode). In the majority of cases, the B-mode appearances of ascites will be hypoechoic. Exudates or aged haemorrhagic ascites may show up as mixed echogenicity in B-mode. A surgical skin marker may be used to mark the preferred spot. Local anaesthetic should be injected under the skin at the needle insertion. The local anaesthetic should be then infiltrated down to the peritoneum.

The clinician can utilize in-plane and out-of-plane techniques for this procedure, although the former is preferable as the needle is visualized throughout its length. The in-plane B-mode visualization of the needle is shown in Figure 9.36.

For diagnostic paracentesis, the clinician may elect to use a needle and syringe to obtain 10–20 mL of fluid (depending on the laboratory samples required), or use a dedicated paracentesis catheter kit if therapeutic drainage is required.

Skin traction is often used prior to needle insertion to ensure that the initial path of the needle is distorted once the traction is taken off (Z-track technique). This can prevent infection and post-procedure leakage.

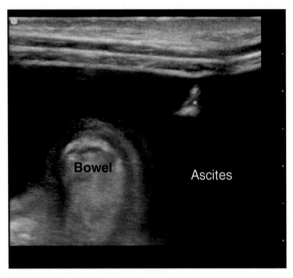

Figure 9.36 B-mode visualization of the needle (*) during paracentesis (in-plane technique).

Complications occur in 1% of cases; however, they are rarely life-threatening. The most common complication is abdominal wall haematomas. Major complications, such as haemoperitoneum and bowel perforation, occur in <1 in 1000 cases.

Coagulopathy is not a contraindication to performing paracentesis, which is reassuring as many patients who develop ascites may be at increased risk of abnormal clotting (abnormally long prothrombin time and thrombocytopenia).

If only the static method is being used, ensure that there is no significant patient movement between the ultrasonic marking of the preferred site and performing paracentesis. As with all the procedures described in this chapter, dynamic ultrasound guidance is preferred.

Ultrasound-guided suprapubic catheter insertion

Purpose

Ultrasound can be used to improve safety when inserting a suprapubic catheter (SPC). This is through identification of the optimal site of insertion, as well as identifying potential hazards. In addition, ultrasound can aid in the insertion of an SPC under direct vision.

Perspective

SPC insertion may be undertaken as an emergency procedure, often in cases where traditional urethral catheterization is unfeasible, due to failure to catheterize (e.g. strictures, prostate enlargement) or in cases of urethral trauma. However, such a procedure is not without complications. The National Patient Safety Agency (NPSA) of the UK published a safety report in 2009. This identified three deaths in the period between 2005 and 2009; there were seven cases of severe harm and 249 incidents related to problems with the use of the SPC. The published 30-day mortality from this procedure is up to 1.8%, although it has been suggested this is under-reported.

The bladder lies in the pelvic cavity, and as it fills up with urine, it distends into the abdominal cavity (i.e. superiorly). Last's Anatomy describes the bladder as being a flattened three-sided pyramid, with the sharp apex pointing forwards to the top of the pubic symphysis. The superior surface is covered by the peritoneum, which sweeps upwards on to the anterior abdominal wall. The distending bladder pushes the peritoneum from the anterior wall; the transversalis fascia is left between the anterior wall and the bladder (see Figure 9.37). The optimal area for suprapubic catherization (SPC) is via the lower anterior wall, going through the transversalis fascia into the distending bladder, thus avoiding going through any peritoneal layers (and viscera such as bowel loops that may lie within).

Bowel injury remains one of the main complications and is increased when ultrasound is not used—the incidence of bowel injury in 'blind' insertion has been

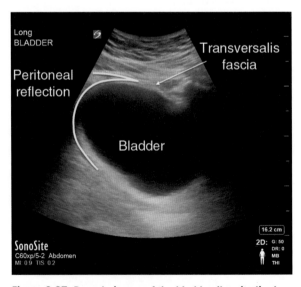

Figure 9.37 B-mode image of the bladder (longitudinal orientation).

quoted to be between 0.15% and 2.7%. This is increased in patients with:

- Obesity;
- Abdominal adhesions from previous surgery;
- Inadequate bladder distension.

Despite the perceived benefits from using ultrasound to identify the anatomy and potential hazards, there is not a large body of evidence to support its use. Nevertheless, urological organisations have recommended ultrasound use, with the caveat that clinicians should be suitably trained. There have been studies describing ultrasound-guided SPC in the ED; Aguilera *et al.* (2002) published a series of 17 consecutive patients who underwent emergent real-time ultrasound-guided SPC in the ED. Ultrasound confirmed urinary retention before drainage in all patients. Continuous real-time ultrasound-guided SPC insertion was undertaken in all patients, with no complications reported.

Performing the scan

Where?

The established site for SPC insertion is the lower midline abdomen, with the site of puncture usually 2–4 cm superior to the symphysis pubis. This should correlate, in an adequately distended bladder, to being inferior to the peritoneal reflection, and thus potential bowel loops. Sites where there are scars or a previous SPC should be avoided.

How?

There are many commercial SPC kits available, of which some utilize the Seldinger method—a puncture needle, a J guide-wire, a skin incision scalpel, a dilator, a peel-away sheath, and a catheter. Other kits may include an obturator needle inserted inside a supplied catheter. The clinician should ensure they are familiar with the kit they intend to use.

The patient should be supine, and the ultrasound machine positioned adjacent to the patient and within reach for the operator to comfortably adjust the settings and apply the probe to the patient's lower abdomen. Due to the depth required to evaluate the pelvic space and adjacent structures, a low-frequency probe, such as a curvilinear or phased array probe, is used. The clinician should perform a preliminary scan in transverse and longitudinal orientations to confirm the presence of a suitably distended bladder and that no bowel or other viscera lies at the intended site of needle puncture. Natural skin creases should be avoided.

Prophylactic antibiotics as per local guidelines should be used.

Local anaesthetic should be injected under the skin at the needle insertion. The local anaesthetic should be then infiltrated down to and into the bladder wall.

The clinician can utilize in-plane and out-of-plane techniques for this procedure, although the former is preferable as the needle is visualized throughout its length.

In the case of a Seldinger-type kit, the needle should be advanced along the predetermined tract and should be seen entering the bladder; at this stage, urine should be aspirated. The guide-wire is then inserted, and the needle withdrawn. A skin incision should be made, if necessary. Following this, a dilator/peel-away sheath should be inserted over the guide-wire. There will be a 'give' as this enters the bladder, and caution should be adopted at this point to ensure it is not inserted unnecessarily deeper. The central dilator is then removed, and urine should be seen to run freely. The supplied catheter is inserted, and the balloon inflated with sterile saline before the peel-away sheath is removed.

It is recommended that patients are observed for at least 24 hours.

The British Association of Urological Surgeons (2010) has described a number of situations when SPC may not be an appropriate option:

- Carcinoma of the bladder;
- Anticoagulation and antiplatelet treatment;
- Abdominal wall sepsis;
- Presence of a subcutaneous vascular graft in the suprapubic region (e.g. a femoro-femoral crossover graft).

In addition, performing SPC insertion when the bladder is relatively empty should be discouraged, as the risk of iatrogenic injury to abdominal viscera is increased.

The risks of SPC insertion include:

- Haemorrhage, including haematuria and intra-abdominal bleeding;
- Infection, including urinary tract infection and infection of the tract site or wound;

- Pain;

- Injury to the abdominal organs;

- General risks associated with long-term catheterization.

Ultrasound-guided lumbar puncture

Purpose

Lumbar puncture is a common and important procedure performed by emergency physicians for a range of indications, including assessment of headache in suspected subarachnoid haemorrhage and meningitis. The key step required for successful completion of this procedure is determining the correct point for spinal needle insertion.

Perspective

Performance of this procedure has relied on a landmark technique for many years. Palpation of the bony landmarks, including the lumbar spinous processes and iliac crest, is used to determine the optimal puncture site. However, suboptimal patient body habitus can often prevent palpation of these landmarks, leading to incorrect needle insertion site and procedure failure.

PoCUS guidance has been shown to both help identify these landmarks, even when impalpable, and also to reduce the number of puncture attempts. A growing number of studies are demonstrating its utility in emergency medicine.

Performing the procedure

As with the landmark technique, patient positioning will contribute towards procedural success. While a patient positioned seated and forward-flexed over a cushioned table maximizes the lumbar interspace opening and reduces lateral curvature, this position is not always well tolerated by the patient (particularly if sedated or in infants). Lying in the left lateral position, while forward flexing, and raising the knees is the common alternative position.

The transducer used depends on the patient's size. With a high-frequency linear transducer, higher-resolution views of the landmarks are visualized; however, in obese patients where the bony landmarks are impalpable due to their depth, a lower-frequency curvilinear transducer is required.

The principle of PoCUS guidance in lumbar puncture is to identify the posterior midline (along which lie

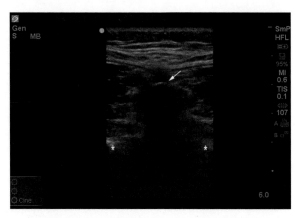

Figure 9.38 B-mode image of the spinous process and transverse processes (transverse orientation).

the lumbar spinous processes) and the midpoint of the lumbar interspace. In order to do this, the transducer is first orientated transversely over the lower lumbar vertebrae. The transducer is then moved cranially or caudally until a spinous process is identified. The spinous process appears as a relatively superficial hyperechoic line or point casting a deep acoustic shadow. The transverse processes (* in figure) can be seen deeper and lateral to the spinous process (arrow in figure) (see Figure 9.38).

Once identified, the transducer is moved laterally or medially in order to centre the spinous process on the screen. Using a surgical marker, a point is then marked on the skin at the centre of the transducer.

The transducer is then moved caudally, and the above process repeated with the next spinous process (see Figure 9.17as 🖼). The two points are then joined to form a line (see Figure 9.17bs 🖼). This is the posterior midline.

The transducer is then rotated to a longitudinal orientation and placed along the posterior midline. The contiguous spinous processes should be identified at the same depth on either side of the screen. It may be necessary to move the transducer slightly from side to side in order to generate this image, if the transducer has moved off the midline (see Figure 9.39). The midpoint of the lumbar interspace (* in figure) is centred on the image and points marked at the centre of the transducer on either side (see Figure 9.18as 🖼). The two points are then joined to form a line (see Figure 9.18bs 🖼).

The intersection of these lines marks the point of needle insertion.

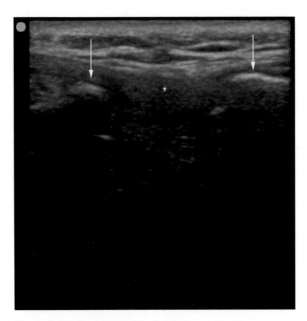

Figure 9.39 B-mode image of spinous processes (longitudinal orientation).

The transducer can be inadvertently placed lateral to the midline, and the space between transverse processes mistakenly identified as the interspace midpoint. Ensure that the depth of the spinous process is the same in both transverse and longitudinal views.

Although ultrasound guidance provides an accurate starting point for needle insertion, the trajectory of needle insertion remains operator-dependent. Keeping the needle perpendicular to the skin surface during insertion remains an important part of this procedure.

Ultrasound-guided abscess drainage

Purpose

As detailed in Chapter 7, ultrasound can be used to identify the presence of an abscess or collection. Ultrasound-guided techniques can also be used to drain a collection.

Perspective

Smith and Bartram described in 1975 using ultrasound for this purpose. The techniques, as previously described, are wholly applicable to draining collections. Interventional radiologists usually undertake the draining of deeper and more complex collections such as pelvic and retroperitoneal abscesses. However, superficial collections are within the capabilities of PoCUS practitioners. The Society for Interventional

Radiology describes success rates for aspiration of fluid for diagnostic characterization of 95%, successful drainage (curative and partial success) of 85%, and complications rates of 10%, which include all types of percutaneous abscess drainage. Hence, any clinician undertaking such a procedure should be adequately trained and ensure that such an undertaking is within their scope of practice. Typical procedures include cutaneous and subcutaneous lesions, especially in cases such as cellulitis that fails to improve with antibiotic therapy. There have been descriptions of peritonsillar abscesses being identified and drained under ultrasound guidance within the ED.

In certain circumstances, the aim of the procedure will be to obtain a sample for culture and sensitivity, rather than definitive drainage. This may optimize the choice of antibiotic therapy.

Performing the procedure

The clinician should be familiar with the anatomy of the area where the abscess or collection is sited. The diagnosing of an abscess or collection is covered in Chapter 7. The patient should be positioned, so that the area of interest is comfortably accessible to the operator. The ability to take appropriate samples, e.g. for culture and sensitivity, should be anticipated.

Local anaesthetic is not always required for simple needle aspiration for diagnostic purposes. However, when used, local anaesthetic should be injected under the skin at the needle insertion. Ensuring the length of the needle is adequate for the patient's body habitus is essential.

The clinician can utilize in-plane and out-of-plane techniques for this procedure, although the former is preferable as the needle is visualized throughout its length.

The relative contraindications for percutaneous drainage include:

- Significant coagulopathy that cannot be controlled or corrected;
- Lack of a safe pathway to drain the abscess or collection;
- Poor patient compliance regarding positioning or co-operation.

There is a risk that infection can be spread beyond fascial planes as a result of such a procedure. There are also potential iatrogenic injuries to adjacent structures; these could include complications such as vascular injury, PTX, bowel perforation, etc.

Miscellaneous ultrasound-guided procedures

Using ultrasound to confirm endotracheal tube placement

Purpose

Can PoCUS help to confirm endotracheal intubation in emergency and resuscitation settings?

Perspective

In emergency settings and during resuscitation, verification of ETT location is important in critically ill patients. Missing an oesophageal intubation can be disastrous. This can happen during emergency situations such as a cardiac arrest or trauma. The incidence of oesophageal intubation can be up to 16% in emergency conditions. PoCUS can assist with early detection of unintentional oesophageal intubation and can help to confirm successful endotracheal intubation. PoCUS has been shown to be reliable for this purpose and, during a cardiac arrest, is more reliable than end-tidal CO_2 detection. PoCUS is included as a method for the confirmation of ETT placement in the 2015 Advanced (Cardiac) Life Support guidelines.

Performing the scan

Confirmation of endotracheal intubation using PoCUS has two components:

1. Direct visualization of the ETT passing through the upper trachea, and absence of oesophageal intubation;

2. Confirmation of anterior lung sliding bilaterally.

Direct visualization

Place a high-frequency linear probe in a transverse orientation, just above the suprasternal notch across the anterior neck. The trachea will appear as a white echogenic curved (oval) structure with a large acoustic shadow.

The oesophagus is usually seen deep to, and to the patient's left side of, the trachea as an oval structure with a hyperechoic wall and a hypoechoic centre. It is usually collapsed (see Figure 9.40). PoCUS can be utilized

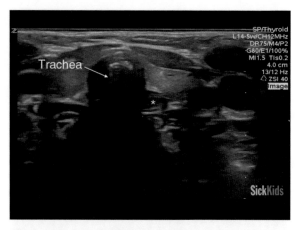

Figure 9.40 B-mode image of a normal 'collapsed' oesophagus (*), seen deep to the left side of the trachea (transverse orientation).

Courtesy of the Hospital for Sick Children, Toronto.

during, or immediately after, intubation. With real time, PoCUS is performed as the ETT is passed. During successful endotracheal intubation, PoCUS will show movement and an increase in artefact and shadowing in the region of the trachea only. Shaking the ETT will show movement of the trachea. Colour flow Doppler can be used to confirm that movement is within the trachea.

In the event of oesophageal intubation, PoCUS will show the ETT in the oesophagus, as demonstrated by an adjacent echogenic round structure with shadowing posterolateral to the trachea. This has been called the 'double trachea sign' (see Figure 9.41). This can be missed if the oesophagus happens to be located directly behind the trachea. Again movement of the tube

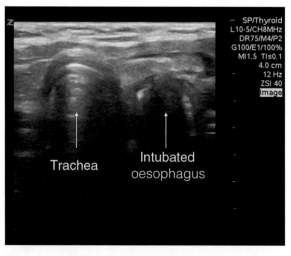

Figure 9.41 B-mode image of oesophageal intubation, demonstrating the 'double trachea' sign.

and use of colour Doppler can help to detect oesophageal intubation.

Confirmation of anterior lung sliding bilaterally

During a cardiac or respiratory arrest, or in the setting of a paralysed patient, detection of bilateral anterior lung sliding during ventilation confirms successful endotracheal intubation. This technique is described further in Chapter 3.

Nasogastric tube placement

Purpose

Traditionally, confirmation of NGT placement is made clinically (auscultation over the stomach, aspiration of stomach contents) or using X-ray. PoCUS can be used to augment this, and it is rapid and non-invasive.

Perspective

Clinical assessment can be unreliable, and relying on X-rays takes time and can cause delays.

X-ray remains the imaging modality of choice for NGT placement. PoCUS of the stomach had a positive predictive value of 97.4% and a negative predictive value of 25% in Kim *et al.*'s study (2014). Gok *et al.* (2015) found that ultrasound of the oesophagus (in the neck) successfully predicted gastric placement of an NGT in 92.8% of cases.

Performing the scan

PoCUS of the stomach can confirm NGT placement. Therefore, a low-frequency curvilinear probe is recommended for this indication. Patient position is usually immaterial, provided that the operator can access the epigastrium and LUQ. Occasionally, one may need to roll the patient in order to shift gas-filled bowel away from the probe.

Begin by scanning over the epigastrium, and slide the probe to the left, maintaining firm pressure in order to move the bowel out from under the probe. If this fails, image the stomach from the LUQ using the spleen as a window.

If empty, the stomach will appear as an area of 'scatter' in the field of view due to stomach gas. If filled with fluid, however, the stomach will appear as a fluid-filled structure (usually with debris and/or bubbles of air scattered within the fluid) (see Figure 9.19s 🖼).

A correctly placed NGT will appear on PoCUS as an echogenic artefact with a clearly defined shadow (see Figure 9.20s 🖼). Gastric placement can be confirmed by instilling saline (or fluid aspirated from the NGT) via an appropriate syringe into the NGT. This will appear as 'swirling fluid' in the stomach (see Video 9.7 🎥). Agitated saline will make the fluid more obvious.

False negative

Gas-filled stomach may make placement difficult to confirm.

False positive

Fluid instilled via an NGT placed too high (in the oesophagus, rather than the stomach) will also appear in the stomach. However, the NGT itself will not be visible.

📖 Further reading

Association of Anaesthetists of Great Britain and Ireland. *AAGBI Safety Guideline: Management of Severe Local Anaesthetic Toxicity*. London: The Association of Anaesthetists of Great Britain & Ireland; 2010. Available at: http://www.aagbi.org/sites/default/files/la_toxicity_2010_0.pdf

British Society of Gastroenterology. *BSG Guidelines on the Management of Ascites in Cirrhosis*. London: British Society of Gastroenterology; 2006. Available at: https://www.bsg.org.uk/resource/bsg-guidelines-on-the-management-of-ascites-in-cirrhosis.html

Harrison SC, Lawrence WT, Morley R, Pearce I, Taylor J. British Association of Urological Surgeons' suprapubic catheter practice guidelines. *BJU Int* 2011;**107**;77–85.

Lindenberger M, Kjellberg M, Karlsson E, Wranne B. Pericardiocentesis guided by 2-D echocardiography: the method of choice for treatment of pericardial effusion. *J Intern Med* 2003;**253**:411–17.

Loubani O, Bowra J, Smith A, Talbot JA, Jarman B, Atkinson P. My patient is short of breath: is there pleural fluid, and will PoCUS help drain it safely? *Ultrasound* 2013;**21**:88–92.

National Institute for Health and Care Excellence. *Guidance on the Use of Ultrasound Locating Devices for Central Venous Catheters*. Technology appraisal guidance [TA49]. London: National Institute for Health and Care Excellence; 2002. Available at: https://www.nice.org.uk/guidance/ta49

Peterson MA, Abele J. Bedside ultrasound for difficult lumbar puncture. *J Emerg Med* 2005;**28**:197–200.

Reddy PS, Curtiss EI, O'Toole JD, Shaver JA. Cardiac tamponade: hemodynamic observations in man. *Circulation* 1978;**58**:265–72.

Tsui BC, Suresh S. Ultrasound imaging for regional anesthesia in infants, children, and adolescents: a review of current literature and its application in the practice of extremity and trunk blocks. *Anesthesiology* 2010;**112**:473–92.

Walker KJ, McGrattan K, Aas-Eng K, Smith AF. Ultrasound guidance for peripheral nerve blockade. *Cochrane Database Syst Rev* 2009;**4**:CD006459.

10

Education and simulation in point-of-care ultrasound

Paul Olszynski, Melanie Stander, Tim Harris, Mark Tutschka, and Paul Atkinson

Summary

There is no formal single international curriculum for PoCUS training. Training should be tailored to meet the needs of the local and national training system and clinical setting. Simulated ultrasound helps with, but does not replace, patient-based PoCUS training. Simulation adds value in low-frequency, high-importance fields.

Consider using simulation prior to clinical practice for procedural ultrasound such as needle guidance.

Enhanced simulation can assist with the clinical integration of PoCUS into broader patient care using simulated patient encounters.

Education

Perspective

The expanding use of PoCUS over the past few decades in critical care and emergency medicine environments has changed the way doctors practise medicine in these settings. The clinician is able to quickly assess and manage patients who present with a wide range of acute illnesses and injuries. An ultrasound examination can be performed rapidly at the patient's bedside; it does not expose the patient to harmful radiation, and the examination is repeatable. There is an increasing body of evidence to demonstrate that implementation of PoCUS in emergency and critical care environments is safe, even with limited training. A more uniform, appropriate, optimal training and credentialing system in PoCUS is a natural progression from the numerous modules and applications that are now accessible.

What exactly are we talking about?

Medjel and Lewiss (2011) help to clarify certain terminology related to competence and training. Competence is deemed to be the recognition of a specific ability or skill. Bustam et al. (2014) described three components of competence in emergency echocardiography, which can be applied to emergency ultrasound in general.

> 'Emergency physicians need to be:
> a) Knowledgeable in the indications,
> b) Competent in the technical skills of image acquisition and in the interpretation of the images, and
> c) Able to integrate the echocardiographic findings into the clinical management of the patient'.

Reproduced from *Emergency Medicine Journal*, Bustam A, Azhar MN, Veriah RS *et al*. Performance of emergency physicians in point-of-care echocardiography following limited training. *Emerg Med J*. 2014 May;**31**(5):369–73, copyright 2014, with permission from BMJ Publishing Group Ltd.

Although a trainee can be deemed to be competent, it does not directly translate into that trainee being granted the credential to perform that ultrasound skill in a clinical setting. A specified credentialing process will result in the recognition of competence. Accreditation is a formal, third-party recognition of competence to perform a specific skill. Certification is represented by a document that reflects the level of training that has been achieved.

Challenges faced

The best method to achieve transition from PoCUS trainee to independent practitioner has not been fully elucidated. Very few studies exist that concentrate on aspects of training requirements and proficiency standards for PoCUS. Assessment of clinical competence in all spheres of medical education, not just ultrasound, remains a hot topic of discussion. A 2014 survey of emergency medicine residency and ultrasound directors found a wide range of assessments and examinations that were in place at different institutions to test for competency. Some of the methods used included objective structured clinical examinations (OSCEs), standardized direct observation tools (SDOTs), multiple choice questions, online interactive examinations, and practical examinations (using human models, simulation or direct observation, or a combination of both). We have proposed that programmes focus on newer methods for training, including simulation and web-based training models. The next section takes an in-depth look into the increased rationale for the use of simulation models in PoCUS training.

The Society of Academic Emergency Medicine's 2012 educational research consensus conference highlighted some important concepts that can be applied to training and competency in PoCUS. Some questions that require future clarity include the frequency of assessments and of observed assessments, which patient encounters should be observed, and how training competence translates to clinical competence. While the outcomes of the educational process for PoCUS are well delineated, the process for getting learners to the end points is not as clear. They conducted a survey among emergency medicine residents attending introductory PoCUS courses in order to attempt to determine the methods that provide the best educational value, as determined by the learners. Small-group formats, video clips, and hands-on scanning, rather than large-group didactic sessions, were felt by the respondents to be the most effective. Researchers have attempted to emulate

templates from medical education in order to delineate the exact learning process that should occur, but due to the very complex nature of achieving proficiency, demonstrating skill, and ultimately being deemed to have passed the credentialing process in PoCUS, a one-size-fits-all approach is bound to fail.

The importance of a standard core curriculum

Henwood *et al.* (2014) published a 2014 article entitled 'A practical guide to self-sustaining point-of-care ultrasound education programs in resource-limited settings'. This text will be very useful for training faculty who are embarking on the journey of implementing an ultrasound training programme, as well as for more established programme directors. The international PoCUS credentialing landscape is varied, with certain national emergency medicine societies involved and, in other places, this responsibility sits with a health authority or an academic institution. A standard core curriculum goes a long way to achieving a high level of quality that is imperative in the ultimate improvement of patient care and will help to decrease liability. It also serves as the foundation to increase research outputs into the training and credentialing arena.

The first model curriculum aimed at physicians training in emergency ultrasound in the United States was published in 1994. Two years later, emergency ultrasound competency was required, as defined by the emergency medicine core content curriculum. Subsequently, the American Council of Graduate Medical Education declared all emergency medicine residents are required to achieve competency in emergency ultrasonography. In 2006, the Canadian Association of Emergency Physicians (CAEP) published the first position statement on PoCUS for Canada. The year 2008 saw the publication of ACEP's specialty-specific emergency ultrasound guidelines. These guidelines were extremely detailed and gave an outline of the exact amount of time that residents should spend in an introductory ultrasound rotation—a minimum of 20 hours of educational sessions should be included, and 150 scans should be completed. It was also suggested that a national examination be administered so that the same standard for competency would be applied to all emergency medicine residents. In the 2000s, in the UK and Canada, PoCUS was established as a core competency for emergency medicine programmes by the Royal Colleges and by the College of Family Physcians of Canada. In 2013, Woo *et al.* developed the Evaluation Tool for Ultrasound skills Development and Education (ETUDE). It was primarily developed to help characterize the diffusion of PoCUS by using Rogers' diffusion of innovation theory (developed in 1962), which examines the spread of innovations in populations. The study was conducted in 2007, and adoption scores were calculated using subgroups of non-adaptors, majority, early adopters, and innovators. Respondents endorsed current and future predicted uses for PoCUS, and several barriers to PoCUS were identified. These types of tools will prove to be useful in the future, as researchers can use them to track trends in their own training programmes on a national, and even an international, scale.

Against this background of varying credentialing and assessment processes in PoCUS, the Clinical Practice Committee of the International Federation of Emergency Medicine (IFEM) tasked the Ultrasound Special Interest Group to produce an ultrasound curriculum guideline for emergency medicine. This comprehensive document serves as a very useful guide to programmes and organizations planning to develop an ultrasound curriculum for emergency medicine, both in countries looking to initiate training in PoCUS and in countries that have a mature PoCUS system in place already.

The introductory phase to training

The traditional method of training has been replicated in many countries and is familiar to most proponents of PoCUS. The training continuum begins with an introductory exposure (see Figure 10.1). This is followed by a period of building and practising the skills that were initially taught. The last component comprises the achievement of competency.

Trainees are required to initially attend an ultrasound course or workshop. Pre-course reading is often offered to the candidates, so that they can become more familiar with the concepts to be presented. Factual recollection can be determined with a pre-course test. Most of the courses presented will introduce the trainee to between four and seven modules that together comprise a Level 1/basic/introductory/core course. The specific modules presented vary from country to country. A needs analysis aligned with the burden of disease of an ultrasound population can help to determine which modules should be presented. The local burden of disease of a region suggested that other modules should be included into the core curriculum, compared to those that were being taught.

Despite the flexibility in the specific anatomical modules presented, there are certain core concepts that remain the same. These include the inclusion of basic physics and instrumentation, the correct ultrasound techniques to perform adequate scans and generate images, and certain administrative aspects that include archiving, clinical governance, and credentialing. The emphasis is placed on small-group teaching with ideal candidate:trainer/machine ratios of 5:1 or less. This ensures that each trainee receives as much hands-on scanning time as possible.

The IFEM curriculum document places emphasis on the identification of PoCUS applications as either diagnostic or procedural. Diagnostic applications can be focused on one anatomical area (e.g. the abdominal aorta) or can include multiples areas in an algorithmic sequence (e.g. the e-FAST scan). Procedural applications included should enhance and improve patient care.

The path to competency

On successful completion of the introductory course, trainees are required to maintain a logbook where they embark on a period of obtaining ultrasound scans under supervision. Much variation exists as to the exact number of total scans that needs to be achieved and the exact breakdown between each module. Despite these variations that exist, a specific

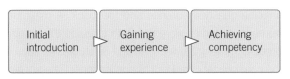

Figure 10.1 The PoCUS training continuum.

Reproduced with permission from IFEM, *Point-of-Care Ultrasound Curriculum Guidelines*, © International Federation for Emergency Medicine 2014.

percentage of the scans should be clinically indicated and a certain number should demonstrate pathology (positive findings).

Predetermined templates are often used to collect scan data, as these can include the date, the patient's details, the type of ultrasound examination being performed, the findings, and the trainee's interpretation of the results. This scanning for purposes of completion of the logbook can take anywhere from a few months to up to a few years, depending on the clinical environment of the trainee (which includes access to an ultrasound machine and the time available to perform scans) and access to ultrasound mentors. These mentors can be affiliated with a clinical department or with a diagnostic imaging department. These scans can be directly observed by an appointed trainer, which enables the student to receive immediate feedback, or the student can record the scans (either by printing them directly or saving them via a digital mechanism which is available on most machines) and these can be assessed at a later stage. Some institutions allow for the completion of the logbook, or an aspect of it, in a non-clinical environment such as an ultrasound finishing school. This allows the trainee access to ultrasound trainers, as well as enabling them to complete a large proportion of their required scans. This setup works well if obstacles to logbook completion include lack of access to dedicated scanning time, lack of access to machines, or even difficulty in obtaining scans that demonstrate pathology.

Completion of the logbook is usually the trigger for the trainee to undergo a formal assessment or summative examination. They are tested on all aspects covered in the initial introductory course. Once the assessment has been successfully completed, the trainee is deemed competent and able to record the results of their scans in the medical record and to make clinical decisions based on their ultrasound findings.

Continual professional development is still an important part of the process, and some organisations do provide guidelines as to the required number of scans that have to be achieved each year in order to maintain credentialing. Peer review and continued audit are important components of demonstrating continued competency. A summary of this training

process, as described in the IFEM ultrasound curriculum document, is presented in Figure 10.2.

PoCUS and focused echocardiography in critical care

Critical care cardiac PoCUS may be performed at different skill levels and is highly operator-dependent. Initially, the practitioner may be content to identify cardiac activity, pericardial effusion, and right ventricular pressure overload to assist in managing cardiac arrest. As experience is gained, the 'fluid, form, function, filling' approach, described earlier in this book, may be more comprehensively applied.

Based largely on recommendations from the American College of Chest Physicians, the Canadian Critical Care Society recently published recommendations 'to guide the dissemination, training and achievement of competency in CCUS among all Canadian critical care providers'. This document defines the core applications of critical care PoCUS to include: basic echocardiography, lung and pleural ultrasonography, guidance for vascular access, and detection of abdominal free fluid. Additionally, the American College of Echocardiography has put forth recommendations that define the core elements of FoCUS to include: assessment of LV dimensions, right and left ventricular systolic function, volume status, pericardial effusion/tamponade, signs of chronic heart disease, gross valvular abnormalities, and large intracardiac masses.

The Canadian Critical Care Society's guidance notes the relative lack of research dedicated to critical care PoCUS training, as well as the lack of validated assessment tools. As a result, the panel's recommendations were driven by consensus and focused heavily on developing local expertise and training initiatives. The authors also suggest a basic training paradigm that includes a period of introductory training, followed by a supervised period of portfolio building with dedicated ongoing quality assurance and feedback. A minimum number of studies were put forth to guide the training process, ranging between ten and 30 studies for each of the core critical care PoCUS applications. Data suggest that a short course can readily teach doctors to obtain basic echo windows and to identify pericardial effusions, and these skills were retained when reassessed at 3 months. The period of training required to make gross

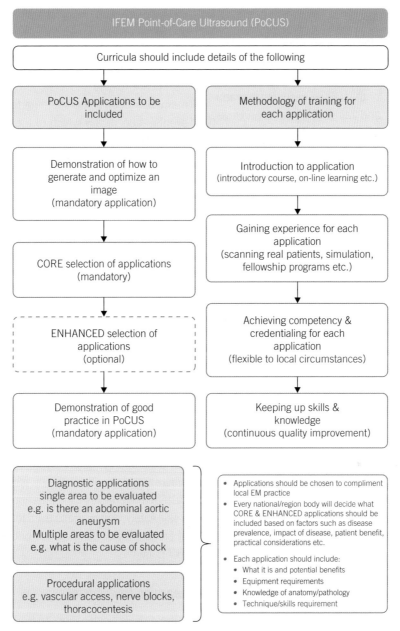

Figure 10.2 The IFEM PoCUS curriculum process.

Reproduced with permission from IFEM, *Point-of-Care Ultrasound Curriculum Guidelines*, © International Federation for Emergency Medicine 2014.

assessments of LV function appears to be short courses over 1–2 days, if the practitioner has some prior ultrasound training. However, competence is hard to define and the number of scans required to become proficient at each ultrasound modality is likely to vary between individuals. Echo seems to be more challenging to perform than abdominal ultrasound. Furthermore, studies suggest that less experience may be required to obtain diagnostic images in patients in cardiac arrest and in the ICU, compared to those in the ED or a pre-hospital location. Some studies suggest that the learning curve generally plateaus after performing 15–25 scans, with increasing operator agreement. However, improvement in even simple PoCUS improves upwards of 100 scans' experience. To perform a more comprehensive study takes dedicated training and regular practice to ensure skill retention. Similar principles apply to critical care PoCUS in other countries.

Ultrasound fellowships

The important role of fellowships in PoCUS needs to be highlighted. This time dedicated to further study and experience should result in improvement across all aspects of PoCUS for the trainee, resulting in graduation as a practitioner and trainer at or near expert level. As Blavias (2002) so succinctly put it, 'Fellowships develop when a unique and discrete body of knowledge or skill set requires additional training for true mastery'. Emphasis is placed on teaching residents and the faculty basic ultrasound skills. Often completion of a formal research project is encouraged. There is a greater emphasis on administrative tasks integral to credentialing and clinical governance. There is a focus on achieving a much higher number of scans (in the couple of hundreds) and increasing knowledge and skill in more advanced ultrasound applications. The majority of respondents to a systematic needs assessment of major stakeholders to define the essential elements for a Canadian emergency medicine PoCUS fellowship training curriculum indicated that they felt there is a clear need for these fellowship programmes.

Simulation in point-of-care ultrasound

Purpose and perspective

Students, residents, and physicians undertaking training in PoCUS and echocardiography may benefit from the use of simulation technologies. There is growing interest and evidence supporting the judicious use of simulation for the development of specific ultrasound skills. The bulk of this evidence is in the realm of procedural ultrasound skills, with a smaller, but growing, subset of evidence in the realms of diagnostic ultrasound training, as well as simulated patient encounters (where the simulated use of ultrasound instructs and tests the trainee in areas of patient assessment, clinical integration of ultrasound findings, and overall management).

Why all the excitement about simulation?

In the short span of a single generation of physicians, western medicine has pushed safety and patient-centric medicine to the forefront of both everyday patient care and medical training. The publication of Leape et al.'s groundbreaking study 'The nature of adverse events in hospitalized patients' fuelled a massive interest in the nature and frequency of healthcare-related adverse events. Of interest to many has been understanding the nature of adverse events—specifically which of these events are due to negligence and which are attributable to some other cause such as expected complications or system failures. The top three offending realms, in order of rates of error observed, were performance, prevention, and diagnosis. While the highest rate of adverse events was identified in the realm of procedural performance, the overwhelming majority of these were not considered to have been caused by negligence. Other factors, such as inadequate training or simply the inherent risks of the procedure, were speculated to be more likely the cause. In contrast, it was in the areas of prevention and diagnosis that negligence was believed to have played the greatest role.

From a medical training perspective, it is no wonder then that medical schools and training programmes began tackling the top three above-mentioned offenders. Whereas negligence may be partly addressed with checklists, brief educational interventions, and the like, improving performance in procedures is a different matter—the ultimate goal being to develop a system that enables clinicians and students to practise a skill safely, and perhaps even to ensure some degree of proficiency or competence prior to performing it on real patients.

Learning from mistakes

If the arrival of safety culture is to be credited, at least in part, for the growth of simulation-based medical education (SBME), another important development is the accelerated and ongoing introduction of new techniques and technologies associated with healthcare delivery. The widespread adoption of laparoscopic surgical techniques in the late 1980s and early 1990s serves as a good illustration of how the rapid growth of healthcare technologies, in the setting of an emerging safety culture, led to the development of simulation-based training experiences.

What Cuschieri described as 'the greatest free-for-all in the history of surgery' was the result of initially uncontrolled expansion and inadequate training in laparoscopic technique and technology. *In vivo* skill development by inadequately trained surgeons (who did not previously possess these skills and were now years out of training) came with a significant cost—increased rates of biliary, vascular, and other gastrointestinal complications—all of this as the Harvard adverse events study was being published and discussed. It became clear to surgical societies that greater attention needed to be placed on skill mastery prior to credentialing and clinical practice.

A landmark study by Scott *et al.* revealed that significant time spent developing psychomotor skills for laparoscopic surgery using task trainers did result in lower complication rates for actual laparoscopic cholecystectomy. This represents some of the earliest literature with robust clinical outcomes supporting the use of SBME, specifically in the area of procedural and psychomotor skill development. In terms of training in laparoscopic surgical techniques, surgical societies began to promote simulation-based training experiences as a means of more safely credentialing surgeons in these newer techniques. It was believed that such findings could be generalized to other laparoscopic skills, and thus credentialing societies developed robust training systems and processes that included simulation-based training on both low- and high-fidelity models.

Support from learning theories

Consider the use of PoCUS in the management of a patient in cardiogenic shock. For the seasoned emergency physician, adding FoCUS to an already familiar shock algorithm is unlikely to be overwhelming. The new task (FoCUS) does not, in this instance, result in an overwhelming amount of cognitive effort. On the other hand, for a trainee who is just beginning to successfully integrate crisis management skills into their biomedical knowledge, while still a novice sonologist, the added challenge of generating and interpreting a focused cardiac scan may result in an excessively high cognitive load.

The cognitive load theory (CLT) proposes a cognitive architecture where working memory is limited and expertise only develops once new knowledge is assimilated, stored into long-term memory, and accessed almost automatically. The implication then is that the sum of all information to be consciously recalled and applied during resuscitation is potentially too large for the novice or even the middle-level trainee. The consequences of this overload may include poorer learning and performance while managing a case (in core resuscitation, as well as PoCUS-related, skills), rushed and substandard image generation and interpretation, and frustration with both the case and ultrasound.

CLT posits that learners can only work with, and incorporate, a fixed amount of novel information at any given time. This is because the process of learning requires the use of working memory, which has limitations when processing novel information. For example, for the novice sonologist, the ability to use an ultrasound machine begins with the recollection of newly acquired information about its many functions and modes. Early in training, it is not uncommon to use improper scan modes or hold the probe incorrectly. Interestingly, CLT also suggests that once something has been learnt and firmly organized in one's mind through the creation of schemas (mental patterns), it becomes a nearly effortless cognitive task, ready to be called upon when needed (much like riding a bike or driving a car with a manual transmission). In short, tasks or topics that are well known can be accessed and applied without significant cognitive effort. CLT's relevance pertains specifically to how it can guide the creation of *simulated* experiences that maximize PoCUS learning.

Another area of particular interest to ultrasound educators relates to 'time on task' and its influence on transfer of learning. The work of Ericsson, Krampe, and Tesch-Romer on the development of expertise and the role of deliberate practice (DP) has brought significant attention to the hours required by any person, regardless of talent, to develop expertise. In their work, Ericsson *et al.* posit that it is through a combination of long hours and deliberate attention to specific aspects of the skill or competence in question that one can achieve expertise. In other words, it is not 'practice makes perfect', but 'perfect practice makes perfect'.

As such, many educators see potential in the ability of well-designed learning interventions, such as various simulation experiences, to shorten the required 'time on task' associated with clinical competence.

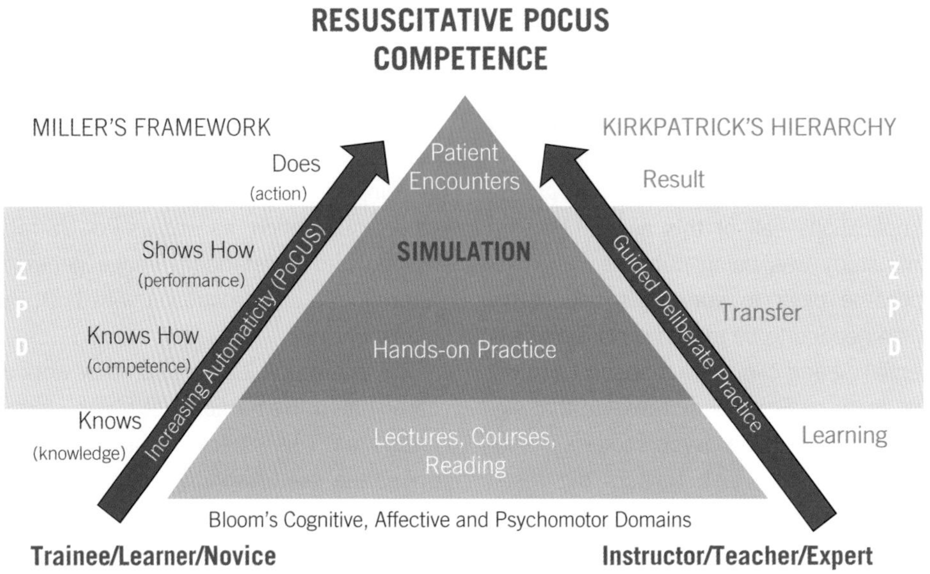

RESUSCITATIVE POCUS COMPETENCE

Figure 10.3 PoCUS simulation.

Data from Kirkpatrick D. Revisiting Kirkpatrick's four-level model. *Training and Development* 1996;50:54–9; and Miller GE. The assessment of clinical skills/competence/performance. *Acad Med* 1990;65(9 Suppl):S63–7.

The concept of layering or 'scaffolding' learning is well established in healthcare professional training. It stands at the root of most applied professions where apprenticeship plays a vital role in training. Its origins are found in Vygotsky's sociocultural development theory. Here, expertise (defined as the ability to complete a task independently) is gained through careful guidance of trainees through their zone of proximal development (ZPD). The ZPD is therefore defined as 'the distance between the actual developmental level (as determined by independent problem solving) and the level of potential development (as determined through problem solving in collaboration with more capable peers)'.

Such guidance is important because it allows for tailored trainee development and addresses factors that may be detrimental to learning (including excessive cognitive loads, performance anxiety, and safety concerns). This can be achieved through careful scenario/case design within a simulated environment (see Figure 10.3).

This being the case, one might wonder when exactly the use of simulation for PoCUS training is most appropriate. As mentioned earlier, the literature suggests that ultrasound-guided procedural tasks (peripheral and central venous cannulation, thoracocentesis, paracentesis, FB extraction, and joint aspiration), as well as invasive scans (pelvic ultrasound in symptomatic first-trimester pregnancy and TOE/TEE), show the greatest promise in terms of improving trainee performance and thus also patient care and safety.

The stage is set

The promising results of the Scott *et al.*'s study and others like it spurred an interest in exploring the roles of SBME in several other clinical and procedural skills. Barsuk *et al.* demonstrated that simulation-based mastery learning in the realm of ultrasound-guided central venous catheterization did decrease the number of needle passes required by trainees during actual *in vivo* performance (an important outcome, as increased needle passes has been associated with an increased incidence of complications, including PTX and arterial puncture). Simulation-based training for ultrasound skill development may offer safer ways of practising and mastering specific skills that will then decrease complication rates and thus improve patient care.

PoCUS as a clinical skill can be divided into two primary applications: diagnostic use and procedural

Components of POCUS competence

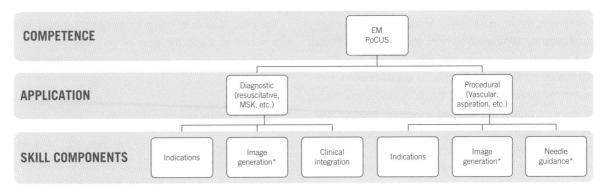

*These skills require simultaneous image interpretation

Figure 10.4 **Components of PoCUS competence.**

guidance. Diagnostic uses include such things as resuscitative, musculoskeletal, and obstetrical ultrasound, and others. Procedural ultrasound includes those procedures that benefit from image guidance and needle visualization. Examples of procedural ultrasound include ultrasound-guided central venous line placement, regional anaesthesia, arthrocentesis, and more (see Figure 10.4).

The two above-mentioned applications (diagnostic and procedural) can be further broken down into several knowledge and skill components. Diagnostic ultrasound is made up of three such components; the first is knowledge of indications and associated rationale for use; the second is image generation skills (which requires simultaneous image interpretation), and the third is clinical integration of ultrasound findings into patient management and care. This last knowledge component (clinical integration) requires knowledge of not only the images that are being generated and interpreted, but also a sound understanding of the patient's clinical condition (the disease in question), as well as the performance of all other tests that have been combined at the bedside to make a determination about the patient's status. Furthermore, it is in the realm of clinical integration where a physician learns how to *choreograph* the use of PoCUS into existing care algorithms.

Procedural ultrasound, on the other hand, requires both image generation skills as well as an *additional* psychomotor skill known as needle guidance (a skill

that requires its own practice to achieve mastery). The clinical integration of procedural ultrasound is addressed through knowledge of indications.

Choosing the skill you wish to teach/practise

With the above skill components in mind, instructors can determine where they perceive a gap or weakness in their training programme (or individual trainees) and proceed to acquire the best equipment to suit these needs and budget.

For example, it is likely that training in endovaginal scanning (with its invasive nature and somewhat unique transducer characteristics) represents a challenge for many ultrasound programmes. In Figure 10.4, the endovaginal scan would be classified as a diagnostic application. Its successful integration into clinical practice requires a unique set of psychomotor skills, combined with appropriate use of protective equipment and patient communication skills. This scan seems appropriate for consideration for simulation. The FAST scan, on the other hand, is non-invasive, employs common and basic probe techniques, and can be taught using normal patient volunteers (the areas of interest in question can be found without the need for positive cases). This represents a scan where use of simulation for image generation training seems less warranted. And yet, despite this reality, thousands of dollars have been spent on shiny, superficially realistic simulators, many of which now sit idle, collecting dust.

211

One possible explanation for this state of affairs relates to the initial wow factor and terminology associated with the introduction of simulation technology. Until recently, simulation technology has been defined and described not by its specific utility or function, but rather by its apparent level of sophistication and realism. As recently as 2014, ultrasound simulators have been primarily classified as either 'high or low fidelity', then further stratified by additional technological specifics like 'static' versus 'dynamic' imaging, and then lastly by the actual skill in question. No wonder then that it seems we (as educators) may have gotten the priorities confused.

Thankfully, Hamstra and colleagues have recently completed excellent work on this important topic and introduced the concept of 'functional task alignment' when discussing and considering SBME interventions. The idea here is to focus on underlying primary concepts of resemblance and alignment (i.e. what the key components of the intended skill are, whether they are represented on the equipment in question, and whether they can be *practised* using the equipment). With this in mind, ultrasound simulation equipment can then be divided into three broad categories, based primarily on identifying the task and then aligning the equipment with that task and desired function: diagnostic trainers, procedural trainers, and simulated patient encounters (see Figure 10.1s 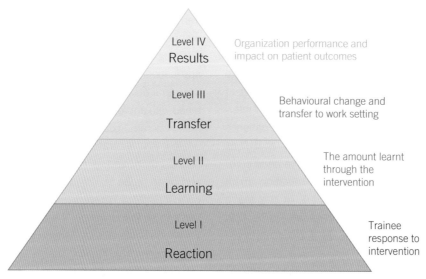).

The next step is to consider the existing evidence with regard to a specific scan or skill and then to determine if proceeding with simulation equipment is warranted.

Stacking the evidence

Much like a clinician's use and reliance on best-evidence clinical practices, today's medical educators are looking to the best evidence in medical education interventions and approaches [witness the advent of best evidence medical education (BEME)]. Kirkpatirck's 'Hierarchy of evidence' has played a major role in the broader context of education and training and has even been modified for medical education. This hierarchy helps educators determine the proven value of an educational intervention by placing the various levels of evidence within a clear order of importance. Placed at the top of the hierarchy are patient and community health outcomes, arguably the most robust impact that an educational intervention could ever have (see Figure 10.5). Many SBME studies strive to achieve evidence levels in the upper levels of the hierarchy. As one might expect, such studies are very difficult and costly to design and execute.

Level IV
Results — Organization performance and impact on patient outcomes

Level III
Transfer — Behavioural change and transfer to work setting

Level II
Learning — The amount learnt through the intervention

Level I
Reaction — Trainee response to intervention

Kirkpatrick's levels of training evaluation

Figure 10.5 Kirkpatrick's hierarchy of evidence.

Data from Kirkpatrick D. Revisiting Kirkpatrick's four-level model. *Training and Development* 1996;50:54–9.

Meanwhile, other educational concerns, such as time to proficiency and non-inferiority comparisons of conventional and novel training interventions, may not be adequately addressed through the exclusive use of Kirkpatrick's hierarchy. When evaluating ultrasound simulation interventions for purchase and implementation within a programme, educators should combine the above-mentioned concerns to determine the net utility of the purchase. This should then be considered within a cost analysis to assist in the final decision.

Lastly, before we proceed with evaluating some of the current evidence regarding ultrasound simulation and its utility, it is important to acknowledge that some of the criteria include a fair degree of subjectivity. For a training programme with significant financial resources, cost–benefit analysis will look very different in comparison to one that is strapped for funding. Controversy can be found even within the relatively small arena of ultrasound simulation where, within the short span of just 2 years, one journal has published two seemingly opposing views on its utility and merit (The *Journal of Ultrasound in Medicine* published two peer-reviewed articles on this topic—Sidhu *et al.*, 2012 and Lewis *et al.*, 2014—with the latter taking a somewhat opposing view to the former).

Procedural ultrasound simulation

Often referred to as procedural trainers or task trainers, this type of ultrasound simulation primarily addresses the skill of image generation/interpretation and probe–needle coordination (also known as the tasks). Such trainers have been shown to benefit trainees through the entire range of Kirkpatrick's hierarchy of evidence (learning, transfer, and results), thus being one of a rare few educational interventions that have been demonstrated to help patients as well. Depending on the level of the trainee, procedural trainers represent a range of complexity and engineered fidelity that can be further suited to the desired task. At the beginner's and intermediate level, where engineered fidelity is not likely of significant importance, 'home-made' trainers are perfectly adequate. Several online resources exist that can assist in the making of these do-it-yourself trainers for comparably very little cost. As expected, with increased complexity and fidelity, often comes increased cost. This may prove warranted in educational sessions where the task requires greater engineered fidelity such as when performing/assessing central line placement under ultrasound guidance while maintaining a sterile technique (here, the desired functional tasks call for equipment that resembles human anatomy, both on the surface *and* under the transducer). Another consideration related to the cost of this equipment is that such trainers do not rely on simulated ultrasound machines but instead depend on the adjunct use of real, clinically applicable ultrasound equipment. Finally, this form of ultrasound simulation has also been shown to be an efficient intervention through studies demonstrating mastery level learning.

Diagnostic ultrasound simulation

Diagnostic trainers offer practice in image generation and interpretation. Current evidence does demonstrate learning and transfer, although this benefit seems to be of greatest significance for novice users. As suggested earlier, such trainers are likely of greatest value when considering invasive scans such as endovaginal ultrasound for the assessment of early pregnancy or oesophageal echocardiography in critical care. For non-invasive scans, such trainers seem to offer little advantage to real practice on volunteer patients in terms of image acquisition. One exception may be found in TTE training where learning the complex anatomic relationships, as well as being able to call on various pathological states, may prove valuable during early training. When one considers the cost of such equipment (and the fact that it is not a real ultrasound machine and thus can only be used in a simulated setting), it becomes evident that outside of a research and development simulation centre, the evaluation is not often in favour of procurement of such trainers.

Simulated patient encounters

This type of ultrasound simulation is relatively novel and, as much as anything, reflects the innovative spirit of ultrasound educators as they strive to improve the clinical integration of ultrasound in everyday patient care. What likely began with the introduction of printed ultrasound images into patient scenarios has now evolved into 'hybrid' simulation scenarios where trainees use either procedural or diagnostic trainers during a simulated patient encounter (see Figures

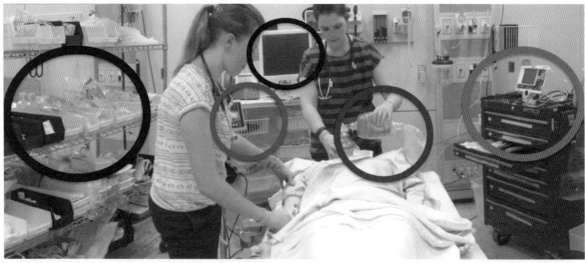

Figure 10.6 Resuscitation point-of-care ultrasound (PoCUS) simulation.

10.6 and 10.7). Such encounters can be virtual or mannequin-based. Here, the primary concept (or task) is clinical integration of PoCUS into broader patient care, which is tied to a specific scan or skill being introduced. Such simulation interventions seem to demonstrate learning and transfer among trainees, including the awareness of important choreographic concerns vis-à-vis the use of ultrasound. Studies have shown that the addition of ultrasound simulation to standard simulation increases trainees' diagnostic accuracy and confidence, albeit within the simulation setting. Because such encounters usually include existing equipment, their associated cost is usually minimal.

Preparing for critical care ultrasound

We can now turn our focus to the use of simulation for the development of critical care ultrasound skills. Use of PoCUS in critical care involves both diagnostic and procedural applications.

Primary diagnostic applications include echocardiography (both transthoracic and transoesophageal), pleural ultrasound, and abdominal assessments (occult blood loss, source of sepsis, volume status). Procedural applications may include ultrasound-guided central

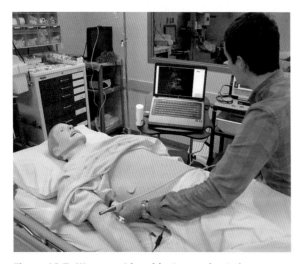

Figure 10.7 Ultrasound in critical care simulation.

venous catheterization and transvenous pacing, arterial pressure monitoring, pericardiocentesis, and thoracocentesis/paracentesis.

For diagnostic applications, there are a growing number of commercially available options. As noted in 'Stacking the evidence', p. 212, the majority of studies on such simulators strive to prove equivalence, or non-inferiority, to more traditional hands-on, real-patient training schemes. Proponents of this approach suggest that scanning real patients can be inconvenient to both volunteers and trainees and that visualization of pathology during image generation practice somehow enhances the learning experience. Trainees consistently express an enthusiasm for such interventions and demonstrate a basic learning achievement (Kirkpatrick's hierarchy levels I and II). There is some evidence that such approaches may shorten the time of training for the novice to intermediate proficiency. Limitations of such trainers relate to the inability to fully explore and engage the full range of sonographic manoeuvres that may be helpful in a given encounter: deep inspiration, rolling to decubitus, and other adjustments that cannot currently be made with existing diagnostic trainers.

The evidence for critical care procedural ultrasound simulation is more robust. Barsuk and colleagues were among the first to demonstrate improved clinical performance among trainees following mastery learning on ultrasound-guided central venous line task trainers. Their work makes the case for the use of simulation for the development and mastery of needle guidance (the psychomotor skill of being able to visualize and guide a needle, as seen on the ultrasound image, in real time). As such, it is hopeful (and likely) that this aspect of any critical care ultrasound-guided procedure is transferable (such as pericardiocentesis).

Of increasing interest is the role that simulated patient encounters can play in helping trainees develop their critical care ultrasound choreography (see Figure 10.2s). The incorporation of PoCUS into resuscitation represents a dramatic shift in bedside care. Established algorithms for various assessments and interventions will need to be re-tuned to this reality. It is with this in mind that resuscitationists are simulating critical care encounters through the use of 'hybrid' simulation. The rapid assessment of undifferentiated shock, the timing of scans in between compressions, and the sequencing of e-FAST during trauma all represent a new choreography that may be best learnt in a simulated environment where risks are low and cognitive/emotional demands are slightly lessened. To date, research into such interventions has, at best, demonstrated transfer in the simulated critical care setting, but not beyond into the clinical realm (at best, Level III of Kirkpatrick's hierarchy).

Conclusion

There is currently no single internationally recognized and accepted training and credentialing system for PoCUS. This is, in part, due to the staggered development of PoCUS across the world, the varied applications in different geographical settings, and the different institutions involved in credentialing and training, as well as the lack of robust research into the determination of ideal teaching strategies for this component of clinical medicine. That is not to say the programmes and techniques that have been developed over the past decades are not of an exceptionally high standard. Rather with concerted efforts to standardize the curriculum and subsequent training, the PoCUS international community will be better placed to conduct studies that examine the precise methods needed to teach this skill—a skill deemed so important that it has become a core part of the fabric that constitutes emergency and critical care physicians of the twenty-first century.

The current evidence suggests that there is certainly a role for simulation in ultrasound training, especially in the realms of procedural ultrasound and simulated patient encounters. It is even foreseeable that some skills (in the domain of procedural ultrasound) will be amenable to assessment of competence through simulation. It is critical that educators carefully evaluate both the trainee skills in need of practice, as well as the merits of these products prior to acquisition, in order to ensure that both trainees and educators are getting maximal benefit for the resources invested.

Acknowledgements

We acknowledge the contributions of Drs Vicki Noble, Hein Lamprecht, and Mike Lambert for their contributions to the IFEM ultrasound curriculum guidelines.

▤ Further reading

Additional further reading can be found in the Online appendix at www.oxfordmedicine.com/POCUSemergencymed. Please refer to your access card for further details.

Arntfield RT, Millington SJ, Ainsworth CD, *et al.* Canadian recommendations for critical care ultrasound training and competency for the Canadian Critical Care Society. *Can Respir J* 2014;**21**:341–5.

Atkinson P, Bowra J, Lambert M, Lamprecht H, Noble V, Jarman B. International Federation for Emergency Medicine point of care ultrasound curriculum. *CJEM* 2015;**17**:161–70.

Atkinson P, Ross P, Henneberry R. Coming of age: emergency point of care ultrasonography in Canada. *CJEM* 2014;**16**:265–8.

Barsuk JH, McGaghie WC, Cohen ER, *et al.* Use of simulation-based mastery learning to improve the quality of central venous catheter placement in a medical intensive care unit. *J Hosp Med* 2009;**4**:397–403.

Brydges R, Carnahan H, Rose D, *et al.* Coordinating progressive levels of simulation fidelity to maximize educational benefit. *Acad Med* 2010;**85**:806–12.

Bustam A, Azhar MN, Veriah RS, *et al.* Performance of emergency physicians in point-of-care echocardiography following limited training. *Emerg Med J* 2014;**31**:369–73.

Ericsson KA, Krampe RTh, Tesch-Romer C. The role of deliberate practice in the acuisition of expert performance. *Psychological Rev* 1993;**100**:363–406.

Girzadas DV, Antonis MS, Zerth H, *et al.* (2009). Hybrid simulation combining a high fidelity scenario with a pelvic ultrasound task trainer enhances the training and evaluation of endovaginal ultrasound skills. *Acad Emerg Med* 2009;**16**:429–35.

Hamstra SJ, Brydges R, Hatala R, *et al.* Reconsidering fidelity in simulation-based training. *Acad Med* 2014;**89**:387–92.

Kirkpatrick D. Revisiting Kirkpatrick's four-level model. *Training and Development* 1996;**50**:54–9.

Labovitz AJ, Noble VE, Bierig M, *et al.* Focused cardiac ultrasound in the emergent setting: a consensus statement of the American Society of Echocardiography and American College of Emergency Physicians. *J Am Soc Echocardiogr* 2010;**23**:1225–30.

Mateer J, Plummer D, Heller M, *et al.* Model curriculum for physician training in emergency sonography. *Ann Emerg Med* 1994;**23**:95–102.

Mayo PH, Beaulieu Y, Doelken P, *et al.* American College of Chest Physicians/La Société de Réanimation de Langue Française statement on competence in critical care ultrasonography. *Chest* 2009;**135**:1050–60.

Medlej K, Lewiss R. I'm an emergency medicine resident with a special interest in ultrasonography: should I take a certification examination? *Ann Emerg Med* 2011;**58**:490–3.

11

Paediatric ultrasound

Jason Fischer and Lianne McLean

Summary

When to scan (clinical indications)

PoCUS can be used in myriad ways in the pediatric population. Some scans can be adapted from the adult approach, but others, such as scanning for skull fracture in head injury or pyloric stenosis in vomiting, are specific to an infant or pediatric population.

What to scan (PoCUS protocol)

In addition to traditional adult PoCUS protocols, pediatric specific applications include focused abdominal scans for appendicitis, intussusception, and pyloric stenosis, among others.

How to scan (key points on scanning)

Techniques that are used in adult scanning can be applied in pediatrics; however, a lighter touch can often be of benefit, with additional supports of parent comfort, positioning, or distraction using toys or music can improve the quality of image acquisition.

What PoCUS adds (clinical reasoning—how results change practice)

In pediatrics, elements of the physical examination can be challenging to obtain in some children as they may have pain or be non-compliant. POCUS can improve our assessment of some physical examination characteristics as well as contributing added information to the clinical picture in children who present acutely or are critically unwell.

Purpose and perspective

The use of PoCUS in the emergency care of ill and injured children has dramatically increased in the last 5 years. Paediatric providers worldwide have rapidly adapted the technology and redefined the management of many paediatric conditions.

A number of diagnostic and procedural applications, including those considered *lifesaving*, have been successfully translated from general emergency medicine and critical care practice and are now used routinely in the paediatric setting (see Table 11.1). The execution of these applications is consistent, despite variations in age, pathology, and injury pattern.

Table 11.1 PoCUS applications translated from general emergency and critical care practice

Diagnostic	Procedural
• e-FAST	• Arthrocentesis
• Focused biliary	• Bladder aspiration
• Focused cardiac	• Central venous access
• Focused lung	• Fracture reduction
• Focused MSK	• Intraosseous needle confirmation
• Focused ocular	• Paracentesis
• Focused renal	• Pericardiocentesis
• Focused testicular	• Pleuracentesis
• Resuscitation	• Peripheral venous access
• Skin and soft tissue	• Ultrasound-guided incision and drainage
	• Ultrasound-guided lumbar puncture
	• Ultrasound-guided regional anaesthesia

For example, the use of e-FAST in paediatric trauma care continues to grow. The identification of free fluid in the abdomen is an important clinical finding, despite the fact that surgical intervention is performed much less frequently in paediatric solid organ injury. Descriptions of these common applications appear elsewhere in the textbook, including assessment of the *scrotum*, identification of *Toddler's fracture*, and arthrocentesis of the *paediatric hip*.

This section will focus on general considerations unique to paediatric PoCUS image acquisition and the growing number of paediatric-specific applications. The future of paediatric PoCUS will also be discussed.

Performing the scan

General considerations in paediatric PoCUS image acquisition

The size and body habitus of most paediatric patients allow for comparatively better anatomical visualization and image acquisition than in adolescent and adult patients. Many key structures, such as the heart, can be consistently imaged with greater clarity and detail (see Figures 11.1 and 11.1s ▣). Other structures not easily accessible in older adult patients, such as an inflamed appendix, can be identified in the majority of paediatric patients (see Figure 11.2). However, in order to fully realize the advantages of scanning a paediatric patient, the provider must take steps to maximize patient comfort.

Scanning children

Patients and caregivers are often anxious in the acute care setting, and providers are encouraged to be patient as infants and small children will often settle down and co-operate once the initial fear of the provider and transducer passes. A clear and age-appropriate explanation of the imaging process is beneficial prior to scanning and should include a brief description of safety and the opportunity to ask questions. Caregivers are often eager to be involved, and clarifying their role during the examination can relieve tension and build trust.

Paediatric patients should always be scanned in a position of comfort, which often means being held by a

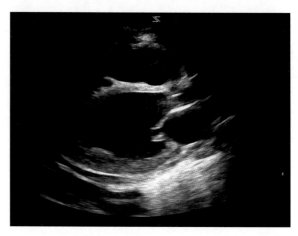

Figure 11.1 Image acquisition of the paediatric patient often allows for comparatively greater sonographic detail in children than in adults. Focused cardiac examination of a paediatric patient with dilated cardiomyopathy is shown as an example.

Courtesy of the Hospital for Sick Children, Toronto.

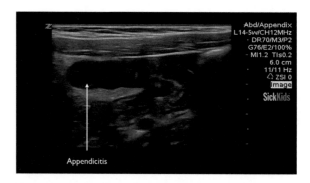

Figure 11.2 Structures, including the appendix, are often more accessible to sonographic visualization in children than in adults.

Courtesy of the Hospital for Sick Children, Toronto.

caregiver. A calm, quiet environment with low lighting is ideal. Warmed gel, that is slowly applied, and an above-ambient temperature in the examination room are important. Only necessary items of clothing should be removed, and extra care should be taken to respect the personal space of the adolescent while scanning.

Age-appropriate distraction is very effective. Videos and songs work well in toddlers, while school-age children often enjoy being involved and welcome an interactive exchange. The use of adjunctive agents, such as intranasal, topical, and parenteral anxiolysis and analgesia, can dramatically improve image acquisition. Feeding paediatric patients, if not clinically contraindicated, can also be helpful.

Paediatric-specific PoCUS applications

PoCUS use has evolved to become more paediatric-specific, with applications now addressing clinical scenarios more common or unique to paediatric patients. Applications in this category include the following.

Appendicitis

Abdominal pain is a frequent presentation of children in the ED. A history of sudden-onset, progressive peri-umbilical, or right lower quadrant pain, associated with anorexia, nausea, vomiting, and pain with sudden movement can be concerning for appendicitis. Many patients require imaging to support the diagnosis and to appropriately direct management.

PoCUS abdominal examination is typically completed using a high-frequency linear transducer in paediatric patients. Prompt visualization of appendicitis can often be achieved simply by asking the patient to point to the area of maximal pain. Alternatively, a provider can begin scanning the right lower quadrant in both the transverse and sagittal planes, using the psoas muscle, iliac vessels, and caecum as anatomical landmarks.

Primary signs of an inflamed appendix include the identification of a non-compressible, blind-ended tubular structure, with absence of peristalsis, measuring 6 mm or greater in diameter (see Figure 11.3). The presence of a large-diameter appendix without the additional criteria cannot be considered a positive sonographic image of appendicitis. Secondary signs, such as a faecolith or adjacent free fluid, further support the diagnosis (see Figure 11.4). Concern for perforation should occur if there is evidence of a complex fluid collection exterior to the appendix or ileus, or evidence of local phlegmon.

The appendix may not be well visualized if it is perforated, positioned retrocaecally, or obscured by overlying bowel gas. Graded compression is used to displace overlying bowel gas by slowly applying downward pressure on the abdomen. Using this graded compression technique, Sivitz *et al.*'s 2014 study found bedside ultrasonography to have a sensitivity of 85% and a specificity of 93%, when compared to clinical and radiological findings.

Appropriate pain control is necessary in order to perform graded compression. It is important to scan the entire appendix in order to ensure complete

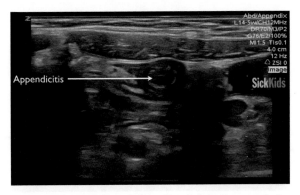

Figure 11.3 A transverse view of an inflamed appendix is shown.

Courtesy of the Hospital for Sick Children, Toronto.

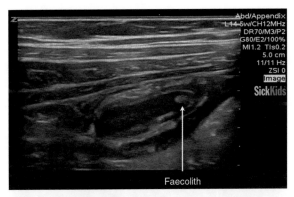

Figure 11.4 A longitudinal view of an inflamed appendix is shown that demonstrates the diagnostic characteristics of a blind-ended tubular structure >6 mm in diameter, with a faecolith.

Courtesy of the Hospital for Sick Children, Toronto.

evaluation, as distal evidence of a large appendix, free fluid, or collection may be present.

Endotracheal tube placement confirmation

Successfully intubating an infant or a child can be challenging in the acute care setting. Tube confirmation is critical with changing vital signs or a difficult intubation. PoCUS confirmation of ETT placement, in combination with other tests such as direct visualization, auscultation, and end-tidal CO_2 detection, can reassure a clinician of a successful intubation at the bedside in real time. A recent study by Tessaro *et al.* demonstrated a sensitivity of 98.8% and a specificity of 96.4% when PoCUS was used to confirm both successful ETT placement and appropriate ETT insertion depth.

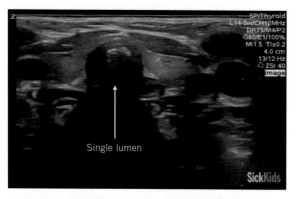

Figure 11.5 A transverse view of the trachea is shown, demonstrating a single lumen, confirming ETT placement within the trachea.

Courtesy of the Hospital for Sick Children, Toronto.

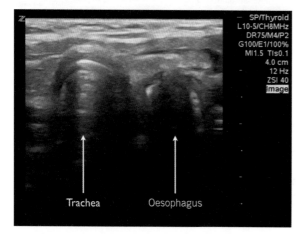

Figure 11.6 A transverse view of the trachea is shown, demonstrating a double lumen, identifying ETT misplacement within the potential space of the oesophagus. (The 'double trachea' sign is caused by air within the trachea and within the ETT in the oesophagus, which normally contains no air).

Courtesy of Dr. Mark Tessaro, University of Toronto.

To perform the scan, a high-frequency linear transducer is placed in the transverse plane over the thyroid cartilage or above the suprasternal notch. Visualization of a single curved echogenic surface with rounded posterior shadowing is suggestive of ETT placement within the trachea (see Figure 11.5). Visualization of double 'tracheal' shadows is suggestive of oesophagheal intubation (see Figure 11.6). Confirmation of a cuffed ETT can be made by inflating the cuff using saline or water, rather than air. On sonography, this appears as a hyperechoic sonographic change from the hypoechoic airway space. Alternatively, lung sliding can be identified bilaterally by placing the transducer longitudinally on the chest wall, confirming that the ETT is not deep to the carina.

Abnormal anatomy (decreased neck length, obesity, congenital malformation) or subcutaneous emphysema may limit visualization of the trachea. Similarly, lung sliding may not be visualized in the context of abnormalities of the lung, including the presence of PTX, mass, deformity, or a history of thoracic surgery.

Lung

Identifying and differentiating lung pathology are important in the care of children presenting with undifferentiated respiratory illness. Imaging is often necessary to support a history or physical examination suspicious for pneumonia. Lung PoCUS provides a detailed view of the pleura and lung parenchyma at the bedside that is safe and radiation-free. This allows the clinician to diagnose viral or bacterial pneumonia in real time and to identify the immediate need for intervention in cases of PTX, pleural effusion, and empyema.

To perform a lung scan in a paediatric patient, the provider uses a high-frequency linear transducer and scans longitudinally in three zones: the anterior chest (at the mid-clavicular line), the mid-axillary line, and the posterior chest wall (paraspinal). Each lung field is scanned, beginning at the apex or axilla and moving in a caudal direction towards the diaphragm. The scan is completed when the diaphragm and abdominal organs are visualized. The transducer should be kept perpendicular to the lung pleura throughout the examination.

The sonographic findings of PTX, pleural effusion, empyema, PE, and various interstitial diseases (pulmonary oedema, pulmonary contusion) all appear the same in children as in adults. However, lung PoCUS is used much more frequently in paediatrics to determine the presence of alveolar consolidation versus viral illness.

The PoCUS appearance of viral illness, viral pneumonia, or chronic lung disease includes increased echogenicity of the pleura, greater than three B-lines in a lung area, or confluent B-lines (see Figure 11.7).

Alveolar consolidation is differentiated from atelectasis by the presence of dynamic air bronchograms and later by *hepatization* of the lung parenchyma (see Figure 11.8). Shah *et al.* found a sensitivity of 86% and a specificity of 89% of PoCUS detection of pneumonia in paediatric patients, when compared to chest

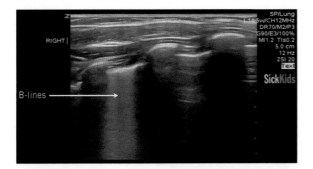

Figure 11.7 B-lines are shown in a patient with a viral upper respiratory tract infection.

Courtesy of the Hospital for Sick Children, Toronto.

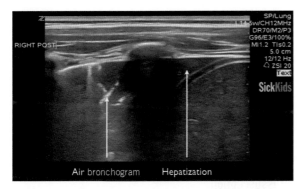

Figure 11.8 Alveolar consolidation with dynamic air bronchograms and hepatized lung parenchyma are shown in a patient with a bacterial pneumonia.

Courtesy of the Hospital for Sick Children, Toronto.

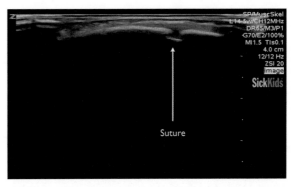

Figure 11.9 Normal appearance of the skull cortex and a cranial suture.

Courtesy of the Hospital for Sick Children, Toronto.

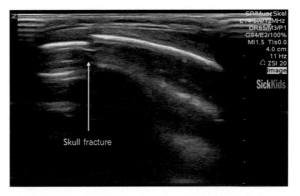

Figure 11.10 Disruption of the cortex in a patient with a skull fracture.

Courtesy of the Hospital for Sick Children, Toronto.

radiography. This study also showed that earlier detection of infectious lung pathology is possible with PoCUS, as specificity increased to 97% when lung consolidation of >1 cm and not visible by radiograph was included.

Skull

PoCUS can be used to accurately identify the presence of skull fractures in paediatric patients. With the presence of a skull fracture, concern is increased for intracranial injury and the need for comprehensive CT imaging. Rabiner *et al.* demonstrated a sensitivity of 88% and a specificity of 97% when PoCUS was compared to CT diagnosis of skull fractures.

Clinical indications for a PoCUS skull examination include the presence of a boggy or tender area on the skull, with or without a step-down deformity. Clinical history may correlate with trauma; however, the provider should always maintain a high level of suspicion

for skull injury, even without a known collateral history, as non-accidental injury can be a cause of skull fractures in neonates.

A high-frequency linear transducer is typically used to visualize the skull. Generous amounts of ultrasound gel should be applied to the area of interest to reduce any pressure or discomfort during the scan. The entire area of interest should then be scanned in a systematic fashion in two planes. All examinations should be extended at least 1 cm beyond the area of interest in order to improve accuracy.

The PoCUS appearance of the skull cortex is a bright, hyperechoic curvilinear line, with age-dependent presence of suture lines (see Figure 11.9) and fontanelles. Understanding of fontanelle and suture line anatomy will help the sonographer differentiate normal suture lines from disruptions in the cortex that are suggestive of a fracture (see Figures 11.10 and 11.2s 🖼). Scanning the contralateral side may provide some

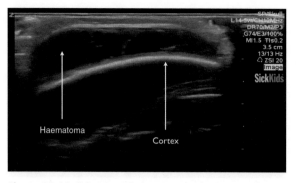

Figure 11.11 **A large scalp haematoma is shown, with an intact bony cortex.**

Courtesy of the Hospital for Sick Children, Toronto.

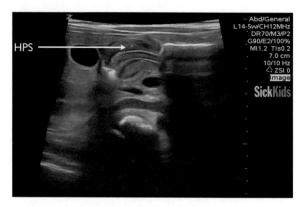

Figure 11.12 **Hypertrophic pyloric stenosis (HPS).**

Courtesy of the Hospital for Sick Children, Toronto.

guidance on normal suture line anatomy. Skull fractures appear as disruptions in the skull cortex, with or without a haematoma, which are seen as dark, hypoechoic areas superior to the skull cortex (see Figure 11.11). Caution is required in young infants as the skull bones may overlap and resemble fractures similar to the appearance seen in Figure 11.10.

Hypertrophic pyloric stenosis

Emergency room providers are often asked to differentiate common non-critical conditions such as gastro-oesophageal reflux from urgent conditions, such as hypertrophic pyloric stenosis (HPS), midgut volvulus, or neonatal sepsis, in a vomiting infant. A history of recent, non-bilious, non-bloody projectile vomiting in a 3- to 6-week-old baby can be suggestive of HPS. PoCUS allows the provider to confirm this diagnosis at the bedside and facilitate appropriate management.

To assess the pylorus, a high-frequency linear transducer is placed in the sub-xyphoid area in a transverse orientation. The gastric wall is identified and then traced both laterally to the right of the patient and distally until the longitudinal image of the pylorus is observed (see Figure 11.12). Measurement of the length and width of the pylorus should be taken in a longitudinal view, with a hypertropic pylorus measuring >14 mm in length and >3 mm in width (see Figure 11.13). Feeding of the patient can occur at this time to assess for obstruction of the gastric outlet. In cross-section, the pylorus can be visualized as a thickened static disc with central muscosal layers, demonstrating a thickened pyloric muscle.

In a small pilot study, Sivitz *et al.* found a sensitivity and a specificity of 100% using this technique, when compared to radiology staff physician assessment. However, care must be taken to avoid measurement during muscle spasm. In addition, a low frequency transducer may be required if the stomach is over-distended and displaces the pylorus posteriorly.

Intussusception

PoCUS can be used to confirm a suspected diagnosis of intussusception in any child presenting with intermittent, sudden-onset abdominal pain, with rapid relief, between the ages of 6 months to 2 years. This rapid bedside diagnosis can expedite care and reduce the risk of bowel necrosis.

Intussusception is best visualized using a high-frequency transducer to scan the abdomen. The provider begins in the right lower quadrant by following the ascending colon from the caecum until the liver is visualized. The transducer is then rotated 90° to follow the transverse colon, and finally rotated another 90° to follow the descending colon to the left lower quadrant.

In transverse view, a positive intussusception appears as a 'target' or 'doughnut' of non-peristalsing bowel, typically measuring >3 cm (see Figure 11.14). In an oblique or longitudinal view, an intussusception appears as a 'pseudokidney' or 'sandwich' (see Figure 11.15). Capturing images of the intussusception in two planes is essential, as thickened bowel loops or other abdominal masses may mimic intussusception.

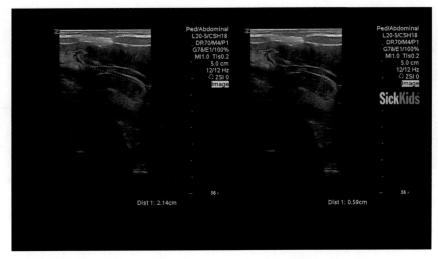

Figure 11.13 Hypertrophic pyloric stenosis measuring >14 mm in length and 3 mm in width.

Courtesy of the Hospital for Sick Children, Toronto.

In Riera *et al.*'s study, the presence of an intussusception was noted with a sensitivity of 85% and a specificity of 97%, when compared to diagnostic radiological imaging. Once an intussusception is identified, colour Doppler can be applied to assess blood flow and possible ischaemia. The appearance of free fluid trapped within the telescoped bowel or absence of blood flow significantly increases the risk of a failed air enema and should be noted.

Ileocaecal intussusception can be effectively ruled out if the ileocaecal valve is located and appears normal on sonographic imaging. Self-reduction of intussusception is not uncommon, so images should be archived in order to eliminate confusion between services or sites. Comprehensive ultrasound is suggested for all children with intussusception outside of the normal age range or clinical presentation to rule out a pathological lead point.

The future of paediatric PoCUS

Paediatric PoCUS has been slow to mature. Early barriers, such as lack of expertise, resource constraints, unrealistic expectations, and bureaucratic inertia have slowed innovation and delayed clinical integration, compared to general emergency and critical care medicine.

That trend is quickly changing. Today paediatric PoCUS applications are not only being adopted for clinical use, but they are also rapidly being integrated into complex shock and trauma algorithms (see Figures 11.16 and 11.17), triage screening tools

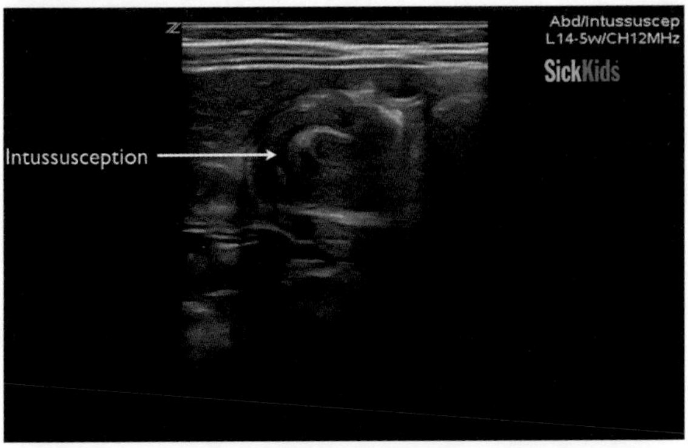

Figure 11.14 A transverse view of intussusception.

Courtesy of the Hospital for Sick Children, Toronto.

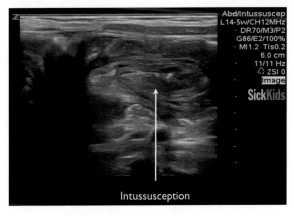

Figure 11.15 A longitudinal view of intussusception.

Courtesy of the Hospital for Sick Children, Toronto.

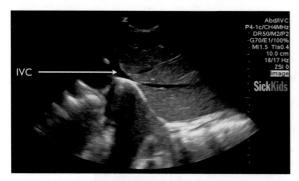

Figure 11.16 Shock algorithms incorporating several PoCUS applications, including the assessment of hydration status. A flat inferior vena cava (IVC) is shown, demonstrating dehydration.

Courtesy of the Hospital for Sick Children, Toronto.

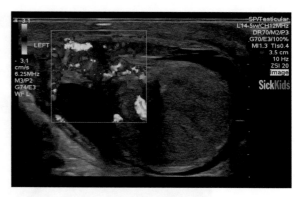

Figure 11.19 PoCUS assessment of a painful scrotum. Epididymitis is shown with associated changes to the left testicle.

Courtesy of the Hospital for Sick Children, Toronto.

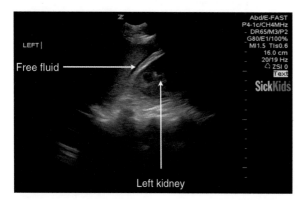

Figure 11.17 A positive e-FAST (Trauma) scan is shown with free fluid in the left upper quadrant.

Courtesy of the Hospital for Sick Children, Toronto.

(see Figure 11.18), and collaborative care pathways with partnering specialties (see Figures 11.19 and 11.20).

Paediatric PoCUS is now growing exponentially worldwide as a result of greater accessibility to ultrasound technology (lower cost, increasing availability, personalization), more paediatric-specific expertise (fellowship-trained leaders), better educational resources (higher quality, open-access), intensified academic focus, and emerging platforms for collaboration.

This expanding user base is quickly reshaping how the technology is used today, but more importantly how it will be used tomorrow.

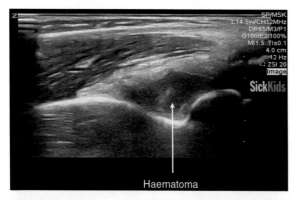

Figure 11.18 PoCUS applications can be used to screen patients at triage. A positive haematoma at the elbow is suspicious for a fracture and necessitates a radiograph.

Courtesy of the Hospital for Sick Children, Toronto.

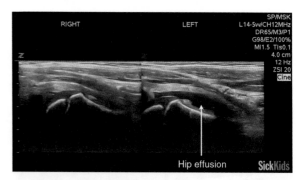

Figure 11.20 Identification of a hip effusion for PoCUS-guided arthrocentesis in the assessment of a suspected septic hip.

Courtesy of the Hospital for Sick Children, Toronto.

⬤ Further reading

Applegate KE. Intussusception in children: evidence-based diagnosis and treatment. *Pediatr Radiol* 2009;**39**(Suppl 2):S140–3.

Cohen HL, Green EB, Boulden TP. The vomiting neonate or young infant. *Ultrasound Clin* 2010;**5**:97–112. Available at: http://www.ultrasound.theclinics.com/article/S1556-858X(09)00091-7/abstract

Fox JC, Solley M, Anderson CL, Zlidenny A, Lahham S, Maasumi K. Prospective evaluation of emergency physician performed bedside ultrasound to detect acute appendicitis. *Eur J Emerg Med* 2008;**15**:80–5.

Kerrey BT, Geis GL, Quinn AM, Hornung RW, Ruddy RM. A prospective comparison of diaphragmatic ultrasound and chest radiography to determine endotracheal tube position in a pediatric emergency department. *Pediatrics* 2009;**123**:e1039–44.

Puylaert JB. Acute appendicitis: US evaluation using graded compression. *Radiology* 1986;**158**:355–60.

Ramirez-Schrempp D, Vinci RJ, Liteplo AS. Bedside ultrasound in the dia gnosis of skull fractures in the pediatric emergency department. *Pediatr Emerg Care* 2011;**27**:312–14.

Riera A, Hsial AL, Langhan ML, Goodman TR, Chen L. Diagnosis of intussusception by physician novice sonographers in the emergency department. *Ann Emerg Med* 2012;**60**:264–8.

Sağlam C, Unlüer EE, Karagöz A. Confirmation of endotracheal tube position during resuscitation by bedside ultrasonography. *Am J Emerg Med* 2013;**31**:248–50.

Shah VP, Tunik MG, Tsung JW. Prospective evaluation of point-of-care ultrasonography for the diagnosis of pneumonia in children and young adults. *JAMA Pediatr* 2013;**167**:119–25.

Sim SS, Lien WC, Chou HC, *et al.* Ultrasonographic lung sliding sign in confirming proper endotracheal intubation during emergency intubation. *Resuscitation* 2012;**83**:307–12.

Sivitz AB, Cohen SG, Tejani C. Evaluation of acute appendicitis by pediatric emergency physician sonography. *Ann Emerg Med* 2014;**64**:358–64.

Sivitz AB, Tejani C, Cohen SG. Evaluation of hypertrophic pyloric stenosis by pediatric emergency physician sonography. *Acad Emerg Med* 2013;**20**:646–51.

Tessaro MO, Salant EP, Arroyo AC, Haines LE, Dickman E. Trachial rapiid ultrasound saline test (T.R.U.S.T) for confiring correct endotracheal tube depth in children. *Rescucitation.* 2015;**89**:8–12.

12

Pre-hospital point-of-care ultrasound

Nils Petter Oveland and Jim Connolly

Summary

When to scan?

PoCUS is an extension of clinical examination used to augment clinical decision-making. If possible, it should be done during transport, and not on site.

What to scan?

Generally, time-critical scans only.

How to scan?

Stay focused and 'goal-directed'; try to answer yes/no questions (e.g. is there a pneumothorax on this side: yes or no?), and use predefined scanning protocols.

What does PoCUS add?

It can improve diagnostic accuracy for the detection of critical illnesses and injuries, resulting in more prompt, accurate treatment; it can assist with the prognosis after a cardiac arrest and help with the consideration of withdrawal of treatment; it may change management and destination, increases safety and success in procedures, and assists monitoring during ground and air transport.

Clinical scenarios

Clinical scenario 1

A general practitioner calls your Emergency Medical Communication Centre with a request for air ambulance support. The doctor is on a home visit to a 64-year-old man with acute abdominal pain. He is pale and has weak pulses and fluctuating consciousness. The air ambulance crew is dispatched and arrives 30 minutes later. The patient is quickly loaded into the helicopter but arrests just before take-off. After two cycles of CPR, he regains spontaneous respiration and a palpable carotid pulse. He appears to have a normal breathing pattern, respiratory rate, and clear chest, with improving Glasgow Coma Scale (GCS), so you assess the risks of intubation to outweigh the benefits at this stage and decide to transport towards the local hospital 10 minutes away. The in-flight examination reveals a distended abdomen. Using a portable ultrasound machine, you measure the abdominal aortic diameter as 5.2 cm (see Figure 12.1), raising the clinical suspicion for a ruptured AAA (see Video 12.1 📹). You decide to change course towards the University Hospital 40 minutes away and alert the vascular surgeon on-call. On arrival, the diagnosis is confirmed by direct transport to CT, and the patient is moved to the operating theatre.

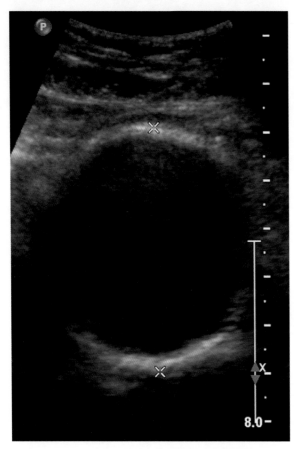

Figure 12.1 *Case scenario*. **Transverse ultrasound scan of the abdominal aorta, showing an increased diameter suggestive of an abdominal aneurysm.**

Purpose

These two cases illustrate some daily challenges faced in the pre-hospital arena:

- The scene constantly changes, and external factors (e.g. weather conditions, noise, distractions, and constricted workplaces) are unpredictable.

- For critically ill and injured patients, time is critical—many deaths are preventable if reversible causes are recognized and treated expeditiously, or the patient is diverted directly to a centre with specific definitive care abilities.

- There are multiple shortcomings in clinical examination both at the scene and during transport. Patients are not always properly exposed and may be combative due to their illness or injury. This, combined with environmental challenges, makes clinical examination less accurate. Nevertheless, clinical examination remains vital, but its shortcomings should be recognized.

All these factors strongly support the introduction of diagnostic adjuncts to augment clinical examination. PoCUS used as an extension of a comprehensive ABCDE resuscitation sequence may represent a solution in this setting.

Clinical scenario 2

A 44-year-old male suffers a cardiac arrest at work. Colleagues start CPR and attach an automated external defibrillator (AED), but no shocks are advised. They continue efforts until you arrive by ambulance some 20 minutes later. Advanced cardiovascular life support (ACLS) is initiated, and the airway secured. The presenting cardiac rhythm is PEA. PoCUS shows a rim of anechoic fluid between the ventricular wall and the pericardium, with some cardiac activity (see Videos 12.2 and 12.3 ◉) The aortic root is dilated at 5 cm, and you are confident the diagnosis is one of thoracic aortic dissection with tamponade. You use PoCUS to assist drainage and get a return of output (see Videos 12.4 and 12.5 ◉) and transfer to a cardiothoracic facility.

Perspective

PoCUS can be performed in almost any clinical setting and are low-risk, rapid, and repeatable. Furthermore, there is increasing evidence that PoCUS outperforms clinical examination alone or in combination with X-ray. This chapter addresses diagnostic and procedural applications of pre-hospital PoCUS and equipment requirements, and highlights the potential for, and barriers to, implementation into both helicopter and ground-based emergency medical services [(H)EMS].

Performing the scans

The current generation of machines are lightweight and utilize sophisticated processors and imaging

Table 12.1 Important key features of ultrasound machines intended for pre-hospital use

Features	Comments
Portable	Size and weight must be minimized
Compact	Ideally fit into pocket or equipment bag
Battery-powered	Long-lasting ± possible to change batteries
Docking	Stations for charging machines/batteries
Robust	Withstand drops from 0.5 to 1.0 m
User-friendly	Simple user interface with minimal buttons
Screen resolution	Screens that adapt to variation in sunlight
Probe exchange	Easy probe change
Standby function	Quick startup time and standby function
Multiple modes	Minimum of standard modes such as B-mode, M-mode, and colour Doppler
Video and image storage	Store still images and videos
Transfer of data	Send images/videos wirelessly

Table 12.2 Pre-hospital ultrasound applications and examinations

Diagnostic	Procedures
• Upper airway	• ETT confirmation
• Lungs	• Vascular access
• Focused echocardiography	• Nerve blocks
• Cardiac arrest	• Difficult line access
• FAST	• Pericardial drainage
• Aorta and gall bladder	
• DVT	
• TCD	
• Optic nerve sheath	
• Ocular scans	
• Bone fractures	
• Tendon ruptures	

software to provide high-quality images, including multiple modes (e.g. B-mode, M-mode, Doppler). They are often laptop-sized (approximately 4–5 kg) or even truly pocket-sized (approximately 0.1–0.5 kg) and are designed for pre-hospital use. Important key features that the user should look for are summarized in Table 12.1.

Diagnostic and procedural applications

PoCUS can complement nearly all the diagnostic questions posed during clinical assessment of ABCDE in the resuscitation sequence (see Table 12.2). Further reading outlining more detailed descriptions of each application (including how to perform the different scans) is provided at the end of the chapter and covered in other chapters of this book.

Airway

Transducer selection: high-frequency (5–14 MHz) linear transducer.

A secure airway and effective oxygenation are key components of resuscitation. Endotracheal tubes (ETT) are considered as definitive airway protection, but rates of oesophageal intubation increase in the pre-hospital setting.

Different techniques are used to confirm correct ETT placement, including direct laryngoscopy, bilateral breath sounds, chest wall movement, and detection of end-tidal CO_2. However, clinical assessment is sometimes inaccurate, and CO_2 often, though not always, is absent or low in arrested and shocked patients.

Ultrasound can help accurately confirm correct ETT placement by direct visualization, as it is passed through the vocal cords and can detect right/left bronchus intubation by indirect visualization of pleural/lung sliding.

For direct visualization, the trachea is imaged with a single transverse view across the trachea and oesophagus (see Video 12.6 ○), watching for inadvertent placement in the oesophagus. This is especially useful during CPR and decreases the need to interrupt compressions and helps when there may be minimal or no CO_2. This method does not exclude right/left bronchus intubation. The latter information is obtained by the presence of pleural/lung sliding on both sides.

PoCUS may assist in the identification of the cricothyroid membrane to guide emergency cricothyroidotomy. This membrane may not always be palpable due to anatomy or disease. A single transverse or longitudinal view can be of value in identifying the location of the membrane/trachea before commencing a surgical airway.

Breathing

Transducer selection: linear (approximately 5–14 MHz) is used for imaging superficial structures (e.g. ribs, pleura).

Micro-convex, convex transducer, curvilinear, or phased array (4–8 MHz) may be used for imaging both superficial and deep structures.

Listening to breath sounds in a noisy environment may be difficult or even impossible (e.g. inside helicopters). In this situation, direct visualization of pleural movement is invaluable. Although PoCUS poorly visualizes the lung parenchyma, dynamic signs (artefacts) originating from the pleural line can help diagnose important pathologies [PTX, HTX, pleural fluid, interstitial fluid, and alveolar consolidation (e.g. pneumonia and lung contusion)].

Pneumothorax

PTXs are difficult to diagnose on clinical examination alone. They are common after blunt chest injury, and failure to diagnose and treat an enlarging PTX, especially during positive pressure ventilation, may prove fatal.

PoCUS can be used to exclude PTX (see Figure 12.2), whereas identifying signs suggestive of PTX is not always specific, with bullae, pleural adhesions, fibrosis, and small tidal volumes offering similar appearances. Excluding PTX can prevent unnecessary field intervention (needle or thoracostomy), with data suggesting the former is performed at a rate considerably higher than confirmed PTXs. Introduction of lung PoCUS to a UK service was associated with an 80% reduction in thoracostomy rates.

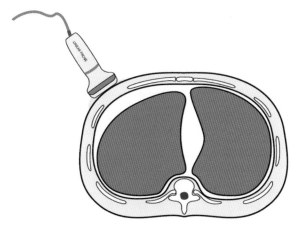

Figure 12.2 Lung ultrasound for diagnosing a pneumothorax; the visceral and pleural layers are separated by air. Thus, the normal lung sliding that occurs with ventilation is absent. The lung point is where the lung detaches from the inside of the chest wall and corresponds to the lateral extension of the pneumothorax.

Lung PoCUS has been shown to be more sensitive (approximately 90%) than clinical examination and conventional supine CXR (approximately 50%), with similar high specificity (>98%) in diagnosing PTXs. This is especially true in the setting of trauma where absence of lung sliding is more likely to be caused by PTX than other differential diagnoses, especially in younger people with no underlying lung disease.

Identifying the 'lung point' (the point at which the visceral and parietal pleura begin to separate as a consequence of intra-pleural air) sign is pathognomonic for PTX, though it can take time to locate or can even be absent if the lung is totally collapsed. Recent studies have shown that the position of the 'lung point' on the chest wall can give an indirect estimate of PTX size (see Figure 12.2).

Monitoring lung point progression in-flight/during ventilation may prove useful to decide when to intervene in patients with known PTXs being transported (see Figure 12.3). A recent Dutch HEMS study concluded that pre-hospital chest PoCUS changed management in one in five patients, specifically reducing unnecessary interventions.

Haemothorax/pleural fluid

The two pleural layers can also be separated by fluid in the form of blood (i.e. HTX) or exudate/transudate (i.e. pleural effusions), both appearing as a black anechoic

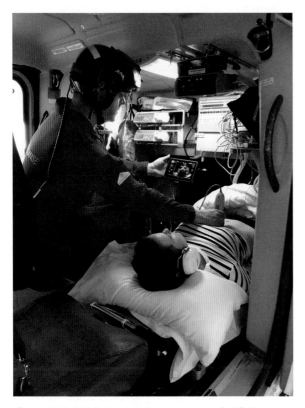

Figure 12.3 Point-of-care ultrasonography in-flight.

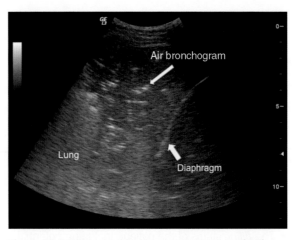

Figure 12.4 Ultrasound image of alveolar consolidation. The alveoli are completely filled with fluid/pus, making the lungs' visual appearance comparable to that of the liver. However, a distinctive feature is the presence of air bronchograms, seen as white hyperechoic dots on the image (thin arrow).

rim around the lungs (see Video 12.7 ▶). The presence of a massive HTX can quickly be confirmed and treated.

Interstitial syndrome

B-line artefacts arise when the ultrasound beam encounters small air–fluid interfaces, such as occurs with acute lung injuries and pathological disease processes in which blood/fluid/pus enter the interstitial tissue (i.e. interstitium), producing reverberation artefacts (see Video 12.8 ▶).

In normal lung, occasional B-lines are seen, but these become more pronounced when there is interstitial fluid (e.g. heart failure, ARDS, pulmonary contusion, infection, or aspirated gastric contents). Most published work is based on three or more B-lines in a single intercostal space as being pathological.

This is useful pre-hospital for assessing dyspnoea and shock, when multiple bilateral B-lines indicate 'wet lungs' (heart failure/infection) and few or asymmetrical B-lines indicate 'dry lungs' (e.g. acute PE or COPD). A hyperdynamic heart with few or no B-lines bilaterally suggests shock is due to hypovolaemia or

sepsis. This can help guide initial therapy and monitor the effectiveness of interventions (as the number of B-lines declines as fluid is absorbed, and B-lines may develop with overzealous fluid resuscitation).

Furthermore, the presence of B-lines also implies the two pleural layers are in apposition and rules out a PTX as the cause of dyspnoea.

Alveolar consolidation

When lung parenchyma is completely consolidated, only small pockets of air remain within the alveoli and the lungs become visible with PoCUS, resembling the liver (termed 'hepatization'). However, a distinctive difference is the presence of air bronchograms (i.e. white hyperechoic dots) within the lung tissue (see Figure 12.4).

This PoCUS pattern is often unilateral and more localized when scanning the lungs, and so indicates a focal process. This may be infection (e.g. pneumonia), PE with infarction, or lung contusion.

Circulation

Transducer selection: phased array (2–5 MHz) or low-frequency curvilinear (approximately 4 MHz) may be used.

One of the most valuable applications is focused examination of cardiac function, pointing to the cause of cardiac arrest and circulatory shock states in both injured and critically ill patients.

Numerous protocols [e.g. SHoC, FATE, RUSH, ACES, FEEL, ELS, EGLS, and cardiac arrest ultrasound examination (CAUSE)] have been developed to define the aetiology of circulatory collapse, particularly to identify reversible causes during ongoing resuscitation. The principles in all these are similar, evaluating (the 4 Fs):

- The pericardial sac for *fluid*;
- The size and shape (or *form*) of the heart;
- The ventricular *function*;
- The *filling* status of the patient, including potential sources of blood loss.

Trauma

In almost half of cases, mortality from trauma is due to uncontrolled bleeding. e-FAST is the most studied example of PoCUS in the pre-hospital setting. Recent research has demonstrated the feasibility of detecting bleeding in the chest, pericardium, and abdomen, using pre-hospital FAST (see Video 12.9 ▣). Field trials show that pre-hospital e-FAST can be performed similarly to ED-performed e-FAST. Furthermore, e-FAST has been shown to not prolong scene time and to alter disposition.

Pre-hospital FAST was found to alter management of patients with abdominal trauma in up to 30% of cases and importantly to reduce time to operative intervention. It is a useful tool for triaging multiple casualties and deciding on the most appropriate hospital; in particular, PoCUS assists in identifying the more urgent priorities.

e-FAST is performed on supine trauma patients on scene or during transportation. It requires little time but should be repeated if initially negative, as continued repetition increases accuracy.

Even in significant injury, e-FAST can be negative. It takes at least 400–500 mL of fluid to become positive, and some patients with multiple injuries may have a very low circulating blood volume due to both external loss and internal losses into other body cavities. PoCUS only identifies fluid in the peritoneal cavity, so any retroperitoneal blood loss will not be identified.

Cardiac arrest

PoCUS can help to diagnose or exclude some of the potentially treatable causes (see Table 12.3). The

Table 12.3 Treatable causes of cardiac arrest

4 'H' causes	4 'T' causes
• Hypovolaemia*	• Tamponade*
• Hypoxia	• Tension PTX*
• Hypothermia	• Thromboembolism*
• Hypo-/hyperkalaemia	• Toxins

Data from the International Liaison Committee on Resuscitation (ILCOR) guidelines.

Reversible causes of cardiac arrest (ILCOR guidelines).

* PoCUS is of use in those marked with an asterisk.

SHoC protocols outlined in Chapter 2 provide a structured approach to PoCUS in cardiac arrest and hypotension/shock, utilizing a *fluid, form, function, and filling* approach.

Regardless of the cause, the most important treatment of any cardiac arrest patient is efficient timely bystander CPR and correcting any cause of the arrest rapidly. PoCUS must be implemented with minimal interruption of CPR via one of three standard echocardiography views (subcostal, parasternal, or apical) and timed to occur with other interventions and the pulse check. This is best achieved by recording a loop that the clinician can play back, especially if inexperienced. The subcostal view is preferable, so as not to interfere with ongoing chest compressions and when automated compression devices are used.

Hypovolaemia is suggested by flattened ventricles in the long-axis view of the heart. The IVC diameter can be a valuable adjunct.

PE is suspected with a dilated right ventricle with a flattened LV septum that creates a D-shape, though other chronic pulmonary and cardiovascular disease processes may also cause right-sided dilatation. Importantly, the right side of the heart may dilate during a prolonged period of cardiac arrest as a physiological change.

DVT in the upper and lower extremities may suggest venous thromboembolism.

(Video 12.10 ▣ shows a femoral vein with thrombus, and Video 12.11 ▣ a normal femoral vein).

Tamponade is identified as pericardial effusion and right chamber collapse (see Videos 12.2 and 12.3 ▣).

Tension PTX is suspected with the absence of lung siding between the pleural layers, accompanied by tension physiology. The diagnosis is confirmed when performing a decompression procedure (see Figure 12.2).

Finally, PoCUS is useful in determining whether the patient has 'true' PEA (where there is an ECG signal, but no detectable cardiac motion) from 'pseudo'-PEA (where there is an ECG signal, no palpable pulses, but coordinated cardiac motion).

A 'pseudo'-PEA is shown from the subcostal view in a real cardiac arrest patient (see Video 12.12 📹) that changed to VF (see Video 12.13 📹) after a few rounds of chest compressions.

The full relevance of this differentiation between 'true' and 'pseudo'-PEA has yet to be determined; however, in studies by Breitkreutz *et al.* and Gaspari *et al.*, coordinated cardiac motion was a strong predictor for improved survival to hospital admission. Furthermore, PoCUS altered management in up to 80% of the cases.

Circulatory shock and intravascular volume status

As with cardiac arrest, PoCUS is invaluable in guiding resuscitation efforts in shocked patients and can help define the cause (see Table 12.4).

Table 12.4 Key elements of pre-hospital ultrasound shock assessment

Rule of thumb— HI MAP	Explanation
Heart	Assess the heart for pathology, chamber dimensions, and contractility
IVC	Assess the diameter and collapse index of the IVC
Morison's pouch	FAST scan for signs of blood/fluid in the thoraco-abdominal cavities
Aorta	Assess the aorta for AAA and dissection
Pneumothorax	Assess the lungs on both sides for PTX (i.e. no lung sliding)

Data from S. D. Weingart, D. Duque, and B. Nelson, Rapid Ultrasound for Shock and Hypotension (RUSH-HIMAPP), 2009, http://emedhome.com/

The FATE protocol consists of four standardized acoustic windows for cardiopulmonary assessment and monitoring. Examination of the heart and pleura makes it possible to diagnose or exclude obvious pathology (e.g. pericardial effusions) and to assess biventricular chamber dimensions and cardiac motion (i.e. contractility). The SHoC-hypotension protocol advises core cardiac, lung, and IVC views, as well as supplementary cardiac views and additional views, where clinically indicated, such as for peritoneal free fluid, AAA, or DVT.

In the pre-hospital setting, treatment of shock is often empirically reduced to fluid resuscitation, based on the erroneous assumption that all hypotensive critically ill and injured patients are hypovolaemic until proven otherwise. Not infrequently, in some patients, fluid resuscitation may be potentially harmful. Focused echo and IVC evaluation can guide decisions regarding inotropic medications/fluid doses.

Measurement of IVC diameter is a rapid, non-invasive method of volume assessment where hypovolaemia is increasingly likely with a small collapsing IVC in spontaneously breathing patients (see Table 12.4 for a useful approach).

Abdominal aortic ultrasound examination

Patients with AAA or aortic dissection may present with a wide range of symptoms.

Pre-hospital abdominal aortic PoCUS examination enables clinicians to confirm these diagnoses in order to mobilize the correct resources at the receiving hospital and take patients to the correct centre (see 'Clinical scenario 1', p. 227).

Any focused PoCUS aortic examination should include the entire length of the aorta and iliac vessels in both the transverse and longitudinal scanning planes. A ruptured AAA may be seen (see Video 12.14 📹). Furthermore, a simple M-mode measure of the aortic root is valuable, as a diameter of above 4 cm should raise suspicion for a dissection.

Disability (neurological status)

Transducer selection: the preferred transducer is a high-frequency (10–14 MHz) linear or a trans-cranial probe.

The role of PoCUS in pre-hospital neurological assessment is limited. Head injuries are the single largest cause of post-traumatic death in civilian practice. A rapid, portable non-invasive test to identify intracranial haemorrhage would be extremely valuable. Today, some emergency medical systems (EMS) have CT scanners, but few are operative. Indirect measurements of raised ICP from ultrasound examination of the ONSD can be used, as the sheath is a continuation of the dura mater surrounding the brain. Studies show moderate correlation between ONSD and raised ICP, but the exact cut-off value is unknown. A direct method is trans-cranial Doppler (TCD) of cerebral perfusion; however, the value in closed head injury has yet to be correlated with outcome and recovery measures.

Exposure/extremities

Transducer selection: high-frequency (10–14 MHz) linear. Higher frequency (up to 20–22 MHz) for small bone fractures, FBs, and tendon pathology.

Fractures

Physical examination is insufficient to exclude pathology. PoCUS can assess displacement, angulation, and comminution and assist in reduction of fractures. Fractures appear as cortical irregularities or steps in the white hyperechoic bone (see Figure 12.5).

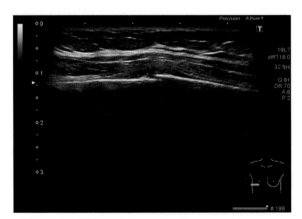

Figure 12.5 Ultrasound of a fracture indicated by cortical disruption of the bone (seen as a discontinuation of the white hyperechoic line in the middle of the ultrasound image).

Other applications

The number of pre-hospital PoCUS applications is increasing. Potential future areas are ocular injuries, soft tissue injuries, and subcutaneous FB identification and removal.

Procedural guidance

Transducer selection: high-frequency (10–14 MHz) linear.

PoCUS guidance replaces the blind insertion of needles into vessels and body cavities. This optimizes the success rate and improves safety, reducing iatrogenic complications.

The following procedures are relevant in the pre-hospital setting:

* Ultrasound-guided vascular access (peripheral and central veins + peripheral arteries);
* Airway intervention;
* Drainage of pleural/pericardial effusion;
* Nerve blocks.

The technique is either static (where PoCUS is used to find the structure of interest, the insertion depth and angle required, and the point of entry on the skin) or dynamic where the needle is visualized in real time during insertion.

The latter can be done 'in-plane' where the whole length of the needle (i.e. the tip and shaft) and the structure of interest (e.g. the vessel) are viewed in a longitudinal plane or 'out-of-plane' in transverse view where the tip of the needle is displayed on the screen as a white dot as it crosses the scanning plane. These techniques are described in Chapter 9.

Challenges of pre-hospital ultrasound

Despite the versatile range of diagnostic and procedural applications, implementation of PoCUS in pre-hospital care has been slow, for reasons summarized in Table 12.5.

Current PoCUS machines are portable and battery-powered, and can be brought to the patient, regardless of location. They are increasingly cheap and robust and give high-quality images. Competition has

Table 12.5 Barriers to implementation of pre-hospital ultrasound

Factor	Brief comment
1. Equipment	Previously PoCUS machines were not designed for 'out-of-hospital' use
2. Regulations	Machines must be tested and approved according to international standards for pre-hospital medical equipment (NS/ISO/IEC60601-1-12:2014. Specifications for pre-hospital medical equipment)
3. Cost	Many (H)EMS cannot afford the equipment
4. Scene time	Increased on-scene times are cited as the main reason for not using PoCUS
5. Weather conditions	Direct sunlight and rain make scanning difficult
6. Space	Constricted working space in wrecked cars or buildings or inside ambulances/helicopters/airplanes makes scanning difficult
7. Lack of evidence	No randomized controlled trials showing improved outcome (morbidity or mortality)
8. Training	Lack of appropriate education /training
9. (H)EMS organization	Staffing pre-hospital varies widely internationally

led to truly hand-carried PoCUS devices, with some weighing <1 kg. More challenging are comprehensive international standards and regulations of medical equipment intended for use in ground ambulances and helicopters/airplanes. This is especially true for air ambulance services where air aviation rules apply.

The most important consideration is that PoCUS should not cause unnecessary scene time delays. However, most applications can be completed in <3 minutes and are performed simultaneously with other procedures, such as vascular access or packaging, and may be the key intervention to direct care. Non-immediate PoCUS, such as e-FAST, may be performed during transport. The key principle is to only perform scans that add value or directly impact immediate management.

Other limitations to pre-hospital PoCUS are the weather and ambient lighting. Scanning in direct sunlight often gives a reflection from the screen that makes it hard to see the grey-scaled PoCUS image (see Figure 12.6). A blackout blind may assist.

Limited workspace sometimes makes it impossible to perform all views (see Figure 12.7).

Physicians working in the pre-hospital arena should undergo the same training as other physicians performing PoCUS in hospitals. Non-physician-based systems will likely limit this to advanced-level providers such as paramedics. Multiple international studies have shown that physicians and non-physician providers can achieve basic PoCUS skills with relative short training courses. Maintaining skills requires continuous practice and good-quality management programmes.

Future direction

Medical history has shown that many procedures and treatments previously only possible in hospital have been implemented successfully in the pre-hospital setting [e.g. advanced airway, thrombolysis, resuscitative thoracotomy, and more recently resuscitative

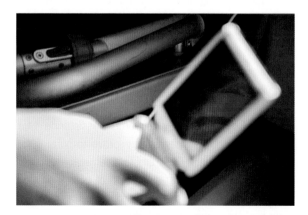

Figure 12.6 Reflection from the ultrasound screen when scanning outside in ambient lighting.

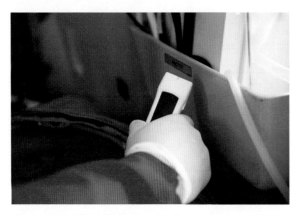

Figure 12.7 Difficulties of performing a complete FAST scan inside a narrow helicopter cabin. The wall hinders positioning of the probe in the upper right quadrant.

balloon occlusion of the aorta (REBOA), and blood transfusion]. Ultrasound machines will likely continue to become smaller and less expensive. It thus seems natural that PoCUS will find an increased role in the pre-hospital setting.

There are many conditions where this may impact care in the future; in acute ischaemic stroke, TCD may provide some assistance. Preliminary results from pre-hospital studies show a high sensitivity and specificity in diagnosing MCA occlusion. Future research should focus on how PoCUS can improve time to thrombolysis intervention that could translate into better neurological outcome.

A growing area of interest is using PoCUS to monitor patients during air transport, as standard monitors can be unreliable during flight. In a helicopter, it is almost impossible to detect a PTX by auscultation. Continuous in-flight thoracic PoCUS is a feasible method to monitor PTX development and progression.

Furthermore, clinicians can use in-flight PoCUS scans to monitor cardiac function after return of spontaneous circulation (ROSC) in cardiac arrest by direct visualization of the heart and detection of carotid blood flow using colour flow Doppler.

Technology allowing real-time assistance for interpreting PoCUS images may prove important for some EMS systems (i.e. remote telementored ultrasonography). Real-time transmission of both the video showing the placement of the probe on the patient's body and the corresponding PoCUS image has been tested in an offshore oil installation, and the study produced clinically useful information in 96.4% of cardiac, and 87.8% of abdominal, examinations and in all lung examinations. This modality is limited only by network availability, as other necessary video conference and PoCUS equipment is readily available 'off the shelf'.

Finally, current research on pre-hospital PoCUS is sparse or of low quality. We know that high-quality images are feasible, and that the resulting information alters management, but there is little to suggest outcomes are improved. Indeed, two recent reviews concluded that there is no evidence that pre-hospital PoCUS improved outcome in trauma and non-trauma patients. We believe that this calls for dedicated research, focusing on the benefits and improved outcomes of performing existing PoCUS applications early in the field.

It is important to remember—lack of evidence for benefit is not evidence of lack of benefit. Future efforts should support the use of pre-hospital PoCUS and improve patient outcome through international research, education, and closer collaboration.

Further reading

Additional further reading can be found in the Online appendix at www.oxfordmedicine.com/POCUSemergencymed. Please refer to your access card for further details.

Brooke M, Walton J, Scutt D. Paramedic application of ultrasound in the management of patients in the prehospital setting: a review of the literature. *Emerg Med J* 2010;**27**:702–7.

El Sayed MJ, Zaghrini E. Prehospital emergency ultrasound: a review of current clinical applications, challenges, and future implications. *Emerg Med Int* 2013;**2013**:531674.

Gillman LM, Ball CG, Panebianco N, Al-Kadi A, Kirkpatrick AW. Clinician performed resuscitative ultrasonography for the initial evaluation and resuscitation of trauma. *Scand J Trauma Resusc Emerg Med* 2009;**17**:34.

Jørgensen H, Jensen CH, Dirks J. Does prehospital ultrasound improve treatment of the trauma patient? A systematic review. *Eur J Emerg Med* 2010;**17**:249–53.

Laursen CB, Rahman NM, Volpicelli G (eds). *Thoracic Ultrasound. ERS Monograph*. Sheffield: European Respiratory Society; 2018.

Nelson BP, Chason K. Use of ultrasound by emergency medical services: a review. *Int J Emerg Med* 2008;**1**:253–9.

Nelson BP, Sanghvi A. Out of hospital point of care ultrasound: current use models and future directions. *Eur J Trauma Emerg Surg* 2016;**42**:139–50.

Rudolph SS, Sørensen MK, Svane C, Hesselfeldt R, Steinmetz J. Effect of prehospital ultrasound on clinical outcomes of non-trauma patients—a systematic review. *Resuscitation* 2014;**85**:21–30.

Index